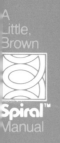

A
Little,
Brown

Spiral™
Manual

Manual of
Surgical
Therapeutics

Fifth Edition

**Departments of Surgery
The Medical College of Wisconsin
and University of Illinois**

**Edited by Robert E. Condon, M.D.
and Lloyd M. Nyhus, M.D.**

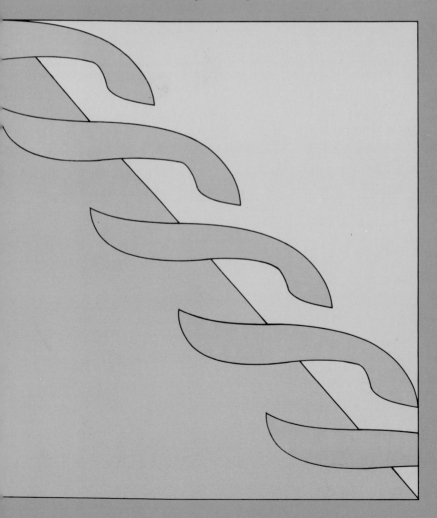

Manual of Surgical Therapeutics

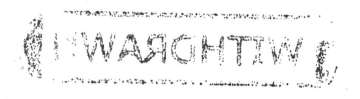

Manual of Surgical Therapeutics

Fifth Edition

Departments of Surgery
The Medical College of Wisconsin
and University of Illinois

Edited by

Robert E. Condon, M.D.
Professor of Surgery and Chairman of the
Department, The Medical College of
Wisconsin, Milwaukee

Lloyd M. Nyhus, M.D.
Professor and Head, Department of
Surgery, the University of Illinois
College of Medicine, Chicago

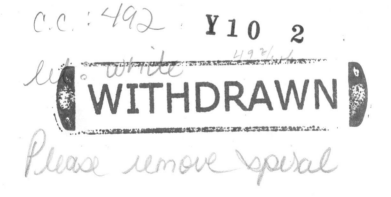

Little, Brown and Company
Boston

Manual of Surgical Therapeutics is
published in the following translations:

Second Edition
Manual de Terapêutica Cirúrgica

Third Edition
Allgemeintherapie in der Chirurgie
Manuale di terapeutica chirurgica
Manual de terapéutica quirúrgica

Fourth Edition

外科診療マニュアル

Preface

Our intention, when we originally developed the *Manual of Surgical Therapeutics* more than a decade ago, was to bring together between the covers of a single volume pertinent information about the nonoperative management of surgical patients. We wanted to keep the volume small enough to fit in the coat pocket of a surgical house officer or student. And we elected to use an outline format, believing that it would make information more rapidly accessible when the book was consulted under urgent circumstances. Because of the constraints relating to size and format, we chose to have each of our expert authors record a single plan of management (or point of view) that had been associated with success in his or her practice. We have followed these principles in each subsequent edition. Therefore, more often than not, the reader will find in this book a straightforward discussion, however opinionated, of a demonstrably successful scheme of management, usually without reference to other viable alternatives.

The value of the *Manual of Surgical Therapeutics* to its intended surgical audience is demonstrated most of all by its presence in the coat pockets of residents, interns, and students, in hospital emergency rooms and nurses' stations, and in the libraries of senior surgeons and physicians around the world. We are gratified at the positive response to successive editions of the *Manual* from our colleagues who have reviewed it and, more important, from those who use it every day. It is our intention to continue to keep this book a valuable reference for all of our wide readership.

In preparation for the revision of each new edition, it has been the practice of our publisher, Little, Brown and Company, to arrange for two senior surgical residents at leading academic institutions to review critically the contents of the preceding edition and to make suggestions for material to be deleted or included in the forthcoming edition. Drs. Gerhard Mundinger and John Macoviak performed these tasks for the fourth edition of the *Manual*, and their pointed and helpful commentaries were transmitted to the authors of each section. For the most part, the suggestions offered by these reviewers have found a place in this, the fifth edition.

For this edition, chapters and sections on general principles in the management of acute injury, together with specific features of the management of chest, vascular, extremity, and hand injuries and infections, have been completely rewritten. Similarly, sections relating to the evaluation of the body's "survival systems," the renal, cardiac, and pulmonary systems, have been completely revised, as have the chapters on fluid and electrolyte therapy, coagulation disorders, and cancer chemotherapy. A new section on stings and bites has been added at the request of many readers. Extensive revisions have been made in the chapters on acute injury, emergency room problems, cardiac arrhythmias, surgical nutrition, surgical infections, and venous disorders of the lower extremities. The entire *Manual* has been reviewed, revised, updated, and rechecked by contributors, old and new.

The *Manual of Surgical Therapeutics* is the work of house officers and attending surgeons from the Departments of Surgery at The Medical College of Wisconsin in Milwaukee and the University of Illinois in Chicago. A few exceptions should be noted: Ronald L. Nichols, author of the chapter on surgical infections, is a former colleague but is now a member of the faculty at Tulane University; Richard Stewardson and Edward Felix, former colleagues, have recently entered private practice. To all of our contributors, whose expertise is recorded in the pages of the *Manual*, we express our gratitude for and appreciation of their efforts and diligence.

v

We want to thank Carol Russell-Hilmer, who did most of the artwork, and William Hamilton, Chief of the Medical Media Service at the Wood Veterans Administration Center, whose work enhances the value of this *Manual*. Our secretaries, led by Mary Ann Seefeldt and Joann With in Milwaukee, and June Svec in Chicago, undertook, with their usual good cheer, the heavy responsibilities of typing and retyping the manuscript and checking the proofs. We are most grateful for and appreciative of their capable help, devotion, and grace under pressure, without which it would not have been possible to complete this edition.

We also wish to express our continued admiration to Fred Belliveau and Lin Richter of Little, Brown and Company, and our thanks to Robert M. Davis who served as the book editor for this edition. It is impossible to thank our wives, Marcia and Margaret, adequately for all their support over these many years. Their good humor and forbearance while our attention has been devoted to professional duties is beyond measure.

Robert E. Condon
Lloyd M. Nyhus

Contents

tracheal intubation. Before an esophageal obturator airway is removed, an endotracheal tube should be inserted to protect the patient from reflux or emesis. With a known or suspected cervical spinal injury, nasoendotracheal rather than oroendotracheal intubation should be attempted. **Transtracheal catheter insufflation** provides emergency airway access to an obstructed airway. A large-bore angiocatheter is inserted through the cricothyroid membrane. Oxygen delivered at high pressure and volume directly from a wall outlet is intermittently insufflated through the catheter and will provide acceptable oxygenation for a short time. **Cricothyroidotomy** (held in disrepute by some authorities) can be accomplished expeditiously and safely. **Tracheostomy** is the traditional transcervical emergency airway procedure. Simpler emergency measures to secure an airway (intubation, cricothyroidotomy) should be done first, after which tracheostomy can be performed electively.

B. Breathing. Abnormalities of respiration involve **ventilation** (movement of air), **exchange** (diffusion of gases across the alveolar capillary membrane), or **transport** of blood to and from the tissues.

  1. Injury to the thoracic cage (soft tissue contusion, rib and sternal fractures, flail chest, ruptured diaphragm), space-occupying pleural lesions (simple and tension pneumothorax, simple and massive hemothorax), parenchymal injuries (pulmonary contusion, laceration, hematoma), or cardiovascular injuries (myocardial contusion, pericardial tamponade, great vessel disruption) produce hypoxia, hypocarbia, and alterations in acid base balance. These lesions can be associated with mediastinal shift, major intrathoracic blood loss, and cardiac dysfunction, and may be complicated by cardiovascular collapse.

  2. Respiratory management

    a. Provide supplemental oxygen. The most important mechanism of oxygen transport is the hemoglobin in erythrocytes. A normal hemoglobin of 15 gm/100 ml provides transport of 20 vol % of oxygen; a hemoglobin of 7 gm/100 ml (hematocrit 21%) carries only 10 vol %, the critical reserve level of oxygen consumption for most tissues, especially the myocardium and brain. Oxygen administered by a properly applied mask or nasal catheter at 8 liters/min will increase inspired oxygen concentration (FIO_2), increase hemoglobin saturation, and improve oxygen delivery to the tissues. Oxygen administered through a T-adapter via an endotracheal or tracheostomy tube will increase the FIO_2 to 40%. Delivering oxygen concentrations above an FIO_2 of 50% is unnecessary in the management of most patients. Pulmonary oxygen toxicity may result if 100% oxygen is administered continuously for 24 hours.

    b. Stabilize chest defects. A sucking chest wound not only produces a pneumothorax but also adversely affects the transtracheal airflow. The defect should be sealed with an impervious dressing (Vaseline gauze and adhesive tape). If the ventilatory defect progresses, tension pneumothorax should be considered.

    c. Assist ventilatory effort. Assistance is indicated when ventilatory effort is marginal, or the respiratory rate, rhythm, effort, or arterial blood gases are abnormal. Ventilatory support is accomplished by mouth-to-mouth, mouth-to-face mask, bag mask, or mechanical administration of **positive-pressure ventilation.** Repeated examination for hemothorax or pneumothorax prior to and during ventilatory support is important. Previously undetected injury may be responsible for the development of a tension pneumothorax when positive-pressure ventilation is employed.

    d. Watch for impaired venous return or decreased pulmonary blood flow. High inspiratory pressure, continuous positive pressure, or use of expiration-retarding devices all may contribute to increased resistance to pulmonary blood flow. Positive pressure is transmitted to the alveolar space, pulmonary capillaries are compressed, and blood flow through the pulmonary circulation is diminished. Decreased return of blood to the left heart causes a fall in cardiac output and may prolong or increase shock, especially in a hypovolemic patient.

e. Evacuate air or fluid-filled pleural spaces. The onset of symptomatic hemopneumothorax may be acute, delayed, or recurrent. The physician must be ever alert to this possibility. **Tension pneumothorax** needs immediate attention; an 18-gauge needle or a McSwain dart and flutter valve is inserted into the anterior second interspace in the midclavicular line until a chest tube can be placed. Major hemothorax may be treated with a closed thoracostomy tube, usually inserted through the fourth to sixth interspace in the midaxillary line (see Fig. 25-19).

C. Circulation. Shock is a state of hypoperfusion, especially of vital organs, which results from a decreased effective circulating blood volume or inability of the heart to pump.

1. Classification. Shock associated with trauma is primarily **hypovolemic.** Associated problems may induce other forms of shock, concurrently or subsequently.

a. Hypovolemic shock is due to loss of blood volume or fluid. Visible blood loss can be verified by a quick check of the floor, cart, bed and bed sheets, clothing, and dressings. Additional visible blood losses via the gastrointestinal tract, GYN system, and genitourinary organs can be quickly assessed by inspection of vomitus, stools, urine, or vaginal discharge, as well as by measuring nasogastric aspirate. **Intrathoracic hemorrhage** should be suspected with blunt and penetrating trauma to the chest. Be suspicious of hidden **intraperitoneal hemorrhage** associated with blunt trauma to the thorax, fractures of the lower ribs, penetrating thoracic trauma below the fifth intercostal space, or any blunt or penetrating injury to the abdomen. **Retroperitoneal hemorrhage** secondary to fractures of the pelvis (1500 ml average), and blood loss associated with **long bone fractures** (500–1000 ml) are other sources of hidden blood loss. Major plasma losses are seen with thermal or electrical burns. Extracellular fluid losses accompany bowel obstruction, peritonitis, and pancreatitis.

b. Cardiogenic shock (pump failure) may be due to myocardial injury (cardiac contusion or penetrating wound) or to failure of flow in and out of the heart (cardiac tamponade, mediastinal shift with tension pneumothroax, major rupture of the diaphragm).

c. Endotoxin shock in septicemia results in peripheral pooling of blood in capacitance (primary venous) vessels, causing a decrease in the effective circulating blood volume without actual blood loss.

d. Neurogenic shock is a decrease in effective circulating blood volume due to loss of sympathetic control of resistance vessels, resulting in dilation of arterioles and venules. Spinal cord injuries and hypotension due to spinal anesthesia are examples of this phenomenon.

2. Physiological responses in shock are directed to improvement in the perfusion of vital tissues.

a. Endocrine response. Release of adrenocorticotropic hormone, antidiuretic hormone, and aldosterone during hypotension results in renal retention of sodium, chloride, and water, increased renal potassium loss, and decreased urine volume. Release of catecholamines (epinephrine and norepinephrine) from the adrenal medulla produces responses mediated through alpha and beta receptors. Alpha receptors are located in peripheral vessels; stimulation produces vasoconstriction, and blockade produces vasodilation.

Beta receptors are located centrally in the heart (β_1) and peripherally in vessels (β_2). Central beta stimulation produces inotropic and chronotropic effects, while peripheral beta stimulation produces mild arterial dilation and venous constriction. Catecholamines maintain blood pressure by decreasing the volume of the vascular space as well as by mobilizing intravascular fluid from peripheral tissues to the central pool. Hyperglycemia during shock is attributed to the glycogenolytic properties of corticosteroids and epinephrine; studies demonstrating depression of insulin secretion in shock imply more intricate relationships.

b. **Metabolic effects.** A normally perfused cell utilizes glucose to form energy through adenosine triphosphate. Without oxygen, glucose is converted to pyruvate and transformed anaerobically to lactic acid, which accumulates and results in metabolic acidosis. Amino acids and fatty acids that normally would enter oxidative pathways for energy production also accumulate in shock, compounding the metabolic acidosis. The oxygen deficit and acidosis eventually interfere with cell membrane function. Intracellular postassium is then lost; sodium and water move into the cell, producing cellular edema.

c. **Cardiorespiratory response.** The intense sympathetic response during shock increases cardiac output by augmenting the rate and force of cardiac contraction in addition to increasing peripheral resistance. Since myocardial perfusion occurs primarily during diastole, tachycardia decreases myocardial perfusion, resulting in myocardial acidosis. Although compensated initially by increasing ventilation to augment carbon dioxide elimination, progressive acidosis combined with hypoxia (both primary and secondary to decreased myocardial perfusion) in prolonged shock results in myocardial depression, irritability, and susceptibility to arrhythmias.

3. **Management of the hypovolemic patient**

a. **Prevent further blood loss.** The most effective measure for controlling visible blood loss is **externally applied direct pressure.** Place a large dressing over the wound, and wrap it tightly with elastic bandages. If it continues to bleed, a second elastic bandage should be applied with greater pressure over the first. If hemorrhage continues, remove the second elastic wrap and apply a third. **Tourniquets and direct clamping of vessels are mentioned only to condemn them.** They are often applied incorrectly and can cause further injury. If a tourniquet has already been applied, obtain direct control of the source of the bleeding and remove the tourniquet. If a clamp already has been applied, it should be left in place until the time of definitive repair.

b. **Pneumatic compression devices.** For selected extremity wounds, an **air splint** may be applied over a bulky dressing. When inflated, it will control many arterial injuries and all major venous hemorrhages. For lower extremity, pelvic, and intra-abdominal injuries associated with major blood loss and hypotension, a **circumferential pneumatic compression garment** (Medical Anti-Shock Trousers [MAST] or Jobst Anti-Shock Garment) may be applied. When maximally inflated, this device provides approximately 100 mm Hg of external pressure, which not only controls hemorrhage but also serves as a splint for pelvic and long bone fractures, increases venous return to the heart, and decreases the flow of blood to the lower extremity. If applied early, before alpha stimulation has caused severe vasoconstriction, these garments will augment the intravascular circulating volume by approximately 100–1500 ml. The garment has recently been added by the American College of Surgeons to its list of **Essential Equipment for Ambulances** and is being recommended for prehospital use for hypotension associated with hypovolemia from any cause but, most notably, with blunt and penetrating trauma to the chest, abdomen, and extremities; fractures of the femur and pelvis; ruptured abdominal aortic aneurysm; and postpartum and postoperative hemorrhage. Respiratory embarrassment has occurred on occasion from compression by the abdominal portion of the garment, but that compartment can be deflated while the two leg compartments remain inflated. Since the garment is used to increase intravascular blood volume by compression of the capacitance vessels, sudden shock may result if the garment is deflated before restoring blood volume. In seriously injured patients, removal of the trousers may have to be deferred until after anesthesia has been given in the operating room. Absolute **contraindications** to use of the garment are obvious pulmonary edema and the presence of isolated head injuries. A relative contraindication is the existence of a source of hemorrhage outside the area controlled by the garment, i.e., from the upper extremity, chest, head, and neck.

c. **Replace fluid losses.** Placing the patient in a modified **Trendelenberg position** will empty the large capacitance vessels. **Retransfusing spilled blood** (autotransfusion), especially that associated with thoracic injuries, should be considered in members of some religious sects, in patients with a rare blood type, and in trauma patients in whom urgent blood replacement is required and local circumstances are conducive to collection and administration. If there is significant blood loss, requiring replacement, **whole blood or components** should be transfused (see Chap. 15).

d. **Crystalloid versus colloid.** There is an ongoing argument regarding the use of crystalloid (normal saline or Ringer's lactate solutions) and colloid (albumin-plasma) solutions in resuscitation from shock. In an acutely hypovolemic patient, **initial volume replacement with crystalloid is adequate and preferred.** Both normal saline and Ringer's lactate are acidic solutions that theoretically might aggravate metabolic acidosis; in practice, this is not a problem. Volume replacement with crystalloid solutions is calculated on a 3:1 ratio of replacement to loss because of the larger distribution space of crystalloid solutions (see Chap. 9). **There is no place for salt-free crystalloid solutions (plain dextrose in water) in primary resuscitation of an acutely hypovolemic patient.**

Albumin and plasma are effective colloid volume replacement solutions. Because of the problem of transudation of fluid into the pulmonary interstitium, with resultant adult respiratory distress syndrome, and concern about costs and transmission of disease, colloid fluids have been reserved for use later in the resuscitative effort if needed. Patients with burns, peritonitis, and pancreatitis may need colloids early. Those with clotting abnormalities will need fresh-frozen plasma to provide coagulation factors. There is little place for regular or low molecular weight dextrans in the treatment of an acutely hypovolemic, traumatized patient.

e. **Treat severe acidosis.** Acidosis may impair cardiac function by decreasing ventricular contractile force; cardiac output decreases, aggravating hypotension. In acidosis, the effects of epinephrine and norepinephrine, as well as those of other cardiotonic drugs, are reduced, the response of both the heart and the peripheral circulation being affected.

Oxygen, ventilatory support, and fluid replacement will permit normal compensatory mechanisms to correct most cases of acidosis. Infuse **sodium bicarbonate** if metabolic acidosis is severe. When multiple transfusions are given rapidly, bicarbonate should be given to counteract the acidotic effect of the citrate in transfused blood. Excessive infusions of sodium bicarbonate may cause base excess and a potential for metabolic alkalosis, hypokalemia, and arrhythmias. Marked hyperosmolarity also can occur and result in a coma, which will confuse post-traumatic neurological evaluation. An organic buffer tromethamine (THAM) may be used instead of sodium bicarbonate but probably has no advantage over bicarbonate in the treatment of metabolic acidosis, and it can cause a decrease in minute ventilation and aggravate preexisting hypoxia in respiratory acidosis.

f. Support the circulation. The majority of trauma victims are previously healthy persons; following volume replacement, cardiac function returns to normal. In patients with prior cardiac disability, hypovolemia and hypoxia further weaken the cardiovascular system and may necessitate support of the heart rate, rhythm, and strength of cardiac contractions. Assured restoration of blood volume must precede cardiac drug therapy. See Table 1-1 for the characteristics of specific drugs.

g. Diuretics should be avoided until a stable normovolemic state has been obtained. Urine production is the best reflection of adequate tissue perfusion. An inadequate urine output usually reflects inadequate volume replacement. Normal urine output (30–50 ml/hr) usually can be attained by providing adequate volumes of intravenous fluids and blood. Until there is reliable clinical evidence that volume expansion has been adequate, diuretics should be avoided. Administration of furosemide (Lasix) or ethacrynic acid (Edecrin) to a volume-depleted patient enhances the risk of ototoxicity due to these drugs. With persistent depression of urinary output in the face of a rising CVP and normal pulse and blood pressure, diuresis may be indicated.

h. Monitoring. During initial resuscitation, major emphasis is directed toward identifying and treating perfusion deficits resulting from pump, volume, or resistance failures. Monitoring of the patient is vital to judge the effects of a given therapy and to determine the need for additional treatment.

(1) The **state of cerebration** reflects the level of hypoxia, perfusion, and injury.

(2) **Urine quantity and quality** indicate the status of hydration and the possible presence of genitourinary tract injury.

(3) **Pulse rate, rhythm, and strength** provide insights into cardiac function and the effectiveness of volume replacement.

(4) The **electrocardiogram** (ECG) identifies arrhythmias and irritability.

(5) **Central venous pressure or Swan-Ganz catheters** provide assessment of myocardial function and the status of volume replacement. Although these catheters are not needed in all patients, they are desirable if there is preexisting cardiorespiratory disease, the patient requires respiratory support, or resuscitation requires large volume replacement.

(a) The CVP catheter may be inserted peripherally through an antecubital vein or centrally through a subclavian or jugular vein; the catheter tip should lie within the right atrium. The pressure noted reflects the status of volume replacement and the ability of the right heart to pump. Initial pressure readings are not as pertinent as are changes noted with volume replacement.

(b) The Swan-Ganz catheter may be inserted in a manner similar to the insertion of the CVP catheter but is advanced through the right heart to wedge in a terminal pulmonary arterial branch. With the balloon tip inflated, the wedge pressure and cardiac output can be measured; wedge pressure reflects more accurately the status of left heart function.

(c) Utilizing the CVP and pulmonary wedge pressures, accurate assessment can be made of volume depletion, volume overload, and myocardial function, thus helping to determine the need for additional volume replacement, removal, or cardiac support drugs.

D. Disability. With the life-threatening problems resolved or controlled, attention is next given to the care and management of fractures, dislocations, and soft tissue injuries. Suspected and obvious fractures and dislocations are splinted. If the patient has been admitted with splints or a pneumatic compression apparatus

Table 1-1. Useful Cardiovascular Drugs

Drug	Initial IV Dose	Principal Actions	Remarks
Dobutamine (Dobutrex)	200 mg in 250 ml 5% D/W at 2.5–15 μg/kg/min	Primarily β_1 stimulator; + inotropic.	Not a mesenteric or renal vasodilator; little peripheral vasoconstriction.
Dopamine (Intropin)	200 mg in 250 ml 5% D/W at 2–5 μg/kg/min	Primarily β_1 stimulator; + inotropic; some β_2 stimulation at usual doses (vasodilation); alpha stimulator at high doses (vasoconstrictor).	Dilates renal and splanchnic vasculature in usual doses via specific "dopaminergic" receptors.
Isoproterenol (Isuprel)	1 mg in 500 ml 5% D/W at 0.25–2.5 ml/min	Strong β_1, moderate β_2 stimulator; + chronotropic and + inotropic.	Little or no vasopressor action.
Epinephrine (Adrenalin)	0.5 mg intracardiac or IV	Strong α and β_1, weak β_2 stimulator; + inotropic, + chronotropic; peripheral vasoconstrictor.	Action impaired in acidosis.
Norepinephrine (Levophed)	8 mg in 1000 ml 5% D/W at 2–3 ml/min	α and β_1 stimulator; + inotropic; powerful peripheral vasoconstrictor.	Visceral vasoconstrictor.
Metaraminol (Aramine)	10–100 mg in 500 cc 5% D/W: titrate dose	α and β_1 stimulator; + inotropic; peripheral vasoconstrictor.	Effects mediated by norepinephrine release.
Methoxamine (Vasoxyl)	3–5 mg IV	Pure α stimulator; powerful peripheral vasoconstrictor.	Deleterious if vasoconstriction already present.
Phenylephrine (Neo-Synephrine)	0.5 mg IV	Pure α stimulator; powerful peripheral vasoconstrictor.	Deleterious if vasoconstriction already present.

Drug	Dose	Action	Indication
Calcium chloride	2.5–5.0 ml of 10% solution. May be repeated at 10 min intervals.	+ inotropic; necessary for excitation-contraction coupling.	Use in asystole if epinephrine is ineffective.
Calcium gluconate	10 cc of 10% solution. May be repeated at 10 min intervals.	+ inotropic; necessary for excitation-contraction coupling.	Use in asystole if epinephrine is ineffective.
Phenytoin (Dilantin)	50–100 mg q 5 min	Similar to lidocaine.	Drug of choice for digitalis-induced arrhythmias.
Lidocaine (Xylocaine)	50–100 mg IV bolus	Elevates fibrillation threshold; ?retards membrane conduction.	Drug of choice for ventricular arrhythmias.
Procainamide (Pronestyl)	100 mg IV over 1 min and repeated every 5 min	Decreases myocardial excitability.	Secondary drug for ventricular arrhythmias that are not digitalis induced; may increase dose up to 1 gm q 5 min.
Bretylium (Bretylol)	5 mg/kg IV	Increases fibrillation threshold; sympathetic block.	For ventricular arrhythmias refractory to all other therapy.
Digoxin	0.25–0.5 mg	Increases myocardial contractility; increases atrioventricular conduction time.	Reduces ventricular response in atrial fibrillation and flutter.
Propanolol (Inderal)	1 mg/min, up to 5 mg	β blocker; decreases sinoatrial node rate; increases arteriovenous conduction time.	For atrial tachyarrhythmias.
Atropine	1 mg	Vagolytic; accelerates discharge rate of sinoatrial node.	For sinus bradycardia.

in place, verify the presence of a fracture by x-rays. If there are no fractures, the splints may be removed. If fractures are present, the splints should remain in place until the patient is ready for definitive care (see Sect. VII).

1. **Tetanus prophylaxis** must be administered to every patient suffering a break in the body's epithelial barrier (skin, mucous membranes).

   a. **Previously immunized persons** who received the last dose of tetanus toxid **within the last 10 years:** Give 0.5 ml adsorbed tetanus toxoid. This booster may be omitted if the wound is clean and superficial.

   b. **Previously immunized individuals** who received the last dose of tetanus toxoid **more than 10 years** previously: Give 0.5 ml adsorbed tetanus toxoid for all wounds.

   c. **Immunization status unknown or inadequate:**

      (1) **Clean, superficial wound** (not tetanus prone): Give 0.5 ml adsorbed tetanus toxoid.

      (2) **All other wounds** (potentially tetanus prone): Give 0.5 ml adsorbed tetanus toxoid plus 250 units human tetanus immune globulin.

E. **Entry.** Once the patient has been resuscitated and vital functions have been stabilized, consideration is given to providing definitive care in an appropriate facility. (The American College of Surgeons has published guidelines for trauma centers based on the availability of support personnel.) In addition to trauma centers, there are centers for the management of spinal cord injuries, burns, replantation of extremities, poisons, and psychiatric illnesses. Arrangements should be made for transfer or hospital admission as appropriate.

Suggested Reading

Blaisdell, F. W., and Lewis, F. R., Jr.   Respiratory Distress Syndrome of Shock and Trauma. In F. W. Blaisdell (ed.), *Major Problems in Clinical Surgery*. Philadelphia: Saunders, 1977. Vol. 21.

Clowes, G. H. A., Jr. (ed.).   Symposium on response to infection and injury. Surg. Clin. *North Am.* 56:1, 1976.

Committee on Trauma, American College of Surgeons.   Essential equipment for ambulances. *Bull. Am. Coll. Surg.* 62:7 October 1977.

Lowe, R. J., Moss, G. S., Jilek, J., and Levine, H. D.   Crystalloid versus colloid in the etiology of pulmonary failure after trauma: A randomized trial in man. *Surgery* 81:676, 1977.

Rhodes, G. R., Shah, D., Scovill, W., Dutton, R. E., Newell, J., and Powers, S. R., Jr.   Cardiovascular function following non-colloid fluid management of severely traumatized man. *J. Trauma* 18:559, 1978.

Shoemaker, W. C., and Hauser, C. J.   Critique of crystalloid versus colloid therapy in shock and shock lung. *Crit. Care Med.* 7:6, 1979.

Siegel, D. C., Cochin, A., Geocaris, T., and Moss, G. S.   Effects of saline and colloid resuscitation on renal function. *Ann. Surg.* 177:51, 1973.

Facial Injuries

Patients with facial trauma may have associated mortal injuries, but facial injuries in themselves rarely cause death. The most common serious injuries associated with facial trauma involve the brain, cervical spine, and eyes. Despite frequently published statements to the contrary, **serious facial injury alone is not an indication for emergency tracheostomy.** Patients with facial injury who require tracheostomy have associated injury of the head, neck, or chest.

The common causes of facial trauma are automobile accidents and accidents occurring in and about the home. The most serious injuries are sustained from automobile accidents, accidents at work, and intentional injuries, especially self-inflicted shotgun wounds. Animal bites can be serious because of regional and central nervous system infection (e.g., rabies).

I. **Classification of facial injury.** To avoid overlooking subtle forms of injury, a scheme of organization of common facial injuries should be kept in mind. The simplest scheme divides both soft tissue areas and facial bones into zones and forms of injury.

   A. **Soft tissue facial injuries**

   1. **Type of injury**

      a. Contusions and abrasions, with or without hematoma.

      b. Accidental tattoo (numerous small foreign particles embedded in the dermis) or retained larger foreign bodies.

      c. Puncture wounds.

      d. Lacerations: simple, beveled, tearing, or bursting (stellate).

      e. Avulsion injury, either with complete loss of tissue or as a flap (undermined laceration).

   2. **Location of injury:** forehead, eyelids, ears, nose, cheek, chin, lips, or intraoral.

   B. **Facial bone fractures**

   1. **Type of fracture:** closed (simple), open (compound), greenstick, comminuted, undisplaced, or displaced.

   2. **Location of fracture**

      a. Upper third of face: frontal bone, frontal sinuses, glabella, and supraorbital ridge.

      b. Middle third of face: nasal bones and septum, maxillary sinuses (antrum), orbital bones, zygoma and zygomatic arch, transverse maxilla (Le Fort I), pyramidal maxilla (Le Fort II), craniofacial disjunction (Le Fort III), alveolar processes, and maxillary dentition.

      c. Lower third of face: mandibular dentition, alveolar process, symphysis, body, angle, ascending ramus, condyle, and coronoid process.

II. **Priorities of treatment.** Although facial injuries may be extensive, the patient first must be evaluated completely, using the priorities that always apply in trauma (see General Principles).

   A. Extensive facial injuries seldom cause great pain. When pain seems to be severe, associated injuries should be suspected.

   B. Most facial hemorrhage can be controlled by direct pressure or ligation of the bleeding vessel. One real danger of facial hemorrhage is **obstruction of the upper airway.** The volume of hemorrhage from facial injuries alone is seldom sufficient to cause shock or to require emergency blood transfusion. Associated cerebral, cervical, or ocular injuries are more apt to be the cause of shock.

III. **The diagnosis of facial injury.** The diagnosis is established by observation, palpation, and x-ray examination.

   A. **Observation.** In addition to obvious soft tissue injuries, **asymmetry** of the face caused by underlying fractures often can be detected early, before the masking effects of soft tissue swelling occur. The eyelids always should be opened to look for ocular injury, and the mouth should be opened to observe for intraoral injury. Dental occlusion should be observed by asking the patient to "bite."

B. Palpation. Observation of facial symmetry is reinforced by palpation of bony prominences. These landmarks may be masked by overlying hematoma or edema. Comparing the height of the malar eminences (zygoma) is especially informative in diagnosing depressed fractures of that bone. Tenderness usually can be elicited at the site of a fracture, but seldom is the discomfort extreme. Systematic bilateral palpation, even in the presence of obvious injury, helps to detect subtle deformities and should be performed in the following order: supraorbital and lateral orbital rims, infraorbital rims, malar eminences, zygomatic arches, nasal bones, maxilla, and mandible.

C. X-ray examination. Gross facial bone fractures can be diagnosed without x-ray confirmation; indeed, some grossly displaced facial bone fractures cannot be visualized well on x-rays.

    1. The most informative x-ray views should be obtained initially: posteroanterior (PA), lateral, and occipitomental (Waters) projections of the facial bones (not skull). After review of these x-rays and as indicated by the nature of the injury, special views of the nasal bones, mandible, and zygoma may be needed.

    2. In addition to routine x-ray studies, laminography (tomography) is useful in diagnosing fractures about the orbit. Sialography may be helpful if laceration of the parotid duct is a possibility and cannot be confirmed by direct observation.

D. Documentation of injury should include a record of the type of injury and measurement of any wounds. A photograph of extensive facial injuries should be taken before treatment begins. Such a photograph can be invaluable in understanding and explaining secondary problems and the nature of final healing.

IV. Triage and treatment of facial injury. Once life-threatening problems have been resolved, soft tissue injuries amenable to repair under local anesthesia are treated first.

A. Complex facial injuries with tissue loss and extensive fractures seldom can be treated immediately, since these patients usually are poor candidates for general anesthesia. When definitive care must be postponed, the simplest accurate tissue approximation will promote a better end result. If necessary, soft tissue injuries can wait without repair up to 24 hr without compromising the final result, provided that bleeding has been controlled and the wounds properly cleansed and dressed. Systemic antibiotics are advisable when delay in soft tissue repair is anticipated.

B. Reduction and fixation of facial bone fractures almost never need to be carried out as an emergency operation, but facial fractures can be difficult to reduce more than 2 wk after injury and should be treated definitively before this time. As facial bones are membranous in origin, healing begins with fibrous union, which usually can be overcome by manipulation and sharp dissection, even if delayed reduction is necessary.

C. Healing in children is accelerated, and reduction of their fractures should be attempted within 7–10 days of injury if possible.

V. Operative care. Repair of facial injuries should be oriented toward anatomical repositioning of soft and bony tissues. If this is accomplished, normal features, symmetry, dental occlusion, and facial functions will be restored.

A. Anesthesia

    1. Patients with acute extensive facial injuries are poor candidates for general anesthesia, often arriving in the emergency room with their stomachs filled with food, alcohol, or blood. Given a reasonably cooperative patient, local anesthesia is unquestionably superior for the management of most facial injuries. Local anesthesia facilitates the surgeon's work, since endotracheal intubation for general anesthesia almost invariably results in restricted access to the patient's face and distortion of the features. Sedation appropriate to the age and condition of the patient will make local anesthesia more successful.

2. Repair of the deep structures of the face and open reduction of most facial bone fractures are best performed under general anesthesia. A weak solution of epinephrine can be infiltrated into the face to facilitate hemostasis and shorten operating time.

B. Operating room. At least a scrub nurse and a circulating nurse are needed to assist in the repair of facial injuries. Attempting soft tissue repair unassisted in an emergency room invites frustration and second-rate results.

C. Tissue loss

1. Extensive tissue losses can await definitive repair until the patient's general condition has stabilized. Repair with adjacent tissue, if it can be moved without distortion of features, is preferred.

2. If skin grafts are needed, full-thickness postauricular grafts serve best to match the color and texture of facial skin.

3. Rotation and transposition flaps often can be used to cover defects immediately following injury, but tubed pedicle flaps, direct pedicle flaps, and island flaps are techniques ordinarily reserved for subsequent reconstructive procedures.

Suggested Reading

Kazanjian, V., and Converse, J. M. *The Surgical Treatment of Facial Injuries* (3rd ed.). Baltimore: Williams & Wilkins, 1974.

Schultz, R. C. *Facial Injuries* (2nd ed.). Chicago: Year Book, 1977.

Head and Cervical Injuries

The most important clinical observation to be made in a patient with a head injury is **change in the state of consciousness since the injury.** Record the present level of consciousness, preferably in terms of what the patient does spontaneously or the stimuli to which he or she responds. Prompt and lucid conversation implies alert consciousness. Memory loss for the accident commonly occurs with concussion. Memory loss for such items as address, occupation, or year means intellectual impairment and represents an early change in consciousness. In progressive stupor leading to coma, lack of a verbal response to questioning occurs sooner than does lack of accurate avoidance of painful stimuli. In coma, there is absence of purposeful movements, either spontaneous or evoked.

I. Head injuries

A. General care

1. Vital signs (blood pressure, pulse, and respiratory rate) are important indicators of a change in the patient's status. Record them frequently and post them in a prominent place; a blackboard on the wall is a help.

2. A good **airway,** oxygenation, and humidification are of the utmost importance, since **hypoxia will increase cerebral edema.** If secretions pool or breathing becomes labored, an endotracheal tube should be inserted or a tracheostomy done. A lateral position with no elevation of the head is superior to the supine position.

3. The patient should be given **nothing by mouth** until it is clear that no operation is to be performed. A nasogastric tube, especially in children, is helpful in reducing gastric dilation.

4. **Intravenous infusion,** preferably dextrose in an electrolyte solution, should be started and a **Foley catheter** introduced if the patient is not alert or if an operation is considered likely. Watch for the development of water excess (dilutional hyponatremia), a common sequela of head injury. Probably 1500 ml/day of oral or intravenous fluid intake is sufficient for the first day or two if no other need for fluid is evident.

5. **Restraint** of the patient in spread-eagle fashion is dangerous. If restraints are unavoidable, the patient should be positioned on either side, alternating the sides every 3 hr, with both legs and arms strapped to the same side of the bed. Very large bandages wrapped in boxing-glove fashion around the hands and up the forearm will prevent pulling at tubings or dressings.

6. **Sedation should be avoided,** since it interferes with the elevation of consciousness. If pain from a coincidental fracture is a problem, small doses of a narcotic can be used if intravenous naloxone is available to counteract it as needed.

7. **Anticonvulsants** are given to all patients who have had a cerebral contusion or an intracranial hematoma. Intravenous phenytoin sodium (Dilantin), 100 mg tid, is given after a loading dose of 500 mg; IM administration is avoided because of poor absorption; IV administration should be no faster than 100 mg/min. Because of precipitation, it must be given at the entry into the venous system and not mixed with an IV solution.

8. **Changes in pupil size or reaction to light** may be caused by pressure on the third nerve or by pontine damage. Dilated or unequal pupils indicate a transtentorial shift resulting from increased intracranial pressure (coning). Constricted pupils that do not react to light are signs of brainstem damage, either primary (e.g., contusion) or secondary to increased pressure.

9. If an immediate **reduction in intracranial pressure** is needed while the operating room is being prepared, give mannitol (400 ml of a 20% solution) or urea (125 ml of a 30% solution) IV. Hyperosmolar solutions are otherwise avoided lest brain shrinkage permit increased bleeding.

10. **Computerized scans** are very useful when the specialized equipment is available. They may permit differentiation of an intracerebral from an extracerebral clot, edema, or contusion and may reveal fractures. Scans rarely give essential information if the patient is very restless, and general anesthesia may be needed in some patients if sedation is inadequate.

11. **Cerebral angiography** is a versatile diagnostic study in the evaluation of craniocerebral injury but may not always be available or without hazard. Lateralizing signs may indicate the presence of an expanding clot but just as often point to cerebral contusion and edema. Angiogram may help define the nature of the injury. Since it is an invasive procedure, it now takes second place to computerized tomography (CT) scanning.

12. **Echoencephalography** is an easily applied noninvasive test that entails no risk to the patient. It may permit determination of the probable pressure of a clot or mass with sufficient accuracy to lead to exploratory bur holes. Rapid deterioration of consciousness may indicate the need for an exploratory operation without any special diagnostic examinations.

B. Definitions and suggestions

1. **Cerebral concussion** means temporary disruption in cerebral activity resulting from injury, reflected in transiently altered consciousness or other temporary loss of neural function (e.g., blindness).

2. **Cerebral contusion** means damage to a portion of the brain and may be characterized by dulled mentation, pink cerebrospinal fluid (CSF), and a sensory or motor deficit. Contused frontal or temporal lobes may have to be resected if sufficient swelling occurs. CT scanning may show clinically undetected contusions.

3. **Linear fractures** of the cranial vault usually are clearly visible in x-rays of the skull. If a linear fracture is present, suspect (1) an **arterial epidural hematoma** in an adult if the fracture crosses any branch of the middle meningeal artery, (2) a **venous epidural hematoma** if the fracture crosses the superior longitudinal or a lateral sinus, and (3) a **diploic epidural hematoma** if there is a large separation of fractured bone fragments in an infant or toddler.

4. **Depressed skull fracture** is an impaction of fragmented calvaria that may result in penetration of the underlying dura and brain. These fragments should be elevated, depending on location, depth of depression, and overlying scalp laceration.

5. **Basilar fractures** may be diagnosed by the leakage of CSF from the nose or ear, more often by bleeding from the ear in the absence of obvious cutaneous cause, or suspected from severe ecchymosis of the eyelids or over the mastoid process (Battle's sign). Broad-spectrum antibiotics are indicated with a CSF leak but not with nasal or aural bleeding alone. The ear canal should not be packed with anything, since it might hinder egress of fluid or blood. X-ray diagnosis is often difficult to establish even with tomography, so an early extensive search is not warranted.

6. **Intracerebral hematoma** may result from severe acute injury or progressive damage secondary to contusion. These hematomas should be removed if they threaten life or well-being.

7. **Epidural hematoma** may be of arterial, venous, or diploic origin. When a change in neural function indicates continued bleeding, craniotomy is performed to evacuate the clot and stop the source of bleeding.

8. **False intracranial aneurysm,** or "pseudoaneurysm," is a cavity with walls composed of clots that are becoming organized with fibroconnective tissue. Such clots must be evacuated and the source of bleeding arrested.

9. In **acute subdural hematoma** there is a variable amount of freshly clotted blood in the subdural space, accompanied by severe contusion of the underlying brain. Usually, it is the severely contused brain that is responsible for the patient's compromised clinical state, not the clot in the subdural space. This type of hematoma has been reported to be fatal in up to 95% of patients; extensive decompressive craniotomy may be lifesaving but with dubious long-term benefits.

10. **Subacute subdural hematoma** implies large amounts of recently clotted blood in the subdural space, with either no contusion of the underlying brain or, at most, punctate cortical hemorrhages and small patches of subarachnoid blood. The clot is responsible for the neurological deficit, and its timely removal almost invariably results in good recovery.

11. **Chronic subdural hematoma** is mentioned in connection with acute head injuries because, although present and asymptomatic for months, it can present very acutely. Fluid similar in appearance to crankcase oil is located within a capsule that in turn is within the subdural space. Bur holes, followed by drainage of the fluid and irrigation of the cavity, almost always results in a cure. Formal craniotomy for removal of fluid and membranes is preferred by some neurosurgeons.

12. **Acute subdural hygroma.** The origin of the blood-tinged fluid present in acute subdural hygromas and the reason why such small amounts cause

severe neurological deficits are not known. The fluid is indistinguishable from CSF. Drainage of the fluid often results in impressive improvement.

C. Clinical evaluation

1. Signs of a progressive increase in intracranial pressure are:

a. Progressive diminution in the level of consciousness.

b. Change in the size and symmetry of the pupils and their reaction to light.

c. Steady slowing of the pulse.

d. Irregularities of respiration.

The presence of one or more of these signs is adequate justification for a **CT scan** or bilateral **carotid angiography.** Cranial exploration is indicated if signs of a clot or lobar contusion are found. If no operable lesion is found, insertion of a ventricular or epidural **pressure monitor** may permit more accurate treatment by withdrawing ventricular fluid or administering IV mannitol.

2. Adult: previous loss of consciousness but now alert. If there is a definite history of head injury and loss of consciousness, the patient should be admitted to the hospital for observation. If the patient is alert at the time of examination, order skull x-rays, with anteroposterior (AP), right and left lateral, and Towne's views. Lateral views are best done across the table to avoid turning the head when the status of injury of the neck is not clear. Generally agreed on **indications for x-rays of the skull** in the emergency room situation include a history of unconsciousness, penetration of the skull, or a previous craniotomy with a shunt tube in place. Physical examination findings justifying skull x-rays include skull depression, a discharge from the ear, CSF discharge from the nose, blood in the middle ear, Battle's sign, raccoon's eyes, the presence of coma or stupor not related to alcohol ingestion, and focal neurological signs.

a. If **no fracture** is seen, 24 hr of observation is probably adequate.

b. If there is a **linear fracture over the convexity** of the skull, especially if it crosses a venous sinus, observation should be prolonged. If the level of consciousness declines, CT scanning, echoencephalography, or cerebral angiography should be done to diagnose hematoma as a prelude to its evacuation.

c. If the **linear fracture crosses the pterion,** longer observation is necessary. Angiography and operation are indicated if the patient becomes obtunded or if a rapid pulse slows to less than 60/min. Displacement of meningeal or cerebral vessels seen in the angiogram, or displacement of the ventricles with accumulation of blood shown in the CT scan, should lead to exploratory craniotomy.

d. If skull x-rays show a **fracture depressed 5 mm or more,** it should be elevated as an elective procedure. If it overlies a venous sinus, the possibility of air embolism from opening the sinus may require use of the Trendelenburg position or positive-pressure ventilation during the operation.

e. If there is **scalp laceration and a depressed fracture,** the patient should be taken directly to the operating room. If there is to be any delay, lacerations should be sutured temporarily in the emergency room. In the operating room, the wound should be irrigated, the edges debrided, the depressed fragments removed and discarded, and the scalp sutured. If the defect is sizable or over a vital area, an elective cranioplasty should be performed later. Some neurosurgeons wash the bone fragments and replace them, using antibiotic coverage.

f. If there is **scalp laceration and a linear fracture,** irrigate and debride the scalp wound and repair the laceration.

3. **Adult: previous loss of consciousness, now irritable or confused**

    a. If there is a definite history of head injury and loss of consciousness in a patient who is irritable or confused, with or without a neurological deficit, order a CT scan and skull x-rays, and observe the patient for several days or a week. Loss of consciousness means there has been concussion and perhaps contusion.

    b. If the patient becomes more obtunded, or more neurological changes develop, consider CT scanning or angiography to determine if a clot or contusion with edema is present. Lobar resection may be needed if the patient's condition worsens.

    c. **Lumbar puncture after head injury is rarely indicated** lest removal of fluid precipitate herniation of parts of the brain to compress the brainstem. It is probably safe if no fluid is allowed to escape when pressure is over 200 mm H_2O in the lateral decubitus position (see Fig. 25-15) and it may be useful if the patient is not too restless to prevent proper estimation of pressure. CT scanning eliminates almost all need for lumbar puncture except to detect meningitis.

        (1) **Pink CSF** implies cerebral contusion, but it may also be pink with subdural hematomas or lobar swelling.

        (2) **Clear CSF** may be present with epidural hematoma.

        (3) **Increased pressure** may be present with contusion or hematoma, with or without blood in the CSF, or with edema.

        (4) **Normal pressure** may be present with concussion or contusion and sometimes with hematoma.

    The presence or absence of a fracture does not correlate with CSF pressure or with the presence or absence of blood in the CSF.

4. **Adult: responsive only to painful stimuli.** Skull x-rays should be taken only if they can be done conveniently and quickly. Echoencephalography is more rapid than angiography and may be repeated frequently. CT scanning is the most useful single test in such a patient and may obviate the hazards of angiography.

    a. If a **CT scan** is done, a contusion or clot may be shown. Compression of both ventricles may indicate massive edema worthy of intracranial pressure monitoring.

    b. If **echoencephalography** shows a **shift of midline structures,** and the patient's condition is stable, cerebral angiography may reveal a hematoma or indicate contusion of the brain. If the state of consciousness is rapidly deteriorating, if the pupils become unequal, or if the pulse rate falls below 60/min, **exploratory bur holes** may supplant angiography as an urgent procedure, especially when CT scanning is delayed or unavailable.

        (1) If there is a **contusion of the temporal lobe,** cerebral angiography will show an elevation of the middle cerebral artery in the AP and lateral projections and sometimes also a shift of the anterior cerebral artery. Treatment consists of resection of the tip of the temporal lobe.

        (2) **Subacute subdural hematoma** is impossible to distinguish clinically from epidural hematoma. If there is no visible medial displacement of the middle meningeal artery in an angiogram to indicate the latter diagnosis, bur holes or craniotomy with removal of the fresh clot is indicated.

        (3) If an **acute subdural hematoma** is present, angiography will show an irregularly outlined filling defect over the surface of the brain, with evidence of intraparenchymal swelling in either the underlying or contralateral hemisphere. Removal of the subdural hematoma through bur holes or craniotomy is the only treatment. Unfortunately, this lesion often is fatal.

b. If **echoencephalography** shows **no shift,** serial observations of clinical signs and repeat echoencephalography are indicated.

c. If CT scanning, echoencephalography, and angiography are unavailable, any sign of clinical worsening indicates the need for cranial exploration by, at least, bur holes.

d. **Lumbar puncture** is rarely necessary in the comatose patient responsive only to painful stimuli; CT scanning and angiography are more useful in detecting masses or swelling, and fluid removal for relief of intracranial pressure is best done via a ventricular catheter.

e. **Corticosteroids** may be used to combat edema, especially when no operable lesion is found. A loading dose of 50 mg dexamethasone is followed by 8 mg q4–6 hr. Proof that corticosteroids, even in megadoses, are effective agents after head injury is still lacking.

5. Infants under 2 yr of age. Unconsciousness at the time of examination is rare in infants. Neurological deficits or changes in pupil size often may not occur, even with major trauma. A rapid pulse secondary to severe blood loss may occur in a child with only a subgaleal hematoma as well as in one with a diploic epidural hematoma. Lost blood should be replaced immediately. If there is intracranial injury without a clot, corticosteroids and mannitol should be used to reduce cerebral edema, preferably with monitoring of intracranial pressure. If a child has only a subgaleal hematoma, it should not be tapped immediately, since it almost always will be resorbed within a 2-wk period. Skull x-rays should be obtained (AP, lateral and Towne's projections). CT scanning is probably the most important radiological procedure in conscious children. Echograms for the detection of an intracranial mass are easier to interpret in children than in adults.

a. If the skull x-rays reveal a **linear fracture,** the child is admitted to a hospital and observed for 48 hr. He or she should then be followed as an outpatient for 3 mo to exclude a chronic subdural hematoma. Subsequent roentgenograms are needed to ensure that the fracture is not enlarging, especially if it is in the parietal region.

b. If the **skull fracture is depressed** more than 5 mm, the child should be admitted to a hospital and the fracture elevated as an elective procedure. If there is a laceration over the fracture, operation should not be deferred.

c. If the **skull fracture is stellate** and there is wide diastasis of the fracture edges, the child is to be observed in a hospital for accumulation of an epidural hematoma.

d. If there is no clear history of trauma, but there is evidence of a bulging fontanelle, split sutures, vomiting, or failure to thrive, or if convulsions are present in any irritable child, one must consider the possibility of a chronic subdural hematoma or a postmeningitis subdural effusion. CT scanning will usually make the diagnosis. Bilateral subdural taps may be performed. Do not aspirate fluid but allow it to flow spontaneously. Do not drain more than 10 ml from each side the first time, since rapid decompression may tear arachnoid venous channels and cause fatal bleeding.

6. Children 2–10 yr of age. The principle to be remembered in this age group is that the level of consciousness, vital signs, and degree of neurological deficit are most compromised immediately after injury, but spontaneous recovery may be rapid and dramatic. General supportive measures (airway, bladder catheter, and IV fluids) are to be emphasized in the immediate post-traumatic period, and CT scanning, angiography, or operation is considered during 2–12 hr of observation.

II. Cervical injury

Injuries to the neck often accompany head injury. Fracture dislocation of cervical vertebrae may result from direct trauma or from deceleration injury. Vertebral column and spinal cord damage often is overlooked in the presence of more obvious injuries to the head, thorax, or abdomen. The comatose or confused patient is not a good subject to examine for neck stiffness, quadriplegia, or a sensory deficit. Diaphragmatic breathing, paralytic ileus, or acute urinary retention may be the only signs of cervical cord damage in the unconscious patient. A pin scratch may be used to elicit a sensory level if there is grimacing or withdrawal on pricking the face. Soft tissue injuries to the neck may complicate the injury to the spine. If trauma or some other problem compromises the airway, this takes precedence over all else; intubation will usually suffice, although tracheostomy may be necessary. Soft tissue x-rays may show subcutaneous emphysema or a deformity necessitating airway attention.

A. The patient who has a **stiff neck but no motor sensory deficit** should have the neck immobilized in a plastic collar, and cervical spine x-rays should be taken. If the x-rays show displacement of one cervical vertebra on another, cranial tongs and traction should be applied. If they show either a teardrop or a compression fracture, the patient should be left in the plastic collar. The lateral views of the cervical spine are best done across the table, without turning the neck and with the arms pulled down to allow visualization of the lower cervical vertebrae. No study of the cervical spine is complete without seeing all the cervical vertebrae. If necessary, a "swimmer's view" is taken to see the bodies of C6 and C7. If this does not clarify the C6 and 7 through T1 area, tomography must be done.

B. Patients who have a **sensory or motor deficit** at the level of the clavicle or involving the upper extremities should be placed immediately in cranial tongs and connected to 15–25 lb of traction. The amount depends on the degree of malalignment of vertebrae. Portable x-rays can be taken with the patient still on the examining table or stretcher or in bed, without turning the patient's head and neck and with the patient in halter or tongs traction. A physician should be present to protect the neck of the paralyzed patient. Lateral turning of the patient from the supine to the prone position may cause sudden death. The supine position is safest, since it allows free diaphragmatic breathing. If possible, a turning frame should be used to turn the patient every 2 hr. Decubitus ulcers are better prevented than treated. If paralytic ileus develops, nasogastric tube suction should be instituted. An indwelling Foley catheter should be inserted to keep the bladder decompressed. The patient should not be allowed to eat.

If the cervical cord injury is at the C5 level, there will be complete quadriplegia and a sensory level at the clavicle, and the patient will breathe only with the diaphragm. Hypoxia may then cause the patient to be confused or delirious. If the injury is at the C6 level, there will be paraplegia and paralysis in extension of both arms. If the injury is at the C7 level, the patient will be able to flex the arms well but extend them only poorly. If extension is preserved, the injury is at or below the T1 level.

C. The patient who demonstrates a **rising sensory or motor level** after cervicovertebral trauma should have a decompressive laminectomy, since he or she may have either an extramedullary hematoma or an extension of intramedullary contusion. Lumbar puncture and manometric studies are not reliable and are not advisable in this situation, but CT scanning or myelography via lateral cervical puncture may be diagnostic. Dexamethasone (4–8 mg, q4h after a loading dose of 50 mg) may be used to combat edema of the spinal cord. Diskectomy and anterior spine fusion may be employed if disk protrusion is responsible for paraplegia with retention of some posterior column sensation.

D. **The newborn child with respiratory difficulty** who does not writhe when pinched or become startled when stimulated may have cervical cord injuries secondary to craniocervical hyperextension during birth. Test for sensory level by slowly passing a pinwheel up the body and watching the face. The child will wince when he or she feels pain, indicating the level of cord damage. X-rays of the spine are usually not helpful. Scalp traction, using 2-in. tape connected to 5 lb of weight, provides excellent immobilization. The tape should be applied to both sides of the scalp, with the center of the tape in the same coronal plane as the external auditory canal. Tracheostomy is often necessary to establish a free airway, and a gastrostomy may be required temporarily to provide nutrition.

E. The infant who develops ileus after a fall or deceleration injury should be tested and treated as outlined in **D.**

Suggested Reading

Adam, G. L. (ed.) *Central Nervous System Trauma Research Status Report.* Bethesda, Md.: Office of Scientific and Health Reports. National Institute of Neurological and Communicative Disorders and Stroke. National Institutes of Health, 1979.

Popp, A. J., Bourke, R. S., Nelson, L. R., Kimbelberg, H. K. (eds.). *Seminars in Neurological Surgery: Neural Trauma.* New York: Raven Press, 1979.

Chest Injury

Chest injury is common, sometimes misunderstood, and occasionally misdiagnosed. If impaired ventilation and circulation are not restored expeditiously, the patient may die. Infection is not an immediate threat, but its prevention is an essential part of adequate therapy. There are **three major steps** in managing a patient with chest trauma: **resuscitation, decision about early thoracotomy,** and **establishing a complete diagnosis.** Nonoperative management of thoracic trauma will suffice for most patients, but thoracotomy is indicated for some and may be urgent (Table 1–2).

I. Initial evaluation and therapy

A. Clear the airway, assist ventilation, and **treat shock.** These three imperative initial steps in trauma therapy have been discussed under General Principles.

B. Look for tension pneumothorax. Air hunger and a hyperresonant hemithorax should immediately raise a suspicion of tension pneumothorax. Needle thoracentesis (see Fig. 25-16), using a medium-bore or large-bore needle thrust into the affected hemithorax, may be a lifesaving maneuver. Air escapes until the excess pressure is relieved. After conversion of tension to a simple pneumothorax, place a chest tube to manage any continuing air leak from the lung (see Fig. 25-17).

C. Look for cardiac tamponade. Beck's triad—falling arterial pressure, rising venous pressure, and a small, quiet heart—indicates the possible presence of cardiac tamponade due to hemopericardium. Although a paradoxical pulse occasionally is felt in a patient with grunting respirations due to chest-wall pain, the presence of a paradoxical pulse should alert one to look for evidence of cardiac tamponade. Hemopericardium rarely is evident on chest x-ray. **Needle pericardiocentesis** (see Fig. 25-18) is the urgent initial temporary treatment of acute cardiac tamponade due to hemopericardium. The catheter is left in place while the patient is taken to the operating room. If the removal of 25–50 ml of blood does not restore arterial pressure, the diagnosis of acute cardiac tamponade is in doubt. Remember that blood in the pericardium may clot and cannot be removed through a needle, and also that heart wounds may occur without cardiac tamponade.

D. Physical diagnosis. Look for clinical signs of respiratory insufficiency (stridor, cyanosis) and for asymmetrical or paradoxical movement of the chest with re-

Table 1-2. Indications for Thoracotomy

Type of Injury	Diagnostic Aids
Open wound into pleural space	Visual inspection.
Failure of initial resuscitation	
Continued bleeding	Record volume of blood loss.
Continued air leak	Unexpanded lung on x-ray; bronchoscopy.
Ruptured diaphragm	Gastrointestinal tract (gas) in chest on x-ray; confirm with contrast x-ray examinations.
Foreign body	Visual inspection; PA and lateral x-ray views.
Traumatic aortic aneurysm	Wide mediastinum on x-ray; depressed left main bronchus; angiography imperative.
Ruptured esophagus	Barium swallow.
Cardiac tamponade	Physical findings relieved by aspiration of blood.

spiratory effort. Subcutaneous emphysema usually indicates a bronchial or pleural tear with a pneumothorax, but it also may indicate a fractured larynx, or tracheal or esophageal rupture, and may require early operative care.

E. **X-ray diagnosis.** Physical diagnosis has severe limitations in defining chest injuries and must be supplemented by x-ray examination. A physician should always accompany the injured patient during x-ray examinations. Upright PA and lateral films are ideal; a portable AP film taken with the head of the bed elevated is better than no film at all. A cross-table film taken with the patient lying on his side (lateral decubitus position) is a compromise but may be essential in planning treatment. Mediastinal changes are often minimal on the chest x-ray of the trauma patient. Their subtlety must not obscure diagnosis of injuries here. Angiography and barium contrast studies should be used freely for definitive diagnosis.

F. **Tracheostomy is not necessary** for the initial treatment of chest trauma. The only indication for an urgent tracheostomy is upper airway obstruction that cannot be removed or managed by intubation.

G. **Endotracheal intubation** with a cuffed tube is the preferred method of establishing and maintaining an airway. The oral or nasal route may be used, but the latter is preferable for the trained operator. Topical anesthesia reduces patient discomfort.

H. **Mechanical ventilation** and **oxygen therapy** are required in most serious chest injuries but are not substitutes for enforced coughing and tracheal suctioning in preventing atelectasis. A manual bag ventilator is useful when the patient must be moved about the hospital. Pressure-controlled ventilators are satisfactory for initial resuscitation. Assistance may be intermittent or continuous, depending on the degree of impairment. A volume-controlled ventilator is necessary for definitive treatment of a flail chest or severely contused lung. Positive end expiratory pressure must be added for the drowned lung syndrome. Patients on ventilators must be carefully observed for increased airway resistance and diminished tidal volume, which are signs of tension pneumothorax.

I. **Arterial blood gas determinations** should be obtained at the first opportunity. Maintain arterial oxygen tension (PaO_2) between 70 and 100 mm Hg, keeping the inspired oxygen concentration (FIO_2) as low as possible. Weaning should be begun as soon as PaO_2 can be maintained without support. Management of progressive or continued respiratory insufficiency is discussed in Chapter 12.

J. A baseline **ECG** is important. Therapy of ischemia and arrhythmias from blunt trauma is outlined in Chapter 3. Cardiac wounds require thoracotomy for correction.

K. Bronchoscopy may be needed if intubation and tracheal suctioning do not remove obstructing secretions or aspirated blood. The flexible bronchoscope is sometimes useful for this task.

L. Strapping of chest-wall injuries with adhesive tape or elastic bandages **is not done,** since it interferes with ventilation. Intercostal nerve blocks also are not part of the emergency armamentarium, though, rarely, they may be useful in later management.

M. Small doses of morphine sulfate, administered intravenously once resuscitation is completed and the patient's condition is stable, relieve pain and allow more adequate voluntary ventilation and coughing.

II. Trauma to the lung and associated structures

A classification of injuries useful in establishing a framework for therapy is listed in Table 1-3. Indications for a thoracotomy are listed in Table 1-2. The management of respirator-supported ventilation is outlined in Chapter 12.

A. Tension pneumothorax may occur with sucking chest wounds but is more often due to lung laceration. The air is prevented from escaping during expiration by collapse of soft tissue, occluding the laceration. When a sucking chest wound is covered with an occlusive dressing, an open pneumothorax may be converted to a tension pneumothorax. In this instance, the patient's condition will worsen, and personnel should be instructed to remove the patch.

1. **High pressure** in the pleural cavity produces collapse of the ipsilateral lung, compression of the contralateral lung, and obstruction of blood flow in the great veins and pulmonary vessels. Myocardial dysfunction due to anoxia produces a further fall in cardiac output. Impaired ventilation is the fundamental disorder.

2. **Relief of tension** must be accomplished at once by inserting a large-bore needle or catheter anteriorly through the second intercostal space in the midclavicular line. Follow by inserting a chest tube (see Fig. 25-17).

B. Pneumothorax occurs when air enters the pleural cavity from an injured lung or through a penetrating thoracic injury, reducing the normal negative (to atmospheric) intrapleural pressure and permitting partial collapse of the lung. Since air is readily compressible, the normal pressure changes essential to ventilation of the lung are damped in pneumothorax. A functional shunt results from the ventilation-perfusion imbalance and adds to the hypoxemia of impaired ventilation. All forms of traumatic pneumothorax are treated definitively by insertion of a chest tube (see Fig. 25-17) connected to underwater-seal drainage. **Prophylatic chest tubes** are advocated by many. In the absence of continued air leak, the chest tube frequently will be blocked early by clot. Since the tube is so easily blocked, surveillance cannot be relaxed even when the tube is used **prophylactically** because of anesthesia or assisted ventilation.

C. Flail chest develops after fracture of several ribs or of the sternum in more than one place.

1. The unstable chest wall segment develops **paradoxical movement,** pushed in during inspiration (intrapleural pressure < atmospheric) and pushed out during expiration (intrapleural pressure > atmospheric). The flail chest may become apparent only after repeated examination. It can cause serious ventilatory impairment if anterior or lateral but may cause little difficulty if posterior. Traction, compression, and operative fixation are no longer recommended.

2. The flail segment causes **hypoventilation.** Atmospheric pressure pushes the unstable area inward during inspiration, diminishing the effect of the decreased intrapleural pressure required to move air into the lungs; i.e., the

Table 1-3. Classification of Chest Trauma

Type of Injury	Typical Source	Effects	Comments
Chest-wall defect	Shearing trauma (shotgun blast, explosion, flying objects, automobile hood ornament)	Circulation deficit; ventilation deficit; pleural infection; pulmonary infection.	Occlusive dressing; chest tube(s); thoracotomy (urgent).
Major blunt trauma	Automobile accident; fall from a height	Ventilation deficit; possible circulation deficit; esophageal or diaphragmatic injury; pulmonary infection (later).	Usually multiple injuries; major resuscitative effort required; need for thoracotomy indicated by failure of resuscitation.
Perforating wound	Bullet	Circulation deficit (life-threatening); possible ventilation deficit.	Frequent associated abdominal injuries requiring celiotomy; need for thoracotomy indicated by failure of resuscitation.
Penetrating wound	Knife	Circulation deficit (usually life-threatening).	Resuscitative measures usually suffice; extent of damage frequently not evident until after 8–12 hr of observation.
Minor blunt trauma	Simple fall	Decreased ventilation and impaired removal of tracheobronchial secretions because of pain; pulmonary infection (later).	Morbidity if not vigorously treated, especially in aged and alcoholic patients.

pressure gradient from bronchus to pleural space across the lung surface is lost. During exhalation, the unstable area is pushed outward, diminishing the effect of the increased intrapleural pressure required to move air out of the lung. Essentially the same mechanism accounts for the ventilatory deficit in open pneumothorax and tension pneumothorax. As with any injured lung, atelectasis leads to arterial oxygen desaturation because of the functional right-to-left shunt and increases hypoxemia.

3. It formerly was thought that failure of the lungs to fill and empty synchronously caused the mediastinum to swing back and forth, and that decreased cardiac output caused by the compromise of venous return resulted from the instability of the mediastinum. The laws of fluid physics confirmed by multiple clinical observations make this concept obsolete. Similarly, in the absence of a rigid mediastinum due to prior disease, the **pendelluft** theory that air enters the compressed lung from the functioning lung defies the laws of fluid physics and should be abandoned. Impaired ventilation is the fundamental disorder.

4. Effective coughing is impaired because of pain and abnormal chest-wall movement, resulting in retention of secretions.

5. Ventilatory support with a **volume respirator** is definitive treatment for most flail defects. It may be needed for 1–4 wk, until the patient is able to maintain PaO_2 without respirator support. The ventilator must be able to deliver sufficient volume at whatever pressures may be necessary to ventilate the lungs. **Contusion of the lung** frequently accompanies a flail chest; although usually apparent on admission, its effects may not appear for 12–24 hr. The ventilatory defect secondary to direct lung injury may be severe. Therapy must be evaluated frequently by measuring ventilation volumes and blood gases.

D. Hemothorax is an accumulation of blood within the pleural cavity. Because blood is not compressible, there is less interference with ventilation in hemothorax than with a pneumothorax of equivalent size, but a large hemothorax can compress the lung and impair ventilation.

1. Needle thoracentesis through an intercostal space is useful in the treatment of a moderate hemothorax. Insert the needle through the fifth intercostal space in the anterior axillary line, the sixth intercostal space in the midaxillary line, or the eighth interspace infrascapularly. Avoid the liver and the spleen. A major hemothorax is drained with a **chest tube** and suction. The chest tube should be placed in a dependent position, the best location being through the sixth or seventh intercostal space in the midaxillary line, directing the tube posterior to the lung (see Fig. 25-19).

2. Hemothorax requires **emergency thoracotomy** and operative control of the bleeding source if adequate blood replacement does not correct shock, or if measured blood loss from the chest tube continues at a rate greater than 250 ml/hr after the first 2 hr or is greater than 1000 ml/24 hr. A large hemothorax that remains visible on the chest x-ray after a chest tube is placed and is functioning is diagnostic of continued bleeding and an indication for early thoracotomy. It is meddlesome to fuss over a small hemothorax. Surprising amounts of blood are absorbed from the pleural space by 4–6 wk after trauma.

E. Laceration of the lung may result from spicules of fractured ribs puncturing the lung or from shearing forces. Pneumothorax and hemothorax of varying degrees always are present and are treated as outlined in **B** and **D,** respectively. The best method of controlling blood and air leaks from lacerated lung is to remove all the air and clot from the pleural space and expand the lung completely via chest tube suction. Continued bleeding or continued air leaks may indicate a need for suture. Resection should be avoided if possible for rapid dissolution of the hematoma and repair is the rule.

F. Contusion of the lung and other thoracic viscera is a common sequela of blunt chest trauma. Contusion of the lung with hemorrhage reveals itself as an area of increased density in the chest x-ray and usually is apparent on admission but sometimes becomes apparent 12–72 hr after injury. Areas of cavitation may appear later. They will heal.

G. Chest trauma patients seem particularly vulnerable to the development of the **adult respiratory distress syndrome.** A falling PaO_2 in spite of increasing FIO_2, a white lung on x-ray examination, and an increase in pressure required to move a given volume of air (stiff lungs) characterize the syndrome. The etiology remains speculative, but excessive IV fluid administration is the most frequently documented event. The excess fluids usually are administered in the emergency room, although the syndrome becomes evident only 48–72 hr later. Prevention is a primary goal. Once the respiratory distress syndrome is present, restriction of fluids, administration of salt-poor serum albumin and diuretics, and the use of positive end expiratory pressure with a volume ventilator are sometimes effective (see Chap. 12).

H. Tracheal or bronchial rupture or laceration produces pneumomediastinum or pneumothorax. Tension pneumothorax may occur. The presence of subcutaneous emphysema, especially in the mediastinum or neck, indicates the possibility of major airway injury. Bronchoscopy is helpful in establishing the diagnosis. Chest tubes should be inserted if a pneumothorax is present. Unless the volume of air leak is small, operative repair of the tracheal or bronchial laceration should be done as soon as the patient's general condition permits.

I. Splinting, due to the pain of rib fractures, results in decreased tidal volume and may lead to atelectasis and pneumonia. A diagnosis of rib fracture may be made if point tenderness and splinting are present; x-ray evidence of rib fractures may not develop for up to 10–14 days. Injection of the involved intercostal nerves occasionally may be used to relieve pain and to **permit a player to finish a game,** but patients are more effectively managed with analgesics, ambulation, and enforced coughing.

J. Chylothorax is a rare complication of chest trauma and is caused by injury to the thoracic duct. Accumulating chylous fluid should be drained by thoracentesis or via a chest tube to prevent fibrothorax and a trapped lung. Most chylous fistulas close spontaneously, and removal of the fluid from the chest is all that is needed. Recurrent chylothorax persisting longer than 3 wk may require direct control of the leak at thoracotomy.

K. Rupture of the diaphragm is seen after blunt trauma to either the chest or the abdomen. The diagnosis is frequently missed even after laparotomy. The chest x-ray most often shows an air-fluid level in the **lower** chest. The torn diaphragm no longer provides a barrier between the thorax and the abdomen. The derangements caused by diaphragmatic rupture or paralysis are the same as those seen in flail chest, except for the absence of pain and splinting. During inspiration (increased negative intrathoracic pressure), abdominal viscera are pushed into the chest, preventing normal inflation of the lung, which then becomes atelectatic. In addition to impairing ventilation, the ruptured diaphragm poses a threat of compromised circulation to the herniated viscera. **Prompt surgical repair of a ruptured diaphragm is imperative.**

III. Trauma to the heart, aorta, and vena cava

A. Contusion of the heart is manifest by ECG changes of epicardial injury or myocardial ischemia and typically is the result of severe anterior chest injury caused by a **steering wheel.** Heart contusion is treated as a myocardial infarction, the details of treatment being dependent on the magnitude of the ECG and serum enzyme changes.

B. Cardiac perforation may involve the walls of the cardiac chambers, the septa, or the valves and can produce cardiac tamponade. While it is true that some small perforations of the heart seal spontaneously and may be treated effectively by observation, all heart wounds should be explored if a cardiac surgical team is available. If the more radical treatment of observation is elected, recurrent cardiac tamponade is an absolute indication for thoracotomy. Pressure and oxygen saturation should be measured in the cardiac chambers during the operation to help delineate the nature of the intracardiac injury.

C. **Cardiac tamponade** should be differentiated from simple hemopericardium. Cardiac tamponade is present when the hemopericardium is of sufficient size to produce Beck's triad of falling arterial pressure, rising venous pressure, and a small, quiet heart. Hemopericardium usually is not evident on a chest x-ray. The basic hemodynamic derangement in cardiac tamponade is impaired filling of the low-pressure chambers on the right side of the heart. Therefore, additional IV fluid therapy in spite of an elevated CVP is rational. Always consider the possibility of cardiac tamponade in chest trauma when the patient fails to respond to appropriate therapy and when a high CVP is associated with shock, decreased pulse pressure, or low cardiac output. **Needle pericardiocentesis** (aspiration) is the initial treatment of cardiac tamponade (see Fig. 25-18). The patient should be transferred immediately to the care of an experienced thoracic surgeon in case definitive therapy becomes necessary.

D. **Injury to the aorta.** Blunt chest trauma, especially of the deceleration type, may lead to aortic rupture, usually just distal to the origin of the left subclavian artery. X-ray changes may be very subtle. A widened mediastinum and depression of the left main bronchus seen on an upright PA chest x-ray must be considered suggestive of aortic injury and should lead to aortography to rule out this potentially fatal injury. Fractures of the scapula, the first and second ribs, and the medial third of the clavicle all suggest severe trauma and should lead to a consideration of aortography. Aortic injuries require emergency thoracotomy with cardiopulmonary bypass or a shunt.

E. **Traumatic asphyxia** is a condition produced by prolonged **compressive** thoracic trauma. Characteristically, the patient is cyanotic only about the face. Cerebral dysfunction almost invariably is present but clears within 24 hr. The significance of this injury is that one should not be misled by the facial cyanosis into giving unneeded ventilatory assistance while overlooking other possible intrathoracic injuries.

Suggested Reading

Blaisdell, F. W., and Lewis, F. R. *Respiratory Distress Syndrome of Shock and Trauma: Post-Traumatic Respiratory Failure.* Philadelphia: Saunders, 1977.

Moore, E. E., Moore, T. B., Galloway, A. C., and Eiseman, B. Post injury thoracotomy in the emergency department: A critical evaluation. *Surgery* 86:590, 1979.

Abdominal Injury

I. General comments

A. Any patient involved in an automobile, industrial, or sports accident should be considered to have an abdominal injury until it is proved otherwise. Serious intra-abdominal injury can occur from very minor trauma.

B. **Patients with blunt abdominal trauma are difficult to evaluate.** The signs of their injury can be delayed, and the consequences of injury, particularly to solid organs, can be difficult to manage.

C. Signs and symptoms of intra-abdominal injury can be masked by injuries elsewhere. The presence of fractured ribs with secondary splinting makes examination of the abdominal wall difficult. A serious central nervous system injury also can mask abdominal findings.

D. Decisions must be made based on **repeated examinations,** especially during resuscitation, since shock may mask abdominal findings. Frequent examinations should be **made by the same person** until it can be ascertained definitely that significant visceral injury, peritonitis, or hemorrhage is not present.

E. **Rupture of a hollow viscus** usually produces signs of peritoneal irritation and loss of bowel sounds. These signs may not be present on initial examination, and some patients with small-bowel and bladder injuries may show surprisingly minimal early signs and must be reevaluated frequently.

F. The patient with **injury of a solid viscus,** such as the liver or spleen, usually presents with hemorrhage. Peritoneal irritation may occur when blood is present within the abdominal cavity. A trauma victim presenting with unexplained hypovolemic shock should be assumed to have an intra-abdominal injury.

G. Organ enlargement, particularly if secondary to other pathological conditions (e.g., lymphoma), makes the organ more susceptible to injury. A distended urinary bladder or pregnant uterus is at increased risk of injury from blunt trauma to the abdomen.

II. Signs and symptoms of abdominal trauma

A. **Pain** following abdominal trauma may result from abdominal wall injury or injury of underlying structures. Pain referred to the shoulder is seen with diaphragmatic irritation secondary to splenic or hepatic injury. Patients who have pain and other findings should not be given narcotics or other analgesics until a decision about the need for an operation has been made.

B. **Localized tenderness** or **abdominal wall rigidity** is a result of peritoneal irritation from blood or hollow viscus content and is usually an indication for exploration. Abdominal guarding during palpation makes evaluation of the abdomen difficult, particularly in anxious or uncooperative patients. This is particularly true if there is associated chest, spinal, or pelvic injury. Repeated gentle examinations are helpful. If rib fractures are present, intercostal nerve blocks will decrease pain and may help in evaluation of the abdomen. Absence of tenderness and rigidity is no assurance that intra-abdominal injury is absent.

C. **Abdominal distention** is always an ominous sign. If it occurs in a patient with a penetrating wound, injury of the liver, spleen, or a major vessel has probably occurred. In blunt trauma, abdominal distention may be due to ileus secondary to retroperitoneal injury, especially involving the pancreas, or to spinal injury.

D. The **absence of bowel sounds** (5 min), particularly in patients with seemingly shallow penetrating wounds, is an indication for exploratory laparotomy.

E. **Inability to resuscitate** a hypovolemic patient with suspected abdominal injury is an indication for rapid operative intervention and direct control of the hemorrhage. If the patient has multiple fractures and a great deal of soft tissue injury, the resuscitative effort must be vigorous before one can conclude that continued intra-abdominal hemorrhage is present.

III. X-ray studies

A. **Routine views.** At an appropriate time during the resuscitative effort, flat and upright abdominal x-rays and a chest x-ray should be obtained. Every effort should be made to obtain an upright chest x-ray. Supine films of the chest are difficult to interpret. Diagnostic features to look for include free air in the peritoneal cavity, retroperitoneal air (especially near the duodenum), elevation of the diaphragm, obliteration of the psoas shadows, displacement of the gastric air bubble, disturbances of normal bowel patterns, and the presence and location of foreign bodies.

B. Intravenous pyelogram (IVP). An IVP should be done on all patients suspected of having an intra-abdominal injury. The infusion of contrast material should be timed so that an acceptable pyelogram is obtained along with the routine abdominal views. The IVP is useful in demonstrating kidney injury and is mandatory to assure the presence of a functioning contralateral kidney if nephrectomy is necessary.

C. Other studies. In patients who present with gross blood at the urethral meatus, a **urethrogram** should be obtained prior to catheterization. In patients who present with gross hematuria, an **IVP** should be done first, followed by a **cystourethrogram.** If the cystourethrogram is done prior to the IVP, extravasation of contrast material may make interpretation of the IVP impossible. Selective **angiography** is useful in patients with blunt abdominal trauma whose initial diagnostic workup is inconclusive. Selective celiac angiography is particularly useful in demonstrating subcapsular splenic injuries. Upper gastrointestinal (GI) tract **barium studies** may be helpful in establishing gastric displacement by an enlarged spleen and in demonstrating a duodenal intramural hematoma. Unfortunately, on occasion, a barium swallow also demonstrates a retroperitoneal rupture of the duodenum. **Ultrasonography** and **CT scanning** can be extremely useful in patients with abdominal injury who have not been operated on and show delayed effects of their intra-abdominal injuries, particularly injuries to the liver and retroperitoneum.

IV. Laboratory examination

A. Although hemoglobin and hematocrit determinations are of little value in the initial appraisal of the patient with blood loss, they can be useful during the observation period to detect continued loss of blood.

B. A leukocyte count in excess of 20,000 mm³ in the absence of evidence of infection is suggestive of significant blood loss and is particularly useful in supporting an early diagnosis of rupture of the spleen.

C. Elevation of serum amylase suggests pancreatic injury or bowel rupture. Elevation of transaminase suggests hepatic injury.

V. Other studies

A. Abdominal paracentesis is a helpful study in determining the presence of blood due to intra-abdominal injury. Peritoneal lavage is the preferred technique (see Fig. 25-19). If one can read newsprint through the effluent within the catheter, the lavage can be regarded as negative. A sample of the effluent is analyzed for red blood cells; more than 100,000 cells/mm³ is an indication for exploratory laparotomy. The effluent can also be tested for bile, leukocytes, bacteria, and amylase. **A negative test is never diagnostic and should be ignored.** Significant intra-abdominal injury can be present in spite of negative results.

Lavage should not be done in patients with gaseous distention or in areas of old scars. In most instances, abdominal x-rays should be obtained prior to lavage to avoid confusion about the origin of free intraperitoneal air.

B. If rectal bleeding is seen or blood is present on the examining finger, the possibility of rectal injury should be evaluated by **proctosigmoidoscopy.**

C. A **nasogastric tube** should be inserted in all patients suspected of having abdominal injury. The presence of blood in the aspirate may mean that an injury to the upper GI tract has occurred.

VI. Emergency management of abdominal trauma

A. Open wounds caused by bullets, shotgun blasts, large knives, or by similar means are an indication for abdominal exploration. If the injury is associated with shock or abdominal distention, the abdomen should be explored immediately. Otherwise, time is taken to perform the examinations listed in **III–V.**

B. **Small open injuries** to the anterior abdominal wall in which penetration of the peritoneal cavity is unlikely can be treated expectantly. If there is any sign of peritoneal irritation, such as tenderness, rigidity, or absence of bowel sounds, the abdomen should be explored. The safest manner of caring for these patients is to explore the injury directly under local anesthesia in the operating room. If there is evidence that the peritoneal cavity has been entered, abdominal exploration under general anesthesia can be carried out. In most instances, it is safe simply to observe patients with stab wounds of the anterior abdominal wall who present without any physical signs.

C. Patients with **blunt trauma** to the abdomen are treated according to the symptoms, signs, and results of other examinations. A positive paracentesis is an explicit indication for laparotomy. If the patient has minimal findings at the time of initial examination, but the suspicion of significant abdominal trauma is still present, he or she should be admitted to the hospital for observation. During this observation period, the patient should be examined frequently by the same examiner; repeat x-ray studies of the abdomen are performed.

Indications for exploratory laparotomy in blunt abdominal trauma include:

1. Persistent abdominal wall tenderness or rigidity.

2. Unexplained, even though minimal, persistent findings on repeated examination of the abdomen.

3. Appearance of signs of shock or blood loss.

4. Positive x-ray or laboratory findings.

D. The use of **pneumatic compression trousers** should be considered for patients who have been exsanguinated and who are not responding to vigorous resuscitation. If pneumatic compression trousers have been applied and inflated in the field, the trousers should not be deflated until such time as immediate operative intervention can be accomplished.

VII. Emergency exploratory laparotomy

A. **Steps prior to exploration.** In addition to the general principles applying to all patients undergoing an operation, the following should be done for patients being explored for possible intra-abdominal injury:

1. Nasogastric suction.

2. Placement of an indwelling urinary catheter.

3. Parenteral administration of antibiotics in patients with signs of GI tract injury, severe shock, or massive trauma.

4. Insertion of a chest tube in patients with rib fractures or with even minimal pneumothorax or hemothorax.

B. The **incision.** An exploratory laparotomy should be performed through a long midline incision. This incision has the advantages of speed of entry and access to the entire abdominal cavity.

C. **The steps of an emergency exploratory laparotomy are:**

1. **Rapid exploration of the entire abdomen** to determine the sites of hemorrhage.

2. Immediate **control of hemorrhage.** If the hemorrhage is due to injury of solid organs, control can be achieved with the use of packs. If the hemorrhage is from a major artery, the injury site should be controlled by vascular clamps. If the hemorrhage is due to injury to a major vein, initial control should be by direct pressure.

3. After hemorrhage is initially controlled and before an operative manipulation

is continued that is liable to be attended by further blood loss, the anesthesiologist should be allowed to catch up with **volume replacement.**

4. Open injuries to the GI tract should be controlled to prevent further contamination of the peritoneal cavity. If a large or expanding retroperitoneal hematoma is present, it may be unroofed and the sites of hemorrhage controlled.

5. Definitive control of hemorrhage should be approached by vascular repair, ligation of vessels, removal of injured organs (spleen), or resection (liver).

6. Repair open wounds in the GI tract and wounds of solid viscera as indicated.

7. If the peritoneal cavity has been contaminated by open wounds, lavage of the peritoneal cavity should be performed with copious amounts of normal saline solution. Consider the use of appropriate intraperitoneal instillation of an antibiotic solution.

8. A formal, complete exploration of the entire abdominal cavity should now be carried out. Included in the exploration should be entry into the lesser sac and visualization of the entire pancreas. If there is any evidence of hemorrhage or edema in this area, the pancreas should be totally mobilized and inspected for injury. A generous mobilization (Kocher's maneuver) of the duodenum should be carried out to inspect the entire posterior duodenal wall.

9. Sites of previously repaired injuries should be reinspected, a final lavage of the peritoneal cavity performed, drains placed only for specific indications, and the abdominal wound closed in layers.

10. If peritoneal contamination has occurred, leave the skin and subcutaneous tissues open.

VIII. Management of specific injuries

A. Abdominal wall. Blunt trauma can cause injury to the abdominal wall without causing intra-abdominal injury. Musculature can be avulsed or major vessels transected. Rigidity, tenderness, and a palpable mass can result, for example, from a rectus hematoma. Any mass within the anterior abdominal wall remains easily palpable when the patient raises the head, tensing the abdominal muscles, whereas this maneuver usually causes an intraperitoneal mass to become less palpable.

B. The **spleen** is the most frequently injured intra-abdominal organ. A ruptured spleen is suspected if there has been trauma to the left side, especially if ribs are fractured.

1. The clinical findings and evidence of **hypovolemia** range from minimal to profound. Pain referred to the left shoulder is common. Other useful findings include leukocytosis, displacement of the gastric air bubble, and presence of blood on paracentesis. In doubtful cases, selective celiac arteriograms can be helpful. Contrast-filled splenic vessels should be seen out to the lateral edge of the abdominal cavity. In the presence of a subcapsular splenic injury, a peripheral avascular rim will be seen on the arteriogram. Delayed rupture of the spleen should be suspected in a patient who has sudden abdominal pain and signs of hypovolemia occurring within 4 wk of an injury.

2. Treatment is abdominal exploration and splenectomy. Control of hemorrhage at the time of exploration can be done by direct pressure with packs or rapid compression of the splenic pedicle. The essential step in the performance of splenectomy is incision of the splenic posterolateral peritoneal attachment. This allows delivery of the spleen into the wound, so that the splenic pedicle can be secured without danger of injuring the tail of the pancreas. If there are no other injuries or specific indications for drainage, the splenic bed need not be drained. Postsplenectomy sepsis with its high mortality can occur at any time following splenectomy. In selected cases, efforts should be made to repair splenic injuries. All postsplenectomy patients should be considered candidates for long-term antibiotic prophylaxis, or administration of pneumococcal vaccine, or both.

C. The **liver** is the largest intra-abdominal organ, and the magnitude of parenchymal damage can range from minimal to almost total destruction.

1. **Minimal injury.** Puncture wounds, lacerations, and low-velocity through-and-through missile injuries to the liver that are not bleeding at the time of exploration and that are in areas of the liver where they are unlikely to lead to injury to major intrahepatic vessels are drained; the capsular wounds are not closed. Simple bleeding wounds should be explored and hemostasis attained by direct suture ligation of bleeding vessels, followed by drainage; the capsule is not sutured. Implantation of foreign hemostatic materials should be avoided.

2. **Major injury.** The key to success is total mobilization of the liver and control of the hepatic vasculature as follows:

   a. Detach the falciform ligament from the anterior abdominal wall down to the anterior aspect of the suprahepatic vena cava.

   b. Incise the left triangular ligament from its left lateral margin to the suprahepatic vena cava.

   c. Retract the right lobe of the liver to the midline, and incise the right triangular ligament, exposing the right lateral margin of the intrahepatic vena cava.

   d. Free the suprahepatic and infrahepatic vena cava adjacent to the liver; incision of the diaphragm usually is not necessary.

   e. Place a tape around the hepatoduodenal structures in the porta hepatis (Pringle's maneuver).

   f. Rapidly assess the extent of injury to ascertain the extent of debridement necessary. This decision is basically logistic, since the amount of bleeding surface in a large, deep laceration may be greater than the surface following resection. Resection must be done if avascular liver tissue is present.

   g. Large mattress sutures to control liver hemorrhage should be avoided, since they create areas of necrotic tissue and may lead to abscess formation.

   h. If hemorrhage is massive or if injury to the intrahepatic inferior vena cava has occurred, the liver can be totally isolated by placing vascular clamps on the suprahepatic and infrahepatic vena cava and using tape control of the porta hepatis. One can also insert a catheter within the vena cava to bypass the venous return from the lower body; this maneuver is somewhat difficult and uses valuable time, and thus total vascular isolation of the liver is much preferred. Occasionally, massive arterial hemorrhage occurs in a through-and-through wound. Ligation of the involved lobar arterial supply is the preferred treatment.

   i. If total mobilization of the liver has been carried out, one usually does not need to extend the midline incision into the right hemithorax. If, however, exposure and continued hemorrhage are problems, there should be no hesitancy in extending the incision.

   j. Massive hemorrhage and hepatic trauma may lead to coagulation problems. Treatment should include administration of fresh blood, fresh-frozen plasma, platelet concentrates, and specific clotting factors (see Chap. 16).

   k. Following resection and control of hemorrhage, adequate soft rubber drains should be placed. The biliary tree is not drained routinely. There is controversy about biliary decompression. Proponents point out that insertion of a T-tube decreases the amount of bile loss through open surfaces of the liver and serves as a vehicle for postoperative detection of hematobilia. More recent evidence indicates that routine biliary decompression is associated with increased morbidity.

D. Pancreas. Unless there has been a significant rise in serum amylase noted prior to operation, injury of the pancreas is usually detected at the time of exploration. Minor contusions that do not involve the major ducts can be drained. Major injuries to the body and tail of the pancreas are treated by resection. Injuries to the pancreas on the right side of the superior mesenteric vessels involving major ductal structures are treated by internal drainage into a Roux-en-Y jejunal loop. Massive injuries to the head of the pancreas may demand a pancreatoduodenectomy, particularly if there has been massive injury to the duodenum.

E. Gallbladder and biliary tract. Injuries to the biliary tract usually are caused by penetrating wounds, although the gallbladder can be devascularized by blunt injury. An injured gallbladder must be excised. Injury to the extrahepatic biliary ductal system usually is detected at laparotomy by the presence of bile staining of tissues. Primary repair of biliary ductal injury is preferred; if the injury is extensive, a bypass such as a choledochojejunostomy must be performed.

F. Stomach. Gastric injuries should be suspected if nasogastric suction reveals the presence of blood. During laparotomy, particularly with penetrating injuries, the lesser sac should be opened, the entire stomach mobilized, and a search made for sites of injury. Particular attention should be paid to the lesser curvature, since injuries in this area are easily missed. Wounds of the stomach should be debrided widely and sutured.

G. Duodenum. Intraperitoneal duodenal injury may be suspected if bile or small-bowel contents are recovered by paracentesis. Retroperitoneal injury to the duodenum is more frequent than intraperitoneal injury. Unless retroperitoneal air is seen on the preoperative abdominal x-ray, injury to the retroperitoneal duodenum will be discovered only when the duodenum is mobilized (Kocher's maneuver) during exploratory laparotomy.

1. The **extent** of the duodenal wall defect following debridement determines the type of repair. Simple lacerations are closed in the direction of the wound. Extensive defects can be closed with a jejunal serosal patch onlay or an isolated jejunal mucosal patch. All duodenal wounds are prone to breakdown. The duodenum should be decompressed internally with transgastric and transjejunal sump suction catheters. The operative area should be drained, and both internal and external drains should remain in place for at least 10 days. Extensive injury to the duodenum and pancreas may require a pancreatoduodenectomy.

2. **Intramural duodenal hematoma** may occur following blunt trauma, particularly in children. The patient presents with vomiting; upper gastrointestinal (GI) contrast studies may show the typical "corkscrew" deformity. Operative evacuation of the hematoma is curative.

H. Small intestine. Small-bowel injury should be suspected in any patient with penetrating abdominal injury. In blunt trauma, small-intestine injury usually occurs at or near sites of mesenteric fixation. Signs of peritoneal irritation usually are present, and small-bowel contents are sometimes recovered on paracentesis. **Treatment** consists of debridement and primary closure. If there are many individual perforations within a short segment of bowel, the entire involved segment is resected. A meticulous search for perforations should be made, with particular attention to the mesenteric border.

I. Colon. Patients with colon injury may present with signs of peritonitis, or upright x-rays may show free air. A *barium enema should never be done in patients suspected of having colon injury.* Preoperatively, vigorous fluid replacement and systemic antibiotics are required. The choices of operative treatment are:

1. **Primary repair.** This is done only if injury is minimal, there are no other significant injuries, no peritoneal contamination has occurred, and treatment is instituted within 3 hr of injury.

2. **Resection.** This is the safer procedure, especially if there is extensive colon injury, significant fecal contamination has occurred, operative treatment has been delayed, or there are associated organ injuries. The ends of the colon are converted to a colostomy and a mucous fistula. Continuity is restored at a second operation.

   Copious peritoneal lavage should be carried out. Septic complications are frequent and should be anticipated.

J. **Female reproductive organs.** Injuries to the female reproductive organs are usually in pregnant women and may cause sudden vaginal hemorrhage following blunt trauma. Hysterectomy or removal of injured adnexa may be necessary. Salvage of a pregnancy depends on gestational age and degree of fetal injury.

Urological Injury

I. General considerations

A. Injury to the genitourinary (GU) tract **rarely occurs as an isolated lesion.** These injuries tend to occur as one aspect of a larger problem in the multiply injured patient. Blunt trauma from automobile accidents and penetrating injuries from bullet and knife wounds account for a majority of the cases. The immediate goal in management of these injuries is to prevent or treat hypovolemic shock and stop major bleeding if the patient's condition remains unstable. A secondary goal is to prevent collection of urine and abscess formation by properly draining urinary extravasations. The long-range goal of therapy should be to minimize functional disability, such as severe stricture formation of the urethra.

B. The role of surgical intervention in the management of renal and urethral injuries has been changing over the past few years. Many urologists now believe that **conservative management** of these injuries results in less long-term morbidity and functional disability.

C. **Complications** of GU injury are: hypovolemic shock, devascularization and loss of renal parenchyma, urinary extravasation with sepsis and abscess formation, and stricture of the ureter or the urethra. There may also be functional disability, such as a loss of significant renal function, voiding dysfunction, and impotence in the male.

II. Diagnosis

A. The **history** may be very useful in helping to establish the diagnosis. Inability to void or severe pain on attempting to void suggests partial or total separation of the urethra. A major problem often encountered in the workup of these patients is that other injuries are so extensive that a careful review of the history is precluded.

B. **Physical examination** should be directed to detection of injuries in three major areas:

1. **Upper urinary tract injuries** are often associated with rib fractures over the involved kidney. An expanding flank mass (found by abdominal palpation) with hypovolemic shock indicates a major renal injury.

2. **Lower urinary tract injuries** are often associated with blunt trauma to the lower abdomen and with fractures of the bony pelvis. Blood at the urethral meatus is an important sign of lower urinary tract injury.

3. **A suprapubic mass** from a hematoma or urinary extravasation and a hematoma in the perineum or scrotum are often found. Rectal examination may reveal a doughy mass in the region of the prostate from a large pelvic hematoma.

C. **The extent of injury** to the external genitalia in both males and females is usually easily assessed by physical examination.

D. **Urinalysis** may be helpful in establishing the diagnosis of urinary tract injury. However, trauma to the urinary tract will not result in gross or microscopic hematuria in all patients. This fact should be kept clearly in mind if the physical examination and other studies reveal a urinary tract injury although the urinalysis is negative.

E. **Plain abdominal x-rays** should be carefully evaluated for loss of psoas shadow, fractures impinging on urinary structures, foreign bodies lying in proximity to the genitourinary systems, kidney outlines, and free air or fluid in the abdomen.

F. **An infusion IVP** should be done in all patients suspected of having a GU injury. An IVP should be performed using the IV line that is set up when the patient enters the emergency room. In shock, the kidney may not be visualized, but the IVP nonetheless remains the single most important radiological study of the urinary tract in trauma. To facilitate visualization of the kidneys, hypovolemia should be corrected with fluid or blood replacement rather than vasopressors, because the latter will diminish renal blood flow and decrease the likelihood of visualization. Drip infusion pyelography using 50–100 ml of contrast medium will provide information regarding the size, shape, and position of the kidneys, may demonstrate urinary extravasation, and, most important, will determine the status of the contralateral kidney and ureter. In the presence of renal injury, the contrast medium may not be excreted into the renal pelvis, but if the main renal artery is intact and not occluded by hematoma, a nephrogram of the injured kidney will almost always be seen. Nonvisualization of the kidney suggests occlusion or transection of the main renal artery and is an indication for renal arteriography.

G. **Retrograde urethrograms** are essential in defining urethral injuries. Retrograde injection of 15–30 ml of sterile contrast medium will define the urethral injury as evidenced by extravasation of contrast material and should precede instrumentation of the urethra. IV contrast material *must* be used for this study, and no lubricating jelly should be injected into the urethra to prevent severe stricture formation if contrast material extravasates at the time of the study.

H. **A urethral catheter** is usually required early in the management of the patient with multiple trauma, to assess renal function and the effect of treatment of hypovolemic shock. However, great care should be taken not to convert a partial tear of the urethra into a complete tear by traumatic catheterization. If there is blood at the urethral meatus or other signs of urethral injury, every attempt should be made to perform a retrograde urethrogram before inserting a catheter. A carefully placed urethral catheter may be all the treatment necessary in many patients with urethral injury with minimal extravasation of urine. If the urine becomes infected after catheterization, an appropriate antibiotic should be started. This is particularly important if extravasation has occurred into a large pelvic hematoma, and there is a risk of infecting the hematoma.

I. **A cystogram** is essential for the diagnosis of ruptured bladder. Installation of 50–300 ml of diluted IV contrast material such as Hypaque should be done through a urethral catheter. AP, lateral, oblique, and postemptying x-rays are all necessary to detect extravasation. An extraperitoneal rupture of the bladder will show extravasated contrast material in the perivesical space; with an intraperitoneal rupture, contrast material is seen in the peritoneal cavity, often between loops of small bowel.

J. Renal arteriography. Arteriograms are needed to assess the extent of renal injury and the possible congenital absence of one kidney if the kidneys are not visualized during intravenous pyelography. Arteriography is also useful for outlining the branches of the renal artery when it is necessary to operate on a fractured kidney with urinary extravasation or massive renal bleeding, or both. The extent of other intra-abdominal injuries, such as tears in the spleen and liver, can often be visualized at the same time.

III. Treatment of external genital injuries

A. Injuries to the penis usually result in loss of penile skin and, in some cases, in partial amputation of the penis. A split-thickness skin graft or burying the penile shaft under abdominal or scrotal skin is necessary to cover the denuded area. Partial amputation is treated by debridement and construction of a new urethral meatus of adequate caliber.

B. Injuries to the introitus and urethra in the female are usually straddle injuries caused by a fractured pelvis. Lacerations are sutured and the urethra is carefully reconstructed to preserve urinary continence.

IV. Treatment of urinary tract injuries

A. Urethral injuries in the male occur in three separate areas: in the pendulous urethra, bulbous urethra below the genitourinary diaphragm, and supramembranous urethra.

   1. Injuries to the pendulous urethra result in hematoma and urinary extravasation inside Buck's fascia and are usually best treated with an indwelling urethral catheter for 10 days to 2 wk.

   2. Injuries to the bulbous urethra most often are straddle injuries. Urinary extravasation and hematoma may be present in the perineum and scrotum and on occasion may be seen on the abdominal and chest walls as the fluid dissects upward beneath Scarpa's fascia. **Treatment** consists of gentle placement of an indwelling catheter or placement of a suprapubic tube into the bladder if the urethral catheter will not pass with ease. Urethral strictures that develop from conservative management during initial treatment are best repaired at a later time. Attempt at primary repair of the injured urethra in the region of the sphincter will lead to an increased incidence of incontinence, impotence, and stricture formation.

   3. Injuries to the supramembranous urethra usually occur as a tear or complete separation at the level of the apex of the prostate and the GU diaphragm. These injuries are almost always associated with pelvic fractures. Large pelvic hematomas develop that are evident on rectal and suprapubic palpation. Treatment consists of placement of a suprapubic catheter into the bladder and secondary repair of the scarred urethra at a later time. Conservative treatment minimizes the problems with primary repair mentioned in **2** and also helps prevent infection of the pelvic hematoma by an indwelling urethral catheter.

B. Bladder injuries occur as extraperitoneal and intraperitoneal tears of the bladder wall. Intraperitoneal rupture must be closed surgically, preferably in three layers. Extraperitoneal rupture can be managed by an indwelling catheter only if the amount of extravasation seen on the cystogram is small. Otherwise, drains should be placed alongside the bladder and in the space of Retzius. Large tears should be sutured as well as drained.

C. Injuries to the ureter most often result from bullet and knife wounds. If only a short segment of ureter has been damaged, a ureteroureterostomy of the debrided and spatulated segments of ureter should be accomplished over a ureteral stent. Loss of a large segment of ureter may be treated by use of a Boari bladder flap to bridge the defect, transureteroureterostomy, or autotransplantation of the kidney.

D. Injury to the kidney may occur either as blunt trauma or as a penetrating injury.

1. **Blunt trauma** results in contusion of the kidney and occasionally in fracture of the parenchyma. Avulsion of the renal artery from the aorta or intimal tears with renal artery thrombosis may also occur with blunt trauma.

2. **Penetrating injuries** usually cause bleeding with formation of a retroperitoneal hematoma. Penetrating injuries may also damage the urinary collecting system and cause urinary extravasation. As previously stated, the IVP and arteriogram are both important in defining the location and extent of renal injury.

3. The **method of treatment** of renal injury depends on three important factors: (a) severity of renal bleeding as evidenced by stability of blood pressure and size of retroperitoneal hematoma; (b) amount of extravasation of contrast material during the IVP; and (c) severity of major renal parenchymal and arterial injury as demonstrated by IVP and arteriograms.

   a. Patients with stable blood pressure, stable size of flank mass, and little or no extravasation of contrast material on IVP should be managed conservatively. If the patient must undergo operation for other intra-abdominal injuries, the posterior peritoneum over the hematoma should not be opened, to prevent increased renal bleeding. Patients who meet the criteria for conservative treatment and have only a renal injury should have bed rest for 5–7 days. Patients should not walk as long as gross hematuria persists after renal injury.

   b. **Fracture of the kidney** with injury to or occlusion of the renal artery or its branches is managed by vascular reconstruction or nephrectomy. Occlusion of the main renal artery for more than 30–40 min almost always results in renal cortical necrosis, and the kidney should be removed. Fractures of the kidney in patients with accessory arteries may occur in a plane between the main artery and the polar vessel, and require partial nephrectomy or revascularization of the parenchyma and collecting system.

      (1) If vascular reconstruction is attempted with renal artery injuries, it should be kept in mind that renal artery branches are end arteries. In general, it is unwise to attempt reconstruction of severe arterial injuries associated with devascularized parenchyma if the patient has a normal contralateral kidney. Patients with a solitary kidney are an obvious exception to this recommendation.

      (2) Grafts of saphenous vein or hypogastric artery may be used for reconstruction. Synthetic graft material should not be used in renal trauma.

      (3) **Autotransplantation** of the kidney with extracorporeal renal artery repair may be the best procedure in patients with injury to a solitary kidney. In such cases, rapid nephrectomy followed by flushing with heparinized Ringer's lactate solution and cooling of the kidney in saline slush will protect the parenchyma from further ischemic injury for up to 8 hr. Autotransplantation can then be accomplished after bleeding is controlled and any other major injuries are repaired.

Extremity and Pelvic Injury

I. **General comments.** Except for hemorrhage from a major vascular wound, trauma to an extremity is not immediately life-threatening. Temporary measures, such as control of hemorrhage by pressure, application of dressings to prevent further contamination, and temporary immobilization of fractures or dislocations to prevent further soft tissue damage, are sufficient initial therapy while attention is being directed to treatment of life-threatening injuries elsewhere in the body.

As soon as hemodynamic stability has been established:

A. Check to make certain **all peripheral pulses are present.** Injury to major arterial or venous vessels may constitute a threat to viability of the limb. Once life-threatening injuries elsewhere in the body are controlled, the nature of vascular, bone, and neuromuscular injuries should be defined by appropriate examination.

B. Examine for **loss of motion** on command, **deformity** of the extremity, and localized or generalized **swelling.** Any of these findings should raise a question of injury to bone, blood vessel, muscle, tendon, nerve, or articular surface.

C. Systematically **search for wounds,** which should be carefully inspected using aseptic precautions. Complete debridement of devitalized tissue followed by primary repair can be carried out if the wound is superficial and uncomplicated. If injury to a nerve, tendon, or major blood vessel is identified or suspected, exploration and repair should be done in the operating room.

II. **Fractures.** Fractures should be suspected if there is deformity, crepitation, swelling, or a transverse loss of function.

A. **Simple closed fractures** are the most obvious consequence of trauma but are not a threat to life and limb. They should be promptly immobilized (a pillow makes a good temporary splint) to prevent further soft tissue injury. When other injuries have been treated and the patient's condition is stable, manipulation and reduction can be carried out. Detailed x-ray studies for fracture fragment position can be deferred until the patient is ready for definitive reduction.

B. **Fractures or dislocations associated with vascular injury or nerve compression** (usually involving the knee, hip, elbow, or shoulder) should be manipulated as soon as the extent of injury has been established. This often restores pulses and eliminates nerve stretch or compression. The principle of initial treatment is to restore vascular and neural integrity.

C. **Open fractures** are those in which a skin wound communicates directly or indirectly with the fracture. They should be treated in the operating room as soon as possible with systemic antibiotics, debridement of nonviable tissue, and copious cleansing irrigation. Bone fragments should not be discarded, since they may be autoclaved and used as grafts.

1. It is best to **leave these wounds open** if there is any question of tissue viability, or if the degree of contamination is in question or is unknown. Primary wound closure may be considered only under ideal circumstances.

2. Definitive reduction, if convenient and not requiring internal fixation, often can be accomplished immediately. When this is not feasible, stabilization may be achieved by temporary splinting or traction. Definitive reduction (with or without internal fixation) should be delayed until the immediate threat of infection has passed.

D. A **pelvic fracture** can be identified by compressing the iliac crests together; with disruption of the pelvic ring, compression will cause pain due to movement of the fractures. Blood loss is usually large because of the vascularity of the pelvic bone marrow, inability to splint pelvic fractures effectively, and the continued bleeding from surrounding soft tissues because external compression cannot be applied. Prompt blood transfusion is essential. Lacerations of the bladder, urethra, and rectum should be sought and treated appropriately. Selective angiography of the aorta and pelvic vessels, and embolization to control bleeding vessels, should be considered if pelvic bleeding is persistent and continuing transfusion is required to maintain hemodynamic stability. Shock persisting after adequate volume replacement requires immediate abdominal and pelvic exploration to control hemorrhage.

Table 1-4. Consequences of Nerve Injuries

Motor Loss	Sensory Loss	Nerve
Upper extremity		
Shoulder abduction	Small patch over deltoid	Axillary
Biceps contraction	Volar radial forearm	Musculocutaneous
Elbow extension	Dorsal radial hand	High radial
Wrist and finger extension	Dorsal radial hand	Low radial
Wrist and finger flexion	Radial two-thirds of hand	Median
Finger abduction	Ulnar one-third of hand	Ulnar
Lower extremity		
Knee extension	Anterior medial thigh	Femoral
Ankle and toe extension	Anterior ankle	Peroneal
	Web space first to second toe	
Plantar flexion toes-ankle	Plantar foot	Posterior tibial
All motor below knee	All sensation below knee except medial ankle	Sciatic

III. Clinical manifestations

A. Motor-sensory examination. Table 1-4 outlines the simple tests that should be carried out to identify specific evidence of nerve injury. When a test is positive, one should consider the possibility of vascular disruption due to the close approximation of nerve and vascular structures in the extremities.

B. Vascular injuries

1. **External hemorrhage.** Blind clamping of a hemorrhaging vessel is **never** done; it often fails to control bleeding, may damage adjacent nerves, and may increase arterial and venous injury that complicates repair. **Pressure** applied at or proximal to the arterial wound will control hemorrhage while preparations to repair the vascular injury are in progress.

2. **Decreased or absent pulses** indicate partial or complete obstruction of flow due to arterial interruption. Spasm may temporarily obliterate pulses; in every such case, objective examinations (e.g., angiography) are required to rule out arterial damage. Doppler flows and ankle pressures are helpful when swelling due to hemorrhage and edema obscures the pulses. Decreased or absent **p**ulses are accompanied by **p**allor, **p**aresthesis, **p**aralysis, and severe **p**ain, (the **five ps** of acute arterial occlusion) in the distal portion of the extremity. Pulses may be absent in elderly patients because of atherosclerosis; a clue may be the symmetrical absence of pulses in the contralateral uninjured extremity. The **absence of pulses and persistence of ischemia in the injured extremity after relief of shock indicate arterial obstruction rather than spasm.**

3. **Initial treatment** in patients with absent or decreased pulses includes:

   a. Correction of shock.

   b. Search for and manipulation of any fracture or dislocation that may be causing arterial occlusion.

   c. Angiography if the pulse deficit persists.

   d. Immediate arterial exploration if obstruction is identified.

4. **Pain** due to ischemia must be distinguished from that due to local trauma. Ischemic pain often is more severe than the pain associated with other body injuries.

5. **Bruit** indicates the presence of an abnormal arteriovenous connection. The vessels should be explored as soon as the situation is recognized, and primary repair should be undertaken. Angiography may be helpful, but it is not mandatory if the presence and location of the lesion are clinically evident prior to operation. Exploration may be delayed if other injuries or their consequences demand priority in treatment, and if there is no threat to the viability of the extremity.

6. An **expanding hematoma** indicates continuing hemorrhage from an artery. Prompt exploration and repair are indicated. Delay may result in shock, nerve compression, or formation of a false aneurysm.

7. **Swollen extremity**

   a. **Compartment syndrome. Pain** is the most significant symptom of ischemic muscle injury. Swelling may be minimal or absent, especially when only the deep compartment of the calf is involved. Swelling, indicating the onset of ischemic muscle injury, is often delayed in onset and is associated with diminished pulses, shiny white skin due to decreased capillary perfusion, hypoesthesia (in the absence of primary nerve injury), and muscle paresis. **Immediate treatment** by extensive fasciotomy, including wide incision of the overlying skin, to decompress completely the involved musculofascial compartments is urgent. Tissue pressure exceeding 30–40 mm Hg, determined by a subfascially placed needle attached to a saline manometer, is a useful guide to the need for fasciotomy. Prophylactic fasciotomy on completion of a delayed arterial repair is often wise.

   b. Soft **diffuse edema** may follow revascularization or may be due to major venous thrombosis. The latter can be confirmed by Doppler examination, venous phlethysmography, or phlebography. Moderate elevation of the limb and toe-to-knee elastic support usually are sufficient treatment for revascularization edema. Anticoagulation with heparin should be employed when venous thrombosis is demonstrated.

IV. Angiography. Angiography demonstrates the site and the nature of the arterial lesion and reveals the status of the distal arterial bed. Direct needle injection into a major vessel proximal to the site of injury is most convenient; catheter angiography from a remote site is the alternative. When the site and nature of the vascular injury are obvious from preoperative clinical examination, angiography is not necessary and may delay treatment. However, it should be routinely used in (a) hemodynamically stable patients with penetrating wounds of the thoracic outlet, (b) when the exact site of injury cannot be clinically determined, and (c) when clinical evidence for vascular injury is equivocal. Penetrating injuries in the vicinity of major vessels should be studied by angiography. It is best to explore penetrating wounds with potential vascular injury if logistics and the patient's condition permit, since arterial injury may be present even though pulses are palpable and evidence of significant hemorrhage is lacking. However, if a good-quality arteriogram is normal, in the absence of direct evidence of arterial, venous, or adjacent nerve injury, surgical exploration is not required for the sole purpose of evaluating major vascular structures.

V. Arterial injuries and their consequences. Extremity ischemia is the invariable consequence of major arterial interruption. Nerve and muscles are the tissues most sensitive to ischemia. Prompt restoration of perfusion is required to prevent gangrene or severe functional impairment.

   A. Laceration. A tear or irregular incision in a vessel is the result of (1) external penetration by a knife, bullet, or protruding metal or glass object in an automobile accident or (2) internal penetration by a bone fragment. Arterial lacerations continue to bleed because the intact portion of the vessel wall prevents retraction closure of the arterial wound. External hemorrhage or an expanding hematoma require urgent intervention. If the patient is not operated upon, and further expansion of the hematoma is blocked by surrounding tissues, a fibrous capsule forms around the contained hematoma. Liquefaction of the center of the clot occurs; communication with the arterial lumen through the laceration produces a pulsating hematoma or false aneurysm. This continues to expand at a variable rate (for weeks or months), causing progressive deformity, pain, and nerve compression. Eventual disruption produces further internal hemorrhage, or external hemorrhage if there is compression necrosis of the overlying skin.

B. Transection is a completed laceration, usually accompanied by moderate or insignificant bleeding, due to symmetrical retraction of the circumference of the transected ends of the artery and formation of a temporary thrombus. Delayed hemorrhage may occur owing to relaxation of spasm of the transected vessel, liquefaction of the thrombus, or dislodgment of the thrombus by arterial pressure. Severe ischemia usually is present but may be variable, depending on the availability of collateral vessels and the degree to which they may have been compromised by associated soft tissue injury. Thrombosis proximal and distal to the injury further obstructs collaterals, often converting mild or moderate ischemia to severe, limb-threatening ischemia within a short time.

C. Perforating or penetrating injuries from small objects or small-caliber missiles may produce arterial occlusion, internal hemorrhage with false aneurysm, or an arteriovenous fistula if the injury is close to a major venous channel. External hemorrhage usually is minimal or absent, owing to the repositioning of the skin and fascia, with obliteration of the injury tract.

D. An arteriovenous fistula produces a variable degree of peripheral ischemia, depending on its size, the degree of reversal of flow from the distal arterial limb into the low-resistance venous system, and whether acute or delayed occlusion of the artery distal to the injury develops. A thrill or bruit becomes evident over a fistula. Cardiac output invariably is increased, and, with large fistulas, progressive cardiomegaly and high-output cardiac failure ensue. Secondary varicose veins become evident in the extremity. The proximal arterial limb feeding the fistula gradually enlarges and becomes tortuous and aneurysmal over a period of a few years. Temporary occlusion of flow through an arteriovenous fistula by external pressure produces an immediate reduction in the pulse rate (Branham's sign).

E. Blunt injury (contusion) may produce partial or complete intimal transection without disruption of the outer media and adventitia. Dissection of the distal intima by arterial flow leads to progressive obstruction and thrombosis. The contused segment, though intact externally, has a characteristically bluish discoloration, owing to the subintimal dissection. Severe ischemia, with a cool, pale, pulseless extremity, is usually evident. However, complete occlusion may not occur for hours or days, with no evidence or only equivocal, evidence of arterial obstruction at the time of initial examination. Full development of ischemic signs may be obscured by other injuries, casts, or failure to continue assessing extremity circulation, which may result in a disastrous delay in arterial repair.

F. Reflex vascoconstriction accompanies injuries adjacent to or directly involving blood vessels and is accompanied by mild to moderate peripheral ischemia. In the absence of arterial disruption or intimal injury, the outcome is spontaneous resolution.

G. Acute ischemic muscle injury, leading to necrosis, fibrosis, and contracture, most commonly involves the flexors of the forearm, as well as any or all the four compartments of the calf. It is most frequently associated with fractures about the elbow and knee and is characterized by increasingly severe pain, intense firm edema, and progressive anesthesia of the hand or foot. The process is due to muscle swelling secondary to prolonged ischemia followed by restoration of arterial flow. Venous flow from the involved muscles, which are encased in an unyielding fascial envelope, is blocked, causing further swelling, increasing pressure within the muscle compartments, and impaired circulation. If the muscle compartments are not promptly decompressed by fasciotomy, necrosis of muscle and nerve ensues, followed by fibrosis, contracture, and a neurological deficit. Involvement of the forearm in this process after supracondylar fracture of the humerus is called **Volkmann's contracture.**

VI. Venous injuries and their consequences. Obstruction may be the result of traumatic thrombosis, laceration, compression due to arterial hemorrhage into a confined space, or distortion by bone or ligament injury. Marked edema and superficial venous congestion usually develop. If venous return is massively obstructed, gangrene may ensue. Obstruction of venous outflow will reduce arterial inflow. As a consequence, an arterial repair is prone to thrombosis in the presence of venous injury, especially in the popliteal area.

VII. Technique of vascular exploration. The objective of vascular repair is to restore unimpeded blood flow to and from tissues peripheral to the injury. Incomplete repair may result in delayed functional ischemia or early thrombosis, threaten limb loss, and require reoperation through a potentially infected field.

A. Prepare and drape the entire involved extremity and adjacent portions of the trunk to permit adequate exposure and effective control of the major vessels proximal and distal to the point of injury. Temporary manual compression of the common femoral or upper brachial artery usually affords sufficient control of hemorrhage to facilitate direct exposure of a more distally injured vessel.

B. A temporary shunt should be used to restore peripheral extremity perfusion promptly if ischemia has been prolonged and to maintain flow through a functioning carotid artery that must be temporarily clamped for vascular repair.

C. After vascular control has been achieved, debride all traumatized and devitalized tissue and thoroughly irrigate the wound.

D. Remove distal propagated thrombus with a Fogarty balloon catheter.

E. Autogenous vein grafts and patches are preferable to prosthetic material; the latter poses the risk of infection in a contaminated wound. Venous grafts should be obtained from the saphenous system of the noninjured leg to avoid compromise of venous return in the event of subsequent deep vein thrombosis of the injured extremity. Arm veins may be employed if the saphenous is unavailable.

F. Simple arterial lacerations, whether partial or complete, can be managed by debridement of the vascular wound edges and restoration of vascular continuity by primary suture, patch angioplasty, or end-to-end anastomosis. The choice of technique depends on the nature of the vascular wound and the size of the injured vessel.

G. Low-velocity missile injuries require somewhat wider debridement than simple lacerations. Vessel continuity can often be restored by direct anastomosis. High-velocity missile injury is deceptive; there is considerable damage beyond that grossly apparent. Wide debridement and restoration of continuity by vein graft are almost invariably required.

H. Contused vessels with intimal dissection and thrombosis over a short segment can be managed by thrombointimectomy and vein patch angioplasty, or by excision and reanastomosis.

I. Extensive arterial injury of any type is best treated by end-to-side vein-graft bypass between healthy vessels proximal and distal to the site of injury. Direct repair in an area of extensive soft tissue destruction should be avoided. Bypass grafts should be passed through healthy tissue planes and anastomoses performed into healthy vessel remote from the injury site.

J. Repair of an arteriovenous fistula is accomplished by interruption of the fistula tract and restoration of both arterial and venous continuity. Management of the arterial injury will depend on its extent and nature, although minor debridement and direct suture are frequently satisfactory. The venous side also should be repaired; avoid ligation unless there is an adjacent and unobstructed collateral vessel to carry the venous outflow.

K. Major venous injuries (caval, iliac, femoral, popliteal, subclavian, axillary) should be repaired by suture or graft interposition, employing the same principles and techniques outlined for arterial debridement and repair. The technique must be extremely meticulous. Dextran may be given during and immediately after operation, although there is no good evidence to support its use in maintaining the patency of repaired veins.

L. Heparin may promote hematoma formation in the vascular repair wound or other sites of injury and should not be used in the immediate postoperative period. Heparin may be used after several days for the treatment of **proven** deep venous thrombosis if there has been no central nervous system trauma, and the danger of bleeding from the operative site or from other injuries is remote. Heparin should be given by continuous intravenous infusion, closely monitored by plasma thromboplastin time or a similar coagulation test. Transvenous insertion of an inferior vena cava filter or balloon, or the application of a caval clip, should be considered to prevent pulmonary embolism when heparin is contraindicated.

M. Coverage of vascular repair must be achieved with viable tissue (skin or muscle) to prevent suture-line infection and secondary hemorrhage. When soft tissue destruction is massive, this may not be possible. Temporary coverage under these circumstances can be accomplished with skin autografts.

Suggested Reading

Heppenstall, R. B.   *Fracture Treatment and Healing.* Philadelphia: Saunders, 1975.

Ledgerwood, A. M., and Lucas, C. E.   Massive thigh injuries with vascular disruption. *Arch. Surg.* 197:201, 1973.

Lim, L. T., Michuda, M. S., Flanigan, P., and Pankovich, A.   Popliteal artery trauma, 31 consecutive cases without amputation. *Arch. Surg.* 115:1307, 1980.

Perry, M. O., Thal, E. R., and Shires, G. T.   Management of arterial injuries. *Ann. Surg.* 173:403, 1971.

Rich, N. M., and Hobson, R. W.   *Venous Surgery in the Lower Extremity.* St. Louis: Green, 1973.

Rockwood, C. A., and Green D. P.   *Fractures.* Philadelphia: Lippincott, 1975.

Smith, R. F., Szilagyi, D. F., and Elliott, J. P.   Fracture of long bones with arterial injury due to blunt trauma. *Arch. Surg.* 99:315, 1969.

Slaney, G., and Ashton, F.   Arterial injuries and their management. *Postgrad. Med. J.* 47:257, 1971.

Whitesides, T. E., Haney, T. C., Harada, H., Holmes, H. E., and Morimoto, K.   A simple method for tissue pressure determination. *Arch. Surg.* 110:1311, 1975.

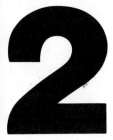

Problems Encountered in the Emergency Room

The Comatose Patient

I. Definitions

A. Normal consciousness is an awareness of the self and the environment, although this can only be estimated from behavior.

B. Sleep is a state of physical and apparent mental inactivity from which the patient can be aroused to consciousness.

C. Clouding of consciousness is a state of reduced awareness, inattention, and distractibility, with lapses in sensory perception and difficulty in following commands.

D. Delirium is characterized by disorientation, fear, irritability, misperception of sensory stimuli, and often florid visual hallucinations.

E. Stupor consists of minimal mental and physical activity, the response to spoken commands is either absent or slow and inadequate, and the patient can be aroused only by vigorous and repeated stimuli.

F. Coma is a state of total unresponsiveness in which the patient appears to be asleep but cannot be aroused by repeated noxious stimuli; there is complete absence of response to the external environment or inner needs.

G. Brain death has occurred when there is no discernible brainstem or cerebral hemisphere function for an extended period, clearly as a result of structural rather than metabolic causes (Table 2-1).

II. Approach to the patient in coma

A. General comments. As in other acute medical illnesses, diagnostic and therapeutic actions must be undertaken simultaneously. The brain must be immediately protected from further serious or irreversible damage.

1. When a patient in coma is first seen, it is imperative to secure a **clear airway,** passing an endotracheal tube if necessary, and to provide adequate ventilation.

2. **Volume replacement** for patients in circulatory collapse from a variety of causes is essential to minimize hypoxic brain damage. One should guarantee cerebral metabolic need by giving 50% glucose IV after first obtaining blood for glucose determination.

3. The **cervical spine must be stabilized** until it is established whether or not an associated fracture is present.

4. **Placement of an indwelling Foley catheter** will decompress the bladder and allow monitoring of urine output.

5. If ingestion of poisons is suspected, the gastric contents should be aspirated and sent for chemical analysis.

Table 2-1. Clinical Criteria for Diagnosis of Brain Death

Nature and duration of coma
  No drugs or hypothermia
  Structural disease or clearly known irreversible metabolic causes
  12-hr duration
Absence of cortical function
  No behavioral or reflex response to noxious stimuli above foramen
    magnum
  EEG isoelectric for 60 min at 5–10 μV/cm
Absence of brainstem function
  Fixed pupils
  No oculovestibular responses
  Apnea unresponsive to CO_2
  Circulation may be intact
  Purely spinal reflexes may be retained

---

6. Patients with pinpoint pupils and obvious injection sites may respond to administration of a narcotic antagonist such as naloxone (Narcan), 1 ml.

B. History. The history is either secondhand or unobtainable. Anyone accompanying a comatose patient to the hospital should not be permitted to leave until he or she has been questioned. Points of interest include: a history of head trauma, especially a lucid interval following an initial period of unconsciousness; ingestion or injection of drugs or other poisons; observed seizure activity; a past history of hypertension, diabetes, heart, lung, or renal disease, or endocrine dysfunction (Table 2-2).

C. Physical examination

1. **General aspects.** Observations of vital signs will include **temperature,** ranging from subnormal (hypothermia) to hyperpyrexia (heat stroke, bacterial infection, or central neurogenic cause). **Heart rate** may reveal the extreme bradycardia of complete heart block or tachyarrhythmia to account for loss of consciousness. The **respiratory rate** and pattern of breathing (considered further in **2.b**) may suggest underlying pulmonary disease with hypoxemia or hypercarbia, or it may suggest pulmonary embolism or congestive heart failure. **Blood pressure** is observed for evidence of shock or extreme elevation, suggesting hypertensive encephalopathy. A rapid but comprehensive survey of the entire patient, with attention to findings seen in the traumatized or acutely ill patient (see Chap. 1), is essential to establishing the cause of coma. Note particularly odors such as alcohol, acetone in diabetic ketoacidosis, the urine smell of uremia, mustiness in hepatic coma, and the gasolinelike odor of hydrocarbon ingestion.

2. **Neurological examination.** Although a complete neurological examination must be done, the following observations give valuable information about the level involved, the pathogenesis, and the course the disease process is taking.

   a. **State of consciousness.** Observe any spontaneous behavior and responses to verbal stimuli, then to noxious stimuli (supraorbital pressure, sternal pressure, compression of nailbeds or nipples). In many circumstances, an accurate description of observed behavior is preferable to a categorical term.

   b. **Pattern of breathing.** Cheyne-Stokes respiration is the most commonly observed breathing pattern in coma resulting from intracranial causes, usually bilateral lesions deep in the cerebral hemispheres and basal ganglia. Metabolic brain dysfunction may also cause Cheyne-Stokes respiration.

Table 2-2. Causes of Coma*

A = Alcoholism: 60% of admissions for coma
E = Epilepsy: 2.4% of admissions for coma
I = Insulin: Too much or too little
O = Opium: Look for narcotic injection sites; tachypnea may indicate respiratory insufficiency due to pulmonary or fat embolus
U = Uremia and other metabolic causes of coma (e.g., hepatic failure, nonketotic hyperglycemia)
T = Trauma: Includes spontaneous cerebrovascular accidents (23% of admissions for coma)
I = Infection: Meningitis, encephalitis, pneumonia
P = Poison: Barbiturates, lead
P = Psychogenic unresponsiveness
S = Shock: Myocardial, bacterial, hypovolemic (blood loss)

*Presented in the form of a mnemonic device to aid the memory: A, E, I, O, U (the vowels), plus T, I, P, P, S.

c. **Size and reactivity of pupils.** The brainstem areas controlling conscious-ness are anatomically adjacent to those serving the pupils. Thus, pupillary changes are a valuable guide to the presence and location of brainstem diseases causing coma. In addition, because pupillary pathways are rela-tively resistant to metabolic insult, the presence or absence of the light reflex is the single most important physical sign distinguishing structural from metabolic coma. Abnormalities seen in comatose patients include:

   (1) **Unilateral Horner's syndrome.** Horner's syndrome consists of pupillary constriction associated with ptosis and anhydrosis. Significantly, uni-lateral Horner's syndrome is often the first sign of incipient transtento-rial herniation.

   (2) **Nuclear pattern.** Interruption of both sympathetic and parasympathetic pathways results in midposition, 4- to 5-mm pupils that are fixed to light, slightly irregular, and often unequal. It occurs most commonly with transtentorial herniation.

   (3) **Pontine pattern.** Interruption of descending sympathetic pathways pro-duces bilaterally small pupils diagnostic of pontine hemorrhage in the absence of drugs.

   (4) **Peripheral lesions.** Compression of the third cranial nerve interrupts parasympathetic pathways, causing unilateral pupillary dilation, par-ticularly in uncal herniation.

   (5) **Pharmacological and metabolic effects.** Atropine produces fully di-lated and fixed pupils accompanied by delirium or stupor. Glutethimide (Doriden) gives midposition or moderately dilated, 4- to 8-mm pupils, unequal and fixed to light. Opiates give pinpoint pupils resembling those seen with pontine hemorrhage. Anoxia or ischemia most com-monly results in wide and fixed bilateral pupillary dilation, but the pupils sometimes remain small or in midposition throughout an episode of profound hypoxia leading to death. Clinically, anoxic pupillary dila-tion that lasts more than a few minutes implies severe and usually irreversible brain damage, although certainly efforts at resuscitation should not be abandoned on this criterion alone.

d. **Ocular movements.** Pathways for vestibulo-ocular reflexes lie adjacent to brainstem areas necessary for consciousness, making it clinically useful to search for both gross and subtle oculomotor abnormalities when evaluating patients in stupor or coma. Examination consists of oculocephalic (doll's head and eye phenomena) and oculovestibular (caloric) reflexes. For the oculocephalic reflex the eyelids are held open and the head briskly rotated from side to side (be absolutely certain that the cervical spine is stable before embarking on this part of the examination). A positive response is controversion conjugate eye deviation. Repeat with brisk flexion-extension; the eyelids may open reflexively when the neck is flexed (doll's eyelid phenomenon). To examine the oculovestibular reflex, proceed after visualization of intact tympanic membranes. Elevate the head 30 degrees above horizontal, so that the lateral semicircular canal is vertical and the stimulus will evoke a maximal response. Place a small, soft plastic catheter in the external canal and irrigate with ice water until either nystagmus or ocular deviation occurs. The normal response in the awake patient is nystagmus, with the slow component toward the irrigated ear. As consciousness is lost, the fast component disappears, and the slow component carries the eyes tonically toward the irrigated ear. Roving eye movements are random disconjugate ones. Their presence rules out psychogenic unresponsiveness and implies intact brainstem oculomotor function. **Abnormal lateral gaze patterns** include:

(1) A sustained involuntary conjugate ocular deviation toward the side of a normal arm and leg. This suggests a hemisphere lesion, except in irritative lesions such as subarachnoid hemorrhage or epilepsy.

(2) Deviation toward a paralyzed arm and leg. This suggests a pontine lesion.

Patients with metabolic cerebral depression usually retain reflex eye movements, whereas destruction or compression of the brainstem produces oculocephalic or caloric reflex abnormalities that localize the lesion.

- **e. Motor function.** Motor and sensory function in patients with clouded or reduced consciousness can be estimated by applying noxious stimuli to various parts of the body and observing responses as appropriate, inappropriate (decorticate or decerebrate), or absent. The type of response gives information about the anatomical distribution of the neurological dysfunction.

D. Laboratory investigations. Details of laboratory testing vary with clinical suspicions and clinical course. However, the following may be helpful in establishing the cause of coma:

1. **Serum glucose.** Hypoglycemia is a common and a serious cause of coma. Insofar as glucose represents the primary substrate for brain metabolism, any protracted period of deprivation may lead to irreversible brain damage.

2. **Serum, Na, K, Cl, CO_2, osmolality, blood urea nitrogen (BUN), Ca.** An obvious electrolyte disturbance may be the cause of coma or may suggest a primary disease process, i.e., adrenal insufficiency, metastatic tumor, or respiratory acidosis.

3. **Toxicology.** Barbiturates, salicylates, or alcohol may be responsible for the coma. Alcohol levels of 250–300 mg/100 ml are required for stupor; levels of 300–400 mg/100 ml are required for coma.

4. **Arterial blood gas determinations** may demonstrate unsuspected metabolic acidosis from ingestion of methyl alcohol, ethylene glycol, or paraldehyde; or they may indicate systemic hypoxemia or the hypercapnea of pulmonary insufficiency. Arterial ammonia level determinations are indicated in suspected hepatic coma, and arterial carbon monoxide level determinations are indicated in poisoning and smoke inhalation.

5. **Electrocardiograms** should be done in cases of suspected heart block with syncope, tachyarrhythmias, or acute myocardial infarction with decreased cardiac output, leading to cerebrovascular insufficiency.

6. **Computerized tomographic (CT) scanning of the brain** is useful for the diagnosis of space-occupying lesions, cerebral infarction, or dilation of the cerebral ventricles.

7. **Lumbar puncture** is performed when primary central nervous system (CNS) infection is suspected. A mass lesion demonstrated on a CT scan or suspected increased intracranial pressure are relative contraindications to the removal of spinal fluid.

8. Electroencephalograms may differentiate coma from psychogenic unresponsiveness and help distinguish among various causes of coma. They are also an essential part of the diagnosis of brain death.

Suggested Reading

Plum, F., and Posner, J. B. *The Diagnosis of Stupor and Coma* (2nd ed.). Philadelphia: Davis, 1972.

Ocular Emergencies

The definitive treatment and follow-up care of eye problems are best undertaken by an ophthalmologist. However, there are two situations, namely, chemical burns and central retinal artery occlusion, in which treatment must be started at once, since minutes count. In addition, there are many situations in which the physician first contacted by the patient must initiate definitive measures.

I. **Conditions in which minutes count**

A. **Chemical burns.** Eyes exposed to acid or alkali must be irrigated immediately with copious amounts of saline solution or tap water. The lids should be everted and the cul-de-sac cleaned with a cotton swab to remove any residual particulate material. This can be facilitated by using a topical anesthetic such as benoxinate hydrochloride (Dorsacaine). No attempt should be made to neutralize the chemical; the heat of neutralization may cause additional damage. Alkali penetrates rapidly into the eye, causing extensive intraocular damage. The irrigation for alkali burns should therefore consist of several liters of normal saline over an hour's time. The efficacy of the irrigation can be monitored by checking the pH of the conjunctiva; the normal pH of tears is approximately 7.4. Subsequent treatment depends on the amount and nature of the ocular damage.

B. **Central retinal artery occlusion**

1. **Signs and symptoms.** There is abrupt, painless loss of vision in one eye due to blockage of the central retinal artery by an embolus or thrombus. When viewed, the fundus arterioles are extremely attenuated. After a short period, there is edema of the retina due to ischemia. The fovea maintains its normal color, so that it appears cherry red in contrast to the whitened retina. A major branch of the central retinal artery may be blocked individually; in this case, only the portion of the retina supplied by that branch is altered, with corresponding visual field loss.

2. **Treatment.** The objective is to move the blockage to a more peripheral and, it is hoped, a less vital portion of the arterial tree. This is accomplished by the following:

a. Carry out digital massage on the eye through closed lids to lower the intraocular pressure. The finger pressure should be removed every 10–15 sec.

b. Decrease aqueous humor production, which also lowers intraocular pressure, by administering acetazolamide (Diamox), 500 mg IV and 500 mg PO.

c. Dilate the retinal arterioles by having the patient breathe into a paper bag to increase the PCO_2.

d. If these measures are not successful within a short time, drain aqueous humor from the anterior chamber. Apply topical anesthesia and topical antibiotic drops, and insert a 30-gauge needle into the anterior chamber. Use extreme caution to avoid damage to the lens. Only a portion of the aqueous humor should be drained.

II. Conditions in which hours count

A. Laceration of the globe is often obvious, but it may be missed if the lids are swollen shut, or if care is not taken when exploring lid and brow lacerations. A seemingly innocent brow laceration may penetrate the globe. To avoid overlooking a serious eye injury, the vision should be tested, the intraocular pressure measured, and a dilated fundus examination performed (avoid dilation of the pupil if the CNS status is doubtful). If a globe laceration is detected, the involved eye should be covered with a patch and protected with a shield. No attempt should be made to investigate the details of the injury in an open eye, since evaluation can best be made by an ophthalmologist with the patient under general anesthesia at the time of the definitive repair.

B. Orbital cellulitis. Periocular infection is potentially very dangerous, since an extension of the infective thrombophlebitis may lead to cavernous sinus thrombosis. The stage of the infection can be assessed by evaluating such signs as proptosis, retinal venous engorgement, and papilledema. If any of these conditions is present, a more posterior and therefore serious orbital infection is suggested. Most cases of orbital cellulitis result from ethmoidal or frontal sinus disease. Broad-spectrum IV antibiotics, warm soaks, and drainage of any sinus abscess are indicated. The patient should be hospitalized.

III. Red eyes. A number of conditions cause red eyes. These conditions must be differentiated from one another, because each requires an entirely different treatment.

A. Acute angle-closure glaucoma is a relatively infrequent cause of decreased vision. Its onset is abrupt and often at night, and immediate diagnosis and treatment are essential if permanent ocular damage is to be avoided. There is usually extreme pain, blurred vision, diffuse redness of the conjunctiva, and little or no discharge. The cornea is "steamy," and the anterior chamber is virtually absent. The pupil is often in a mid-dilated position. The intraocular pressure is elevated, often to a very marked degree.

Treatment consists of constricting the pupil with 4% pilocarpine drops given q5min for 30 min and then hourly until a response is noted. Acetazolamide, 500 mg PO plus 500 mg IV, is given. If this is not successful in breaking the attack in a relatively short time, intravenous mannitol is administered in doses of 1.5 gm/kg body weight as a 20% solution. An operative procedure, placing a hole in the iris to allow normal aqueous flow, is necessary after the acute attack has been brought under control. The pupil should be kept constricted with pilocarpine until the operation can be carried out.

B. Acute iritis is a relatively common cause of a red eye that may be difficult to distinguish from acute conjunctivitis. Vision is usually somewhat blurred, and there may be sensitivity to light. Associated pain is not generally as intense as with angle-closure glaucoma. An important feature is the frequently reduced size of the pupil on the involved side. The conjunctival injection is most marked around the edge of the cornea. The cornea is clear, and there is little or no discharge. The anterior chamber is generally of normal depth. There are inflammatory cells in the anterior chamber, but slit-lamp magnification may be necessary to observe them. The intraocular pressure is normal or even somewhat low unless the condition has been present for a significant period, in which case secondary glaucoma may ensue. Prompt and vigorous dilation of the pupil is essential to prevent adhesions of the iris to the lens, with subsequent cataract formation or glaucoma. Topical corticosteroid drops are used to decrease the inflammatory response.

C. Acute conjuctivitis is the most common cause of a red eye. It may be allergic, bacterial, or viral in origin. There is usually a discharge, which varies with the different causative agents. A conjunctival smear often is useful in making the diagnosis. Vision is essentially normal, and there is burning and itching rather than true pain. There may be some light sensitivity, but it is usually relatively mild. The conjuctiva is diffusely red, while the cornea, anterior chamber, and pupil are unremarkable. Most cases of acute conjunctivitis are treated as bacterial infections, with broad-spectrum antibiotic drops. This is generally a safe practice as long as the cornea is not ulcerated. Corticosteroids should not be used until a bacterial or viral origin is ruled out. The use of combination antibiotic-corticosteroid medications as the initial therapy is to be discouraged.

IV. Foreign bodies and ocular trauma

A. Conjunctival foreign bodies often cause a great deal of pain, especially if the cornea is abraded. The foreign body may be lodged under the lids, in which case the lid must be everted to identify the offending material. A topical anesthetic (benoxinate hydrochloride or proparacaine hydrochloride [Ophthaine]) is useful to allow an adequate examination. Topical fluorescein should be applied to the cornea to identify any corneal abrasions. Fluorescein stains areas of denuded cornea green, while normal epithelium is unstained. The fluorescence can be best viewed using a Wood's lamp or a slit lamp with a cobalt-blue filter. No further treatment is necessary if a corneal abrasion is not present.

B. Corneal foreign bodies embedded in the cornea usually can be removed with a cotton swab after application of a topical anesthetic. If this is unsuccessful, a spud or 25-gauge needle may be used to lift the foreign body from the cornea. Magnification with a loupe or slit lamp is generally necessary and is best carried out by an ophthalmologist. Rust rings may be present surrounding a metallic corneal foreign body. These rings are generally best ignored unless they are present centrally. Following removal of the foreign body, the eye should be treated with an intermediate-acting dilating drop, such as 5% homatropine solution, to remove ciliary spasm, and a topical antibiotic ointment to prevent secondary infection. The eye is then covered with a tight patch using two eye pads, and the cornea is rechecked in 48 hr. Topical anesthetics should never be given to the patient to use at home since they retard corneal reepithelialization and may facilitate the development of a bacterial ulcer.

C. Corneal abrasions. The surface epithelium of the cornea may become abraded, resulting in exquisite pain and lacrimation. The diagnosis is made with fluorescein (see **A**) and treated as after the removal of a corneal foreign body (see **B**). Abrasions, especially with vegetable matter, may lead to fungal ulcers of the cornea.

D. Blunt trauma. Many types of intraocular injuries may be caused by blunt trauma, and their recognition is important. Among the more common injuries are:

1. Hyphema, or blood in the anterior chamber. The patient should be sedated and placed on absolute bed rest to facilitate reabsorption of the blood and, more important, to prevent rehemorrhaging which is often devastating to the eye.

2. Traumatic iritis, treated as suggested in **III.B.**

3. **Iridodialysis.** The iris is torn at its insertion into the ciliary body.

4. **Glaucoma.** Traumatic glaucoma may be delayed in onset. The patient should be warned regarding this possibility as a late complication.

5. Dislocated lens or cataract.

6. Vitreous hemorrhage.

7. Retinal edema and hemorrhage.

8. Retinal tears and subsequent retinal detachment.

9. Choroidal rupture.

10. Papilledema.

11. **Scleral rupture** often occurs under one of the recti muscles and may be overlooked. If any suspicion exists concerning the possibility of a scleral rupture, the conjunctiva should be reflected and the extraocular muscle mobilized to rule out an underlying rupture. The intraocular pressure determined by a tonometer usually is low with a scleral rupture, but this is not invariable, since the wound may be temporarily sealed. Hyphema is often present. An unusually deep anterior chamber should alert the examiner to the possibility of a scleral rupture.

12. Optic nerve injury.

E. **Intraocular foreign body.** There should always be a high level of suspicion regarding the possibility of an intraocular foreign body, which is occasionally overlooked, with unfortunate results.

1. When the history suggests even the vague possibility of an intraocular foreign body, further investigation is indicated, including a thorough ophthalmological examination as well as x-rays of the orbit. If the foreign body is believed to be lodged in the anterior portion of the eye, a bone-free radiological examination with dental film is often useful. Many objects capable of penetrating the globe unfortunately are not radiopaque, and a normal x-ray thus does not necessarily rule out the presence of an intraocular foreign body. Foreign bodies can sometimes be identified with the aid of ultrasonography. Once an intraocular foreign body is diagnosed, the patient should be placed on IV antibiotics.

2. Topical antibiotic drops should be applied to the eye, the eye covered, and the patient referred to an ophthalmologist for prompt surgical removal of the foreign body.

Suggested Reading

Gombos, G. *Handbook of Ophthalmologic Emergencies.* Flushing, N.Y.: Medical Examination Publishing Co., 1973.

Paton, D., and Goldberg, M. *Management of Ocular Injuries* (2nd ed.). Philadelphia: Saunders, 1976.

Epistaxis

I. **General comments**

A. Epistaxis is usually intermittent and easily treated, but it may be persistent and refractory to simpler forms of therapy, with considerable loss of blood. It is estimated that 10% of the population has nasal bleeding during a lifetime.

B. **Trauma, hypertension, and arteriosclerosis are the common systemic causes of nosebleed.** Blood dyscrasias, tumors, inflammation, foreign bodies, and so on, are causes listed in texts, but it is unusual to identify any of them in patients with epistaxis.

C. Bleeding may arise from the **anterior** or **posterior** part of the nose. The clinical signs and the details of required treatment of these two types of hemorrhage are outlined in **II** and **III**. The site of origin is most frequently anterior in children and posterior in older adults.

D. In general, **treatment** of epistaxis involves the use of packing, cautery, or vessel ligation. Systemic drugs, such as carbazochrome (Adrenosem), conjugated estrogens (Premarin), and vitamin K, are not of value.

E. Analgesics and antipyretics may interfere with platelet function and cause increased bleeding. Aspirin does this most often, causing abnormalities in platelet aggregation and increased bleeding time.

F. When systemic disease is suggested as the etiological factor by family history or bleeding at other sites, the following hematological screening tests are indicated to identify the disorder: bleeding time, partial thromboplastin time, platelet function, and prothrombin time.

II. Anterior nasal hemorrhage

A. An intermittent or continuous flow of blood is noted from one side of the nose.

B. The most frequent (in 90%) site of bleeding is on the medial side of the naris in the anteroinferior portion of the nasal septum, known as Little's or Kiesselbach's area. Here, a confluence of blood vessels lies beneath the mucous membrane.

C. A pulsating eroded arterial vessel is sometimes seen, but continuous venous bleeding is more common.

D. Anterior nasal bleeding is first temporarily controlled by packing and pressure. A compressed dental roll moistened with 5% cocaine or a 1:1000 epinephrine solution is inserted well into the inferior nasal vestibule, and external pressure is applied to the lateral walls of the anterior nose ("pinch") for 5 min.

E. If the bleeding continues, an injection of 1–2 ml 1% lidocaine containing 1:100,000 epinephrine is indicated. The anesthetic is infiltrated into the mucosa around the bleeding point with a 25-gauge hypodermic needle. The vestibule is then repacked.

F. Cautery of the bleeding point is carried out once bleeding is under control. The mucosal ulceration is exposed with the aid of a headlight or mirror and nasal speculum. Chemical cautery can be applied with a silver nitrate stick or a small, cotton-tipped applicator moistened with 50% trichloracetic acid. The bleeding point is circumferentially cauterized. If bleeding recurs, packing is repeated and then withdrawn, and cautery is applied again. Chemical cautery is ineffective unless the bleeding is controlled before application. Electric cautery is more effective and, if a suction-tip electrode is used, can be applied during active bleeding.

G. The treated area is then covered for 24 hr with petrolatum (Vaseline) or iodoform gauze impregnated with antibiotic ointment.

III. Posterior nasal hemorrhage

A. Blood flows posteriorly into the pharynx and also may flow anteriorly out the naris. With profuse posterior hemorrhage, blood may issue from both nares. The patient may expectorate blood, aspirate and cough up blood, or swallow blood and later expel it by emesis.

B. The posterolateral nasal fossa, beneath the inferior turbinate, is the second most frequent site of origin of nasal hemorrhage. The vessels in this area are known as the nasopalatine plexus of Woodruff. The bleeding is often profuse and difficult to manage.

C. In posterior nasal hemorrhage, an initial injection of 2–3 ml 1% lidocaine with 1:100,000 epinephrine into the greater palatine foramen is recommended. The foramen lies just medial and posterior to the last molar tooth and can be palpated as a dimple in the hard palate. Bleeding will subside or diminish in 75% of patients and facilitate postnasal packing.

D. Balloon tamponade is the second step in treating posterior nasal bleeding. A #14 or #16 Foley catheter is passed along the nasal floor on the bleeding side until the tip is visible in the posterior pharyngeal wall below the soft palate. The balloon is partially inflated with 10 ml of air or saline solution, and the catheter is withdrawn until resistance is noted. Then another 5 ml of air or saline solution is added to the balloon, the catheter is withdrawn further until taut, and the posterior choana is occluded. The nose anterior to the balloon is then packed. Finally, gauze or an ophthalmic patch is draped over the catheter, and an umbilical clamp is applied to it, occluding the anterior nose. A vaginal tampon can be substituted for the balloon to occlude the posterior choana.

E. In profuse nasal hemorrhage, bilateral posterior nasal packs may be necessary to control the bleeding. The patient is admitted to the hospital, sedated, and carefully observed for signs of hypoxia and for recurrent bleeding. The obstruction of the nose by the pack, enforcing mouth breathing, combined with the palatal edema that often develops, leads to hypoventilation and decreased PaO_2. Supplemental oxygen is administered as required. Posterior nasal packs should be removed in 24–48 hr. Prophylactic antibiotics are recommended to prevent sinusitis and otitis media.

F. Major vessel ligation is required for recurrent or intractable posterior nasal hemorrhage.

1. For posteroinferior nasal bleeding, the branches of the internal maxillary artery are interrupted via an approach through the posterior wall of the maxillary sinus. Alternatively, the external carotid artery can be ligated above the level of the superior thyroid artery. External carotid ligation is less likely to control bleeding because of excessive collateral circulation.

2. For persistent hemorrhage from above the level of the middle turbinate, the anterior and posterior ethmoidal arteries are ligated. These vessels are approached through a curvilinear incision on the medial orbital rim; by a subperiosteal dissection they are located on the superior medial wall at the junction of the orbital plate of the frontal bone with the orbitalis ossis ethmoidalis of the ethmoid bone.

3. In post-traumatic nasal hemorrhage with intracranial rupture of the internal carotid artery, neurosurgical intervention is occasionally necessary.

Acute Genitourinary Problems

I. **Acute urinary retention.** Acute urinary retention is a sudden complete inability to urinate. Subjective symptoms range from suprapubic discomfort to severe, agonizing pain.

A. Causes

1. In children, common causes in addition to glomerulonephritis include neuromuscular vesical dysfunction, posterior urethral valves, vesical neck contracture, hypertrophy of the verumontanum, meatal stenosis, ureterocele, hematocolpos, hydrocolpos, marked phimosis, foreign body in the urethra, and urethral diverticulum.

2. In adults, common causes include the following:

a. Prostatic causes include benign prostatic hypertrophy, cancer, acute prostatitis, abscess, and infarction.

b. Urethral causes include stricture, trauma, tumor, foreign body, infection of Bartholin's and periurethral glands.

c. Neurological causes include such conditions as trauma, tumor, inflammation of the spinal cord, peripheral neuropathy, and pelvic surgery.

     d. Pharmacological causes include narcotics, anticholinergics, alpha-adrenergic agents, ganglionic blocking agents, phenothiazines, diazepam, methyldopa, and other false neurotransmitters.

     e. Other causes include pelvic masses, pelvic inflammatory disease, and psychogenic and postoperative disturbances.

B. The **diagnosis** is based on the character of onset or recurrences; relation of retention to trauma, instrumentation, or surgery; neurological findings; previous urethral pathology; infections elsewhere in the body; history of ingestion of alcohol, anticholinergics, antidepressants, tranquilizers, or decongestants; and physical findings of a distended bladder by palpation and percussion.

C. Management

    1. General measures include hydration, sedation, and antibiotics in the presence of sepsis.

    2. Obtain a retrograde urethrogram to determine urethral patency.

    3. If the urethra is patent, pass aseptically a #F 14-16 coudé Foley catheter and connect it to a closed drainage system.

    4. If a pathological condition of the urethra is present or the catheter fails to pass, do a suprapubic puncture, inserting a polyethylene catheter, or perform a suprapubic cystostomy.

    5. Admit the patient to the hospital for a definitive diagnostic workup, treatment, and observation for sepsis and postobstructive diuresis.

II. Hematuria. Hematuria can be gross or microscopic, initial, total, or terminal and may or may not be associated with pain. Initial hematuria occurs at the start of urination and usually indicates disease of the urethra. Terminal hematuria occurs at the end of urination and indicates disease of the posterior urethra or bladder neck. Total hematuria persists throughout the voiding and indicates a pathological condition in the bladder neck or at a higher level.

A. The **origin** of hematuria in approximately 50% of patients is the bladder or urethra and in 50%, the kidney or ureter.

B. The most **common causes** of hematuria of bladder origin are neoplasia, bladder stone, and specific, nonspecific, and radiation cystitis. Benign prostatic hyperplasia is the most common cause of bleeding of prostatic origin. Associated renal colic and hematuria suggest that the origin of bleeding may be the kidney and upper ureter.

C. In the case of **asymptomatic microhematuria,** extensive urological investigation discloses a significant lesion in 10% of patients, and a neoplastic lesions in 3%. A compromise plan of workup, including a plain x-ray of the abdomen, intravenous urogram, and urine cytological examination, is suggested for this group of patients.

D. In the case of **gross hematuria,** age is an important element. It is rare in infancy and childhood, when it usually is due to infection, obstruction or, rarely, malignancy of the genitourinary tract. In young adults (up to 40 years), gross hematuria is a manifestation of infection; rarely, is it due to malignancy. The most common causes of gross hematuria in the patient 40–60 yr of age are infection, malignancy, and stones. In the male over 60 yr of age, benign prostatic hyperplasia is the most common cause of hematuria.

    In a large series of approximately 6000 cases of gross hematuria, the kidney was the source of bleeding in 42.8%, the bladder in 29.7%, the prostate in 14.2%, the ureter in 8.7%, and the urethra in 4.6%. The causes of gross hematuria were inflammation (31.4%), neoplasia (27.9%), foreign body (20.0%), tuberculosis (9.4%), trauma (3.8%), and others (7.5%).

E. The **differential diagnosis of hematuria** includes the following:

1. **Primary glomerular disease,** including idiopathic recurrent hematuria, Buerger's disease (mesangial IGA nephropathy), resolving postinfectious glomerulonephritis, membranoproliferative glomerulonephritis, extracapillary proliferative glomerulonephritis, and focal glomerulonephritis.

2. **Secondary or hereditary glomerular disease,** including systemic lupus erythematosus, polyarteritis, endocarditis, Alport's syndrome, Fabry's disease, Goodpasture's syndrome, and malignant hypertension.

3. **Nonglomerular renal disease,** including hypersensitivity nephritis, sickle cell trait, polycystic kidney disease, medullary sponge kidney, trauma, neoplasia, lymphoma, leukemic infiltrate, vascular anomalies, papillary necrosis (e.g., analgesic abuse), and renal infarcts (embolic or thrombotic).

4. **Nonrenal causes** include cystitis, prostatitis, urethritis, genitourinary tract tuberculosis, congenital anomalies (e.g., ureterocele, vascular malformation), varices of pelvis and ureter, neoplasms of the collecting system, ureter, bladder, prostate, or urethra, trauma, ureteral stone, foreign bodies, allergic cystitis, disease of adjacent organs (e.g., appendicitis, salpingitis, diverticulitis), and a group of miscellaneous causes: exercise; coagulation disturbances; ingestion of chemicals (methenamine, turpentine, carbolic acid, cantharidin, sulfonamides, anticoagulants, cyclophosphamide); scurvy, smallpox, malaria, yellow fever, and congestive heart failure.

F. **Diagnosis and evaluation** is based on age, sex, familial history, a precise history and physical examination, careful examination of a three-glass urine test, bacteriological and cytological examination of the urine, intravenous urography, and cystoscopy if necessary. Hemoglobinuria, obstructive and hepatocellular jaundice, porphyria, and ochronosis all can be ruled out by microscopic examination of urine, which invariably shows red cells in true hematuria.

G. **Assessment**

1. **Absence of infection but presence of casts and protein in the urine with a normal urogram.** The patient requires a nephrological workup that includes: BUN, serum creatinine, sedimentation rate, alkaline phosphatase, calcium, uric acid, antinuclear antibody, C3 complement, serum protein electrophoresis, and a 24-hr urine for creatinine, protein, and electrophoresis.

2. **Absence of infection and presence of poor, partial, or nonvisualized kidney.** The patient should be admitted to the hospital for evaluation of the integrity of the kidney vasculature and the possibility of obstructive uropathy.

3. **If any abnormalities are present** (masses, filling defects, foreign bodies, obstructive uropathy, positive cytology), the patient should have a complete urological evaluation.

4. **In the presence of recurrent infection and normal urogram,** a micturation cystourethrogram and nuclide cystogram should be done after treatment of the infection. If the results are normal, the patient needs periodic examinations, urine cultures, and possibly prophylactic chemotherapy.

5. **The patient with reflux and infection** needs close follow-up and may require long-term prophylactic chemotherapy and reconstructive surgery.

H. **Management**

1. **Acute symptomatic measures,** such as relief of pain and obstruction, evacuation of clot from the bladder, bed rest, and transfusion if needed.

2. **Definitive treatment** will depend on the ultimate diagnosis.

III. **Pain.** Pain impulses from the kidney, ureter, and testes are carried in visceral afferent fibers of sympathetic nerves; bladder pain impulses are carried via parasympathetic nerves. Sympathectomy (T7–L3) abolishes renal and ureteral pain without much effect on bladder pain.

A. Causes

1. **Flank pain** related to the upper urinary tract localized in the flank or lumbar region may be sharp, dull, or consist only of a sense of discomfort; the pain may be intermittent or constant. Flank pain due to increased tension of the renal capsule or pelvis may be caused by inflammatory renal disease, pyelonephritis, perinephric abscess, renal abscess, pyonephrosis, obstructive uropathy at any level from any cause, renal or ureteral stone, renal vascular occlusion, renal artery aneurysm, or the ovarian vein syndrome.

2. **Nonurological or neurological flank pain.** A careful history and clinical examination may lead to a diagnosis of radiculitis; nerve root compression due to arthritis or disk disease; neuroma in a flank scar; herpetic neuritis; disease of the colon, stomach, or liver; scoliosis; lumbodorsal hernia; twelfth rib joint arthritis; or back pain (the "soft bed" syndrome).

3. **Renal colic pain** is a sharp, stabbing, agonizing pain associated with sweating, fainting, nausea, vomiting, shock, and sometimes collapse. The pain is maximal in area of the posterior flank and radiates along the course of the genitocrural nerve, so that pain can be felt in the testes, ovary, bladder neck, and urethra. Renal or urethral colic is due to rapid distention of the ureter and renal pelvis above the level of obstruction, which causes violent hyperperistalsis and paroxymal spasms as the kidney attempts to expel urine, stones, blood clots, sloughed tumor, or renal papillae.

4. **Bladder pain** usually is due to infection and presents as a dull, continuous discomfort in the suprapubic area and may be referred to the distal urethra. Pain is severe and agonizing in acute retention, but there is little or no pain in cases of chronic overdistended bladder.

5. **Urethral pain** is often associated with burning, dysuria, strangury, and terminal urinary spasm. Posterior urethral pain usually is referred to the distal urethra and perineum. The cause of pain often is infection or a foreign body in the urethra.

6. **Prostatic pain** in acute prostatitis is characterized by a sudden onset of low back pain and discomfort or fullness in the perineum or rectum, associated with fever, chills, urgency, nocturia, dysuria, retention, malaise, arthralgia or myalgia, and an extremely tender, indurated, warm, swollen prostate gland. In chronic prostatitis, pain in the low back, perineal discomfort, and painful ejaculation with varying degrees of irritative voiding symptoms occur.

B. Diagnosis

1. The **history** should include particularly the location; character (sharp, dull, mild, severe, intermittent, constant); duration; relation to other symptoms, especially during micturition; radiation; or any disease predisposing to hematuria; renal vascular occlusion; papillary necrosis; calculous diseases; obstructive uropathy, or inflammatory genitourinary disease.

2. The **physical findings** may include costovertebral angle and suprapubic tenderness, a mass, ileus, urethral discharge, tender or swollen prostate, and a palpable foreign body in the urethra.

3. **Laboratory examinations** include urinalysis, urine culture, complete blood count, serum electrolytes, BUN, and creatinine, to detect infection, hematuria, proteinuria, crystalluria, electrolyte imbalance, and renal failure.

4. **X-rays** of the abdomen will demonstrate calculi in 94% of patients with a stone, obliteration of psoas shadow, abnormal renal outline, soft tissue mass, calcification of renal mass, and ileus. An infusion intravenous pyelogram and tomogram may demonstrate poor or delayed visualization or nonvisualization of the kidney, hydroureteronephrosis, renal masses, and filling defects in the collect-

ing systems. In the case of nonvisualization and absence of obstruction, immediate renal arteriography or venography (or both) is required.

5. **Sonography** of any renal mass detected during the physical examination or by urography is necessary to differentiate solid from cystic masses. It is also helpful to assess renal anatomy, biopsy localization, cyst aspiration, antegrade pyelography, perinephric collections, and retroperitoneal, adrenal, and pelvic masses.

C. The **differential diagnosis** includes acute appendicitis, intra-abdominal testicular torsion, acute diverticulitis, intestinal colic, and dissecting or ruptured aortic aneurysm. A pathological spinal condition may mimic flank pain and renal colic and should be considered in the differential diagnosis.

D. **Management**

1. **General treatment** includes hydration, symptomatic relief of pain after the diagnosis is made, and antibiotics in the presence of sepsis.

2. A ureteral stone less than 4 mm in diameter will pass in 90% of patients and should be caught by straining the urine. A stone larger than 5 mm may necessitate open surgery or transcystoscopic stone manipulation.

3. A patient with complete ureteral obstruction and sepsis needs immediate ureteral catheterization or open surgery to relieve or bypass the obstruction.

IV. **Urinary tract infection.** The incidence of symptomatic infection in children before the age of 10 yr is 3% for girls and 1% for boys. Approximately 1.2% of schoolgirls and 4% of females between the ages of 16 and 65 have asymptomatic bacteriuria (as compared with 0.5% of males). It is estimated that 10–20% of women have bacteriuria at some point in their lives. The role of the emergency room physician is to prescribe therapy for the patient with an uncomplicated urinary tract infection, as well as to recognize, diagnose, and classify patients at serious risk of complications, including patients with neurogenic disease of the lower urinary tract or obstructive uropathy, pregnant women; males with chronic prostatitis; patients with congenital urinary tract abnormalities, perinephric abscess, renal failure, foreign bodies (e.g., stone), or nephropathy with papillary necrosis due to diabetes; and analgesic abuses. These patients all require a complete urological evaluation and supervision.

A. **Classification.** Urinary tract infections are divided (Stamey) into four categories: first infection, unresolved bacteriuria during therapy, recurrent reinfection, and bacterial persistence.

1. **First infection.** The infecting organism is usually sensitive to most antimicrobial agents; only 25% of patients will develop a recurrent urinary tract infection.

2. **Unresolved bacteriuria during therapy** is usually due to inadequate therapy but may be due to bacterial resistance to the drug, selection of resistant mutants, rapid reinfection, azotemia, or the presence of staghorn calculi.

3. **Recurrent reinfection** despite the absence of any structural abnormality in the urinary tract may occur with a new organism.

4. **Bacterial persistence or relapse** is the presence or reappearance of the same organism in the urine 5–10 days after successful treatment. Common causes of relapse are struvite stones, structural abnormalities, and chronic prostatitis.

B. The **diagnosis** is based on the symptoms, signs, and physical and laboratory findings, including examination of the genitalia, perineum, rectum, flanks, and abdominal organs; measurement of blood pressure; and assessment of a urinalysis, urine culture, BUN, serum creatinine, electrolytes, x-rays, and radionuclide and urodynamic studies.

1. **Upper urinary tract symptoms** include fever, chills, flank pain, frequency, urgency, and hematuria. Signs include costovertebral angle and flank tenderness and flank mass.

2. **Lower urinary tract symptoms** include frequency, urgency, dysuria, straining at micturition, dribbling, slow stream, hematuria, urinary retention, low back and perineal pain, suprapubic discomfort, scrotal pain, and (rarely) fever. Signs include suprapubic tenderness, urethral discharge, tender boggy prostate, distended bladder, scrotal swelling and tenderness.

3. **Laboratory findings.** Urinalysis: pyuria ($\geq$ 5 WBC/high-power field, clumps or casts of WBC). The presence of fresh WBCs and a high ratio of leukocytes to epithelial cells are suggestive of infection. Absence of pyuria does not exclude infection; approximately 50% of women with asymptomatic bacteriuria do not have pyuria. The presence of bacteria in midstream urine in a woman is not always a sign of urinary tract infection; it could be due to improper specimen collection or storage. The absence of bacteria also does not exclude infection, because urine has to contain 50,000–100,000 bacteria/ml in order to see 1 bacterium/high-power field. Significant bacteriuria in a properly collected, transported, and cultured midstream urine is the presence of 100,000 bacteria/ml (or for a bladder puncture, 10,000 bacteria/ml). In patients with frequent voiding, infection may be present with a count as low as 100 colonies/ml.

   In females with recurrent urinary tract infections and bacteremia, 20% of the urine counts are less than 100,000.

4. **Causative organisms.** The common organisms responsible for urinary tract infections are *Escherichia coli* (responsible for approximately 80%), *Klebsiella, Proteus, Enterobacter, Pseudomonas, Serratia* (rare), and *gram-positive cocci* (very rare).

5. **Localization of bacteriuria.** The site of infection may be determined by ureteral catheterization, bladder irrigation with neomycin, segmented cultures in males, detection of antibody-coated bacteria, determination of C-reactive protein, and serum antibody titers.

6. **Roentgenography.** To detect congenital abnormalities, obstructive uropathy, calculi, foreign bodies, and fistulas or to assess the degree of parenchymal damage or the rate of kidney growth is important in patients with recurrent or asymptomatic infection. Plain x-rays of the abdomen, an intravenous urogram, a voiding cystourethrogram, and a nuclide cystogram must be done.

   A **plain x-ray of the abdomen** may detect an opaque stone, soft tissue mass, obliteration of psoas shadow, curvature of spine, fractured bone, and the size, shape, and location of the kidneys. Anatomical malformations are detected in 25–50% of children and 51% of pregnant females with infection. Obstruction is found in 5–10% of boys and 1% of girls. An abnormal voiding cystourethrogram is seen in 43% of girls with bacteriuria, 20% of whom have ureteral reflux. The yield of x-rays in evaluation of females with recurrent reinfection is very low.

7. **Urodynamic evaluation** of the lower urinary tract may be necessary in patients with obstruction or neurological disease.

8. **Sonography and transillumination** of the flank and abdomen may be indicated in the presence of masses in these areas.

C. **Natural history of infection.** Spontaneous cure lasting 1 year is seen in only 10% of patients. Treatment with effective antibiotics in proper dosage eliminates infection in nearly all patients with a first infection and in over 95% of patients with recurrent infections. Half of patients with treated symptomatic infection and 80% of patients with asymptomatic bacteriuria (irrespective of the number of previously treated urinary tract infections) will develop one or more attacks of recurrent infection.

   Renal scarring occurs in 5–13% of female children with recurrent symptomatic urinary tract infections without obstruction and in 13–26% with asymptomatic bacteriuria. There is a higher incidence in boys. A small number of these patients will subsequently develop hypertension and renal failure.

D. Treatment includes chemotherapy, follow-up radiological and urological investigation, and manipulation if necessary.

1. The first uncomplicated infection can be treated by a 7- to 10-day course of ampicillin, sulfamethoxazole-trimethoprim, sulfonamide, nitrofurantoin, cephalosporin, or methenamine mandelate without any further workup. Lack of clinical response to treatment (decreased temperature in 2–3 days, clearing of urinary sediment in 4–5 days, return of concentrating ability in 3 wk) usually indicates obstructive uropathy or bacterial resistance.

2. Patients with recurrent infection or bacterial persistence need prophylaxis after successful treatment to maintain urine sterility. Effective antimicrobial agents include ampicillin (500 mg bid), sulfamethoxazole-trimethoprim (½–1 tablet at bedtime), nitrofurantoin (50–100 mg at bedtime), methenamine mandelate (0.5–1.0 gm qid), and ascorbic acid (2–12 gm/day) for 2–6 mo.

3. Patients with obstruction, stones, anatomical abnormalities, or abscess require surgical intervention while on therapy.

E. Acute bacterial prostatitis

1. **Symptoms.** Sudden onset of fever, chills, back pain, perineal and suprapubic discomfort, urgency, frequency, dysuria, hesitancy, slow stream, urinary retention, arthralgia, myalgia, nausea, and vomiting.

2. **Signs.** Rectal examination shows a severely tender, swollen, indurated prostate gland.

3. **Laboratory findings.** Due to the risk of bacteremia, prostatic massage is not recommended; if it is done, the prostatic secretion is packed with WBCs and large oval fat bodies. Culture of prostatic fluid grows large numbers of bacteria. Acute cystitis is a common secondary finding, and the pathogenic organism can be cultured from the urine.

4. **Treatment.** The patient has to be hospitalized. An intravenous or intramuscular aminoglycoside and intravenous ampicillin or carbenicillin are administered until the results of sensitivity tests are available. Usually after 1 wk of intravenous treatment, an antimicrobial such as sulfamethoxazole-trimethoprim or tetracycline can be continued orally for 4 wk as outpatient therapy.

F. Perinephric abscess is usually secondary to an **underlying disease,** such as pyelonephritis, renal stone, obstructive uropathy, trauma, hydronephrosis, tuberculosis, polycystic renal disease, renal papillary necrosis, or carcinoma. Perinephric abscess may be **hematogenous** in origin; the common sources are dental or tonsillar abscess, furuncles, acute prostatitis, and prostatic abscess. Extension of infection from neighboring organs is an uncommon mechanism. Approximately 25–30% of perinephric abscesses are diagnosed at autopsy. Patients are often sick 2–3 wk before consultation.

1. Common **symptoms** are fever, flank or costovertebral pain, palpable flank mass, chills, nausea, vomiting, and weight loss. Spasm of the psoas and paravertebral muscles leading to scoliosis, flank and costovertebral tenderness, and aggravation of pain while walking and alleviation by flexing the ipsilateral thigh are often present. A flank mass is palpable in more than 50% of patients.

2. Common **laboratory findings** include leukocytosis, anemia, pyuria and albuminuria in two thirds of the patients and bacteriuria in one half of the patients. Plain x-rays may reveal abscence of psoas shadow, scoliosis, obliteration of the renal outline, gas bubbles in the abscess cavity, or an opaque stone. Intravenous urography may demonstrate underlying renal disease, fixation of

the kidney, hydronephrosis, obstruction of the ureter, calyceal abnormalities, displacement of a kidney and ureter, or extravasation of contrast media. Retrograde pyelograms are indicated in instances of poor visualization or nonvisualization of the kidney. The chest x-ray may reveal elevation of a diaphragm, pleural effusion, basilar pulmonary infiltration, or atelectasis on the side of abscess.

3. **Treatment** includes surgical drainage plus adjuvant antimicrobials.

V. Priapism. Priapism is a persistent and painful abnormal erection unaccompanied by sexual desire. There is a high rate of permanent impotence if priapism is not properly treated within 72 hours. Primary priapism is due to prolonged sexual stimulation. Secondary priapism is due to an underlying disease, such as sickle cell disease, leukemia, polycythemia, carcinoma metastatic to the penis, pelvic thrombophlebitis, retroperitoneal bleeding, drugs (heparin, phenothiazine, hydralazine, testosterone), penile trauma, prostatitis, spinal cord injury, or CNS involvement by syphilis or tuberculosis. **Treatment** includes sedation, warm enemas, spinal anesthesia to the T8 level, corporal irrigation with 10% heparin or saline using a large needle to aspirate sludged blood, and intermittent penile compression with a blood pressure cuff. If these measures fail to relieve the erection, creation of a venous shunt to drain the corpora may be needed.

VI. Paraphimosis. Paraphimosis consists of compression and strangulation of the glans penis by the retracted prepuce. Treatment is by manual digital reduction. If this fails, surgical release of the constricting band by a dorsal or lateral slit or circumcision is needed.

VII. Scrotal masses. Scrotal masses require immediate attention. They should be explored in children because of the high incidence of testicular torsion in this age group.

A. Common causes

1. **Newborn.** Torsion, hydrocele, hernia, hematocele.

2. **Prepubertal child.** Torsion of a testis and its appendage, scrotal hernia, epididymitis; rarely, tumor of the testis.

3. **Adolescent and young adult.** Epididymitis, tumor of the testis, varicocele, hydrocele.

4. **Middle-aged and elderly.** Epididymitis, scrotal hernia, hydrocele, spermatocele; rarely, tumor.

B. Differential diagnosis (Table 2-3). Physical examination plays an important role in the differential diagnosis of a scrotal mass. The testes should be palpated, with special attention to size, shape, mobility, consistency, position, and relative weight. Any hard area within the testis is assumed to be malignant. The epididymis should be palpated between the thumb and forefinger; it is normally located posterior to the testis and is flaccid and slightly sensitive to palpation. When acutely inflamed, it becomes thickened, severely tender, and tense.

A globular translucent mass above the testis but separate from it is a **spermatocele.** A peritesticular cystic mass that transilluminates and surrounds the testicle except posteriorly is a **hydrocele.**

C. Torsion of the testis presents as testicular pain of sudden onset with radiation to the lower abdomen; rarely, it is associated with nausea, vomiting, fever, or urinary symptoms. Examination reveals a swollen, tender, hyperemic scrotum; the testis is elevated, and the epididymis is rotated laterally or anteriorly. Evaluation of the blood supply of the testis by Doppler ultrasound or testicular scan may be helpful. When torsion is suspected, prompt exploration and orchiopexy is necessary. Contralateral orchiopexy as prophylaxis is indicated in cases of intravaginal torsion.

Table 2-3. Differential Diagnosis of Scrotal Masses

	Torsion		Tumor	Hernia		Epididymitis	Hematocele	Hydrocele	Spermatocele	Varicocele
	Extravaginal	Intravaginal		Reducible	Incarcerated					
History of trauma	−	−	±	−	−	±	+	−	−	−
Pain	−	+	−	±	+	+	±	−	−	±
Fever	−	±	−	−	±	±	±	−	−	−
Nausea	−	±	−	−	±	−	−	−	−	−
Abnormal color	+	+	−	−	−	±	±	−	−	+
Decreased pain by elevation of mass	−	−	−	−	−	+	−	−	−	+
Consistency	Firm, rubbery	Firm, rubbery	Firm, hard	Soft, crepitation	Irregular, doughy	Rubbery, hard	Compressible	Cystic	Cystic	"Bag of worms"
Position of mass	High	Horizontal	Normal	Normal	Normal	Normal	Normal	Normal	Postero-superior	Postero-superior
Orientation of epididymis	Normal	Abnormal	Normal	Normal	Normal	Normal	Normal indeterminable	Normal indeterminable	Normal	Normal
Cremasteric reflex	−	+	+	+	+	±	+	+	+	+
Transillumination	Opaque	Opaque	Opaque	Lucent, opaque	Opaque	Opaque	Opaque	Lucent	Lucent	Opaque
Urinalysis	−	−	−	−	−	±	±	−	−	−
Abnormal CBC	−	−	±	−	±	+	±	−	−	−
Testicular scan	+	+	±	−	−	±	±	−	−	−
Treatment	Operation	Immediate operation	Immediate operation	Elective operation	Immediate operation	Medical management	Operation	Operation if symptomatic	Operation if symptomatic	Operation if symptomatic

Vaginal Bleeding and Other Gynecological Problems

An understanding of the physiological process of menstruation is helpful in managing patients with vaginal bleeding. Every physician who works in an emergency room should be capable of performing an adequate pelvic examination; a female nurse or attendant should be present at all times. The differential diagnosis of the acute abdomen (see Chap. 5) requires that the physician be constantly aware of pathological conditions in the pelvis.

Abnormal uterine bleeding may be an early symptom of cervical cancer. Every patient having a pelvic examination must have a Papanicolaou smear even if there is bleeding. All patients with perimenopausal or postmenopausal bleeding must have a dilation and currettage to exclude endometrial carcinoma.

I. Traumatic lesions

A. Perineal or vaginal lacerations are the result of direct trauma. Hymenal tears may bleed profusely and require suturing under local anesthesia. Coital vaginal injuries are uncommon in premenopausal women but are more common after the menopause, owing to atrophy of vaginal mucosa. Vaginal lacerations bleed profusely and require initial control with a tight vaginal pack, replacement of blood loss, and suturing under general anesthesia. If the lacerations are in the periurethral region, an indwelling catheter should be placed.

B. Perineal or vulvar hematoma occurs as the result of blunt trauma or a straddle-type fall. Usually, the hematoma involves the vulva and perineum; rarely, it extends into the vagina. Rarely, avulsion, transection, contusion, or laceration of the urethra occurs. These injuries result in excruciating pain. Most patients may be treated by bed rest, ice packs to the perineum and vulva, and an indwelling catheter if urinary retention occurs. If the hematoma extends rapidly, it may require evacuation and placement of drains under general anesthesia.

C. Foreign bodies in the vagina or in the urethra are most commonly seen in young children. Rarely, a foreign body such as a tampon may be forgotten in adult females. The foreign body results in vaginitis and an offensive, malodorous, occasionally bloodstained discharge. Often, the foreign body can be identified and gently removed in the examining room.

II. Rape. Rape is labial penetration by the penis without consent, using force, fear, or fraud.

A. Immediate care of physical injuries. Victims of rape may experience a variety of traumatic injuries ranging from laceration of the hymen, vulva, or vagina to rupture of the cul-de-sac.

B. Prevention of venereal disease. A serological test for syphilis is performed. Cultures for gonorrhea are taken from the cervical canal, urethra, and rectum. If indicated, a throat culture is taken. Antibiotic prophylaxis of gonorrhea consists of procaine penicillin, 4.8 million units IM, and probenecid, 1 gm orally. If the patient is allergic to penicillin, an appropriate alternative antibiotic should be prescribed. Follow-up is mandatory to evaluate the gonococcal cultures and serology and to provide any additional needed treatment.

C. Prevention and alleviation of psychological damage requires tact and gentleness on the part of the examining physician. Rape is a particularly demoralizing kind of assault. Psychiatric referral and careful follow-up of the patient often are indicated.

D. Medicolegal examination involves recording the following:

1. History of events surrounding the assault.

2. Patient's emotional state.

3. Menstrual history, including use of contraception.

4. Coital history other than the rape incident.

5. Condition of the patient's clothing. Look for blood or seminal stains, and collect any hairs or foreign fibers as evidence.

6. Physical findings, including the results of inspection of all body surfaces. Describe in detail any evidence of trauma, such as bruises, abrasions, or lacerations.

7. Pelvic findings, including the results of examination of any dried secretion from the perineum and thighs. Record any evidence of trauma, especially to the introitus. Take carefully labeled smears for spermatozoa from the vulva, vagina, and cervix, and also take a Papanicolaou smear. Examine a fresh drop of vaginal aspirate for motile spermatozoa. Seminal fluid in the vaginal aspirate may be tested for acid phosphatase (Phosphatabs Acid). Finally, perform a careful bimanual examination.

E. **Prevention of pregnancy** may be offered as Premarin, 20–25 mg daily, or ethinyl estradiol, 1–5 mg daily, for 5 days. All patients should be checked after 21 days for possible pregnancy if no menstrual bleeding has occurred. The option of therapeutic abortion also may be offered to these patients.

III. **Bleeding due to abortion.** Abortion is the termination of pregnancy prior to 20 wk of gestation or when the fetus weighs less than 500 gm. The incidence of spontaneous abortion is between 10 and 15% of all pregnancies. The exact incidence of induced abortion is not known.

A. **Threatened abortion** is associated with vaginal bleeding or bloody vaginal discharge and may be accompanied by cramps and backache. The cervix is closed and not effaced. Speculum and vaginal examinations are made to exclude any local cause of bleeding. Bed rest and avoidance of coitus are advised. In most cases the bleeding will cease and the pregnancy will continue. If bleeding persists, the patient should be advised that she may abort. The effectiveness of progestational agents in preventing abortion is controversial.

B. **Inevitable abortion** is associated with rupture of the membranes and the presence of cervical dilation. Rarely, the membranes seal, but the usual course is progression of the abortion, accompanied by bleeding. The patient should be hospitalized and have blood typed and cross-matched, and an IV infusion of oxytocin (10–20 units per liter IV fluids) started to aid completion of the abortion. Intravaginal prostaglandin E_2 or $F_2\alpha$ may be used in place of the oxytocin infusion to facilitate completion of the abortion in selected cases. If the passage of tissue seems to be incomplete, the products of conception should be evacuated by sharp or suction curettage under anesthesia.

C. **Incomplete abortion** is the most common disorder of early pregnancy requiring treatment. Surgical intervention is nearly always necessary. The history is one of severe uterine cramps accompanied by considerable bleeding and, frequently, by the passage of the products of conception. On pelvic examination the cervical os is found dilated and effaced, and tissue is found in the cervical canal or vagina. Blood is typed and cross-matched, an IV infusion with oxytocin is started, and evacuation of the products of conception by sharp or suction currettage is done when the patient's condition is stable. Ergonovine, 0.2 mg IM or IV, is administered after curettage to keep the uterus firmly contracted.

D. **Complete abortion** occurs in early pregnancy, prior to 10 wk, when the fetus and the placenta are passed as an intact conceptus. The patient has contractions and bleeding, and the uterus, when examined, feels firm and contracted, with a tightly closed cervix. If cramps and bleeding persist, this type of abortion is managed by dilation and curettage and evacuation of any residual products of conception from the uterine cavity.

E. Septic abortion. The gravid uterus and adjacent parametria are extremely vulnerable to infection. On sterile pelvic examination, if the tenderness is limited to the uterus, the infection probably is contained within the uterine cavity. Parametrial thickening or tenderness associated with lower abdominal tenderness, guarding, rigidity, or rebound indicates pelvic peritonitis.

   1. The patient should be hospitalized. Cervical specimens should be taken for aerobic and anaerobic culture and a Gram stain examined. If the temperature is above 38.3°C (101°F), blood for culture should be drawn. Blood should be typed and cross-matched and IV fluids started. A central venous catheter is mandatory in severe infections. An indwelling catheter is required to monitor urine output. Appropriate antibiotics should be started, preferably by the IV route (see Chap. 14).

   2. Unless massive hemorrhage dictates the need for immediate evacuation of the uterus, it is best to prevent and control the spread of infection by an intensive 24-hr antibiotic treatment prior to dilation and curettage.

   3. If there is suspicion of prior intrauterine manipulation, an x-ray of the abdomen should be obtained to look for evidence of uterine perforation (presence of subdiaphragmatic air) or the presence of a foreign body or gas in the subcutaneous tissue. If the diagnosis of perforated uterus is made, exploratory laparotomy is required to exclude traumatic injury to the bowel and other viscera.

   4. In the presence of extensive pelvic infection or uncontrollable hemorrhage, hysterectomy may be a lifesaving procedure.

IV. Ectopic pregnancy. Ectopic pregnancy means implantation outside the uterine cavity. Almost all ectopic pregnancies (95%) occur within the fallopian tube. The clinical picture of ectopic pregnancy is rarely typical. The physician must "think ectopic" when faced with the triad of amenorrhea, abnormal uterine bleeding, and pelvic pain.

A. Signs and symptoms. The first symptom usually is a delay in menstruation lasting a week or two, followed by vaginal spotting. Amenorrhea of longer duration may be followed by frank vaginal bleeding. Passage of a decidual cast may occur as a result of a falling hormonal level. Cramplike pain occurs in the pelvis or lower abdomen on the affected side. With rupture of the tube, pain is severe and steady, associated with a feeling of faintness or actual syncope. Pallor, sweating, tachycardia, and hypotension are due to intra-abdominal bleeding. There is diffuse abdominal tenderness, with guarding. Percussion reveals shifting dullness and crown tympany. Pelvic examination may reveal a tender adnexal mass and fullness in the cul-de-sac. There is pain on moving the cervix, which may be softened and blue, and there may be slight uterine enlargement.

There is a mild leukocytosis without fever, and there may be anemia. Radioreceptor assay for pregnancy is of value in suspected ectopic pregnancy. A negative pregnancy test does not exclude an ectopic pregnancy. An ultrasound examination of the pelvis may be helpful in establishing the diagnosis of an early intrauterine pregnancy and thereby in excluding an ectopic pregnancy. The diagnosis may be supported by the free flow of blood at culdocentesis when hemoperitoneum is present. Confirmation of the diagnosis usually requires evaluation of the adnexa by laparoscopy, culdotomy, or laparotomy.

B. Treatment of an ectopic pregnancy is aimed at controlling the intra-abdominal hemorrhage. Usually, a salpingectomy is performed, with excision of the cornual portion of the involved tube.

C. Differential diagnosis. Conditions that may be confused with an ectopic pregnancy are:

1. Ruptured corpus luteum cyst.

2. Intrauterine pregnancy with threatened or incomplete abortion.

3. Pelvic inflammatory disease.

4. Torsion of an ovarian cyst or fallopian tube.

V. Acute pelvic inflammatory disease

A. There are **two types** of acute pelvic inflammatory disease:

1. **Gonorrheal infection** ascends from the cervix along the endometrium to produce an acute salpingitis; pelvic peritonitis follows when purulent exudate escapes.

2. **Pyogenic infection** occurs in puerperal and postabortive states, as well as in postoperative infections of the genital tract.

B. **Signs and symptoms.** Acute symptoms may appear during or after a menstrual period. Fever, leukocytosis, and tachycardia are present. There is severe pain in the pelvis and lower abdomen, accompanied by tenderness, guarding, and abdominal distention. Urinary frequency and dysuria may occur. On pelvic examination, leukorrhea and marked tenderness bilaterally are observed, especially on motion of the cervix. Tubo-ovarian masses (abscesses) may be palpated in some patients. The urethra and Skene's glands may also be inflamed. Aerobic and anaerobic cultures should be taken from the endocervix, and a specific search for gonococci should be made by examining a gram-stained smear. If gonorrhea is suspected, anorectal and pharyngeal cultures should be taken.

C. **Treatment.** The patient is kept at bed rest. Fluids are given IV. Vigorous parenteral antibiotic therapy is instituted. Usually, the infection subsides. If rupture of a tubo-ovarian abscess occurs, generalized peritonitis and septic shock may ensue. An immediate operation then is essential; hysterectomy and bilateral adnexectomy are almost always necessary.

VI. Infections with an intrauterine device (IUD). An **acute pelvic infection** may develop. If mild, it can be treated with appropriate antibiotics with the IUD in place. If the infection is more serious, the IUD should be removed, aerobic and anaerobic cultures taken from the endocervix, and antibiotic treatment for aerobes and anaerobes instituted.

The **early symptoms** of a **progressive pelvic infection** occurring with an IUD in place are: foul-smelling leukorrhea, bloating, intermenstrual bleeding, dyspareunia, and abdominal and pelvic pain. Finding a unilateral, tender adnexal mass on pelvic examination suggests that the patient has a unilateral tubo-ovarian abscess, pyosalpinx, or ovarian abscess. The bacteria in these tubal abscesses most often are synergistic *Bacteroides* and **streptococci.**

In patients with a unilateral tubo-ovarian abscess, the IUD must be removed, aerobic and anaerobic cultures taken from the endocervix and uterus, and appropriate parenteral antibiotic therapy instituted immediately. The majority of patients with adnexal abscess formation will require surgical treatment, such as unilateral salpingo-oophorectomy. Rarely, infection may be bilateral and require total hysterectomy and bilateral salpingo-oophorectomy.

Hand Injuries and Infections

I. **Anatomy.** Knowledge of the anatomy of the hand and forearm is essential in order to perform a proper examination and make an accurate diagnosis, as well as to avoid damage to uninjured and uninvolved structures in both operative and nonoperative treatment.

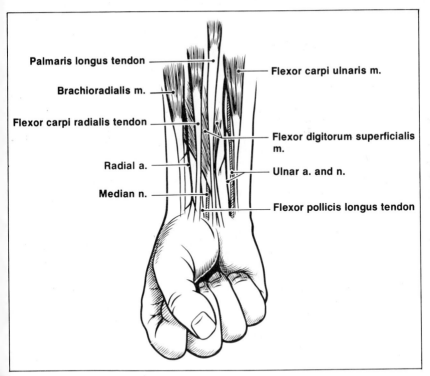

Figure 2-1. The volar aspect of the wrist.

A. Volar surface of wrist. See Figure 2-1

1. Lacerations here are common, and the structures injured vary significantly. The prerepair examination with an awake, cooperative patient is critical in determining what is intact and what has been cut in whole or in part.

2. The palmaris longus and the flexor carpi radialis tendons are in the center of the volar surface. The median nerve lies beneath these tendons.

3. On the ulnar side is the flexor carpi ulnaris tendon. Just beneath and radial to it are the ulnar artery and nerve.

4. The radial artery is radial to the flexor carpi radialis tendon.

5. In the deeper central wrist are the nine tendons of the flexor digitorum superficialis (4), flexor digitorum profundus (4), and flexor pollicis longus (1).

B. Dorsum of wrist and hand. See Figure 2-2

1. Because the structures here lie just beneath the skin, they are frequently cut.

2. At the wrist, there are six compartments for the extensor tendons. From radial to ulnar, the tendons in each and their insertions are:

   a. Abductor pollicis longus (base of first metacarpal) and extensor pollicis brevis (base of proximal phalanx of thumb).

   b. Extensor carpi radialis longus and brevis (bases of second and third metacarpals).

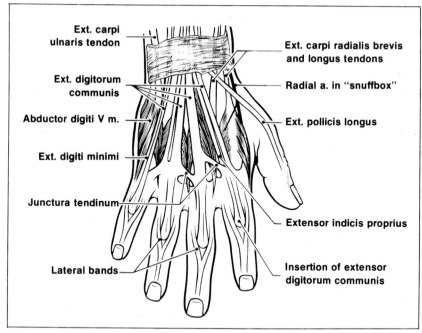

Figure 2-2. The dorsum of the hand and wrist.

    c. Extensor pollicis longus (base of distal phalanx of thumb).

    d. Four extensor digitorum communis tendons and the extensor indicis proprius (bases of proximal and middle phalanges, not the distal phalanx).

    e. Extensor digiti quinti (bases of proximal and middle phalanges of little finger).

    f. Extensor carpi ulnaris (base of fifth metacarpal).

  3. Note that there are two extensor tendons to the index and little fingers and only one to the middle and ring fingers.

  4. The long extensor to the thumb angles obliquely from the wrist to the thumb and overlies the insertion of the two radial wrist extensors.

  5. The superficial radial nerve (sensory) is on the radial side of the dorsum of the wrist and hand. It is frequently cut and should be identified and repaired to provide some sensation to the area and to avoid painful neuromas.

C. Palm of hand See Figure 2-3

  1. In the center of the proximal palm is the carpal tunnel, which contains the four superficialis and four profundus tendons, the flexor pollicis longus tendon, and the median nerve. These structures are protected here by the thick transverse carpal ligament that forms the roof of the tunnel.

  2. The ulnar nerve and artery are more superficial than the radial artery and the radial and median nerves. The ulnar nerve divides into three branches: a proper digital to the ulnar side of the little finger; a common digital to the radial side of the little finger and the ulnar side of the ring finger; and a motor branch, which runs through the origin of the hypothenar muscles to lie deep to

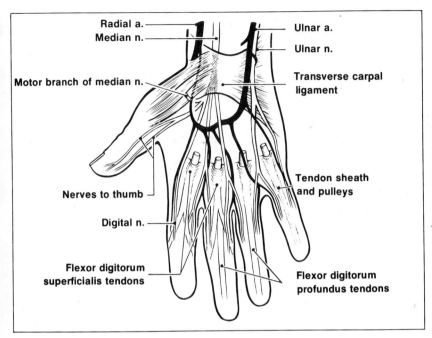

Figure 2-3. The palm of the hand.

the flexor tendons and innervate the hypothenar muscles, all interossei, the lumbricals of the ring and little finger, and usually both heads of the adductor pollicis.

3. Distal to the carpal tunnel, the tendons and median nerve branches are covered only by the palmar fascia as far as the distal palmar crease. Beyond this crease the tendons lie within a fibrous tendon sheath.

4. The motor branch of the median nerve leaves the main trunk at the distal edge of the transverse carpal ligament to innervate the thenar muscles. The median nerve also innervates the lumbrical muscles to the index and middle fingers.

D. Fingers

1. At the level of the web space, the superficialis tendon divides into two slips. These circle the deeper profundus tendon and then reunite to continue to their insertion on the base of the middle phalanx. The superficialis flexes the proximal interphalangeal (PIP) joint.

2. The profundus tendon goes through the two slips of the superficialis to its insertion on the base of the distal phalanx. The profundus flexes the distal interphalangeal (DIP) joint.

3. On the dorsum, the long extensor tendon inserts on the base of the proximal phalanx and also on the base of the middle phalanx and extends the metacarpophalangeal (MCP) and PIP joints. The DIP joint is extended by the two lateral bands, which are the tendons of the interossei and lumbricals. These unite beyond the PIP joint to insert on the base of the distal phalanx.

II. Injury. Following injury, a hand may be seriously disabled. This holds true if treatment is appropriate—and even more so if the initial care rendered and the follow-up thereafter are not correct. The first person caring for an injured hand may determine its ultimate usefulness.

A. History

1. Time and place of the accident.

2. Agent and mechanism of injury.

3. Amount and type of first aid given.

4. Right or left hand dominance.

5. Occupation.

6. Age.

7. General health.

B. Examination

1. General

a. The patient should be supine on a cart or table with the arm extended.

b. When there is an open wound, the examination should be carried out with sterile technique, including cap, mask, and gloves.

c. The initial examination determines the structures injured and the need for further treatment. All but the simplest procedures should be performed in the operating room with adequate anesthesia, assistance, lighting, and instruments, including a tourniquet, which is frequently necessary.

2. Sensory function. See Figure 2-4

a. Must test prior to injecting the wound with local anesthetic.

b. Use a sharp needle.

c. Test for sensation in areas supplied by all nerves that may have been injured.

d. Test the dorsum of the first web space for superficial radial nerve sensation.

e. Test both sides of the volar aspect of each finger for digital nerve sensation.

f. Record with a diagram all areas of decreased or absent sensation.

3. Motor: flexor tendons

a. Test for profundus function by holding the PIP joint in full extension and asking the patient to flex the distal phalanx.

b. Test for superficialis function by holding all fingers except the one being tested in full extension (especially all DIP joints) and asking the patient to flex the PIP joint of the finger not held.

c. Test for flexor pollicis longus function by holding the thumb MCP joint in extension and asking the patient to flex the distal joint.

d. Test for wrist flexor function by asking the patient to flex the wrist against resistance as you palpate the tendons.

4. Motor: motor branch of median nerve

a. Ask the patient to abduct the thumb as far from the palm as possible and rotate it to touch the little finger (first show the patient with your own hand what you want him or her to do).

b. Repeat by resisting the motion of the thumb with your finger as you palpate the thenar muscles with a finger of your other hand.

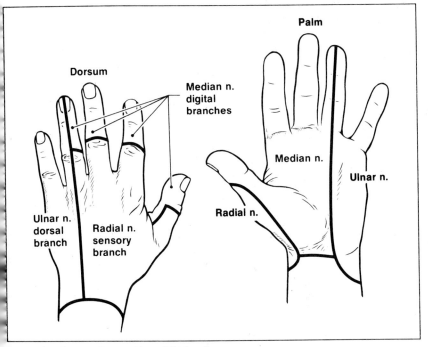

Figure 2-4. Sensory innervation of the hand.

c. Be wary of "trick" movement, i.e., some abduction of the thumb by the abductor pollicis longus, with "opposition" by flexion with the flexor pollicis longus.

5. Motor: motor branch of ulnar nerve

a. Ask the patient to spread the fingers apart with the fingers fully extended (tests interossei).

b. Have patient hold a piece of paper in the web space between the thumb and index finger. Try removing the paper (tests adductor).

c. The motor branch may be intact and the sensory branch or branches cut, or vice versa. Be sure to test both sensory and motor function and record both. The same holds true for the median nerve.

6. Motor: extensor tendons Ask the patient to extend all fingers and the thumb fully.

7. Vascular

a. If bleeding from a wound is brisk, do not attempt to clamp the bleeding vessels. The vessels may be damaged further, making reanastomosis impossible without a vein graft. Adjacent structures (e.g., digital nerves, ulnar nerve) may also be damaged by the clamp. Bleeding can be controlled by placing a blood pressure cuff on the upper arm and inflating it to 250–300 mm Hg while a compression dressing is applied.

b. The hand and fingers should be pink and warm. If they are not, the arteries have been damaged and require prompt exploration to restore blood flow.

c. Test by applying pressure to the fingernail. It should blanch and promptly refill. If it takes longer than 1 sec, the blood supply to the finger is compromised.

8. Bone and joint

a. Suspect injury if the appearance is distorted.

b. Palpate gently for movement at the suspected fracture site.

c. Test for ligament injury by active and passive motion of the joint.

d. X-rays (anteroposterior, lateral, and oblique) for fractures and stress x-rays for ligaments. In children, x-rays of the normal hand are needed for comparison because of the presence of epiphyses.

e. Be suspicious of wrist dislocations and fractures. These are often difficult to diagnose and require precise x-ray study.

C. Treatment

1. General

a. The goal of treatment is to maximize function. Joint stiffness must be kept to a minimum, as must the adhesions that form around tendons and limit their ability to glide. Prompt healing is essential and requires careful wound preparation and delicate tissue handling.

b. The injured hand should not be subjected to repeated examinations. If the initial examiner suspects an injury to any deep structure, he or she should ask for consultation from the surgeon who will carry out the definitive repair. Nerve or tendon injuries can be determined by the testing techniques described. Exploration of the wound after injection of a local anesthetic is not necessary. This may produce more damage and increases the possibility of infection.

c. Simple lacerations involving only the skin can be repaired in the emergency room if facilities are adequate.

d. Most other injuries involving bones, tendons, nerves, vessels, or complex skin lacerations require the facilities of the operating room for repair. *Do not attempt to treat complicated hand injuries in the emergency room.*

e. The primary objective in treating hand injuries is to ensure that the patient is no worse off than before treatment. Complicated injuries should be managed by a surgeon with experience and skill in the treatment of hand injuries. **The obligation of the physician who first sees a patient with a major hand injury is to examine the hand, control bleeding, clean the wound, apply a dressing, splint in the safe position, elevate the hand, and obtain consultation.** This may require transferring the patient to another facility.

2. Preparation

a. Remove any clothing that may interfere with access to the hand and arm. Remove watches and rings.

b. The entire hand and forearm around the wound should be thoroughly scrubbed with soap and water. Dirt and debris should be removed and the wound thoroughly irrigated with saline. This is much less painful for the patient if the wound has been anesthetized, but this must be done only after the examination has been carried out.

3. Anesthesia

a. Repair of simple lacerations can be carried out in the emergency room, with infiltration of the local anesthetic directly into the wound or with a digital nerve block. **All nerve blocks at or proximal to the wrist should be done in the operating room.**

b. Anesthetic solutions containing epinephrine should not be used for digital nerve blocks, since the resulting vasoconstriction may result in gangrene of the finger and amputation.

c. Plain 1% lidocaine (Xylocaine) is commonly used. A #25 needle is fitted on the syringe, placed in the skin of the web space, and directed proximally at an angle of 20 degrees from the long axis of the digit being anesthetized. A maximum of 3 ml of the anesthetic solution is injected around the digital nerve. No more than this is used in order to avoid mechanical compression of the vessels. A similar approach is used to anesthetize the nerve on the opposite side of the finger.

d. For the nerves on the radial side of the index finger and the ulnar side of the little finger, the solution is placed proximal to the distal palmar flexion crease and 5 mm from the border of the hand.

e. The digital nerves to the thumb lie on either side of the flexor pollicis longus tendon at the MCP joint flexion crease. The anesthetic solution is placed here.

f. If an injury involves the dorsum or the lateral borders of a finger, the nerve branches that supply this area are anesthetized by placing the anesthetic solution transversely across the dorsum of the finger, just beyond the MCP joint.

4. Tourniquet

a. A tourniquet makes wound closure easier if the wound is bleeding.

b. For repair of finger lacerations, a small tourniquet may be used. A ¼-in. Penrose drain is placed around the base of the finger and held with a hemostat. **Rubber bands are never used because they may be forgotten and incorporated in the bandage;** this has resulted in gangrene and required amputation. The Penrose drain tourniquet should not be used for more than 20 min.

c. For repair of more proximal lacerations as well as for finger lacerations, a tourniquet around the upper arm may be used. **A blood pressure cuff is preferred** rather than a pneumatic tourniquet, for with the latter, exceedingly high pressures may be applied unknowingly and cause severe damage. The blood pressure cuff is inflated to 250 mm Hg, and the rubber hoses are clamped with large hemostats next to the cuff to avoid the possibility of leaks in the tubing or connections. The blood pressure cuff can be tolerated by most adults for 20–30 min. It probably should not be used in young children because it often increases their anxiety and restlessness.

5. Repair

a. Strict attention to fundamental principles is essential to prevent infection. Aseptic technique must include appropriate sterile draping, removal of all foreign material, debridement of devitalized and contaminated tissue, good hemostasis, and closure without tension.

b. **Primary closure may be unwise** if the wound has foreign material in it and is seen after 6 hr. In a "clean" wound, e.g., most glass or knife cuts, this interval may be longer, but antibiotics should be used.

c. If primary skin closure cannot be achieved without tension, coverage may require a skin graft or flap. Such procedures should be done in the operating room, with the possible exception of a graft for a fingertip amputation. Primary or early delayed closure is especially important to avoid necrosis if tendon or bone is exposed.

d. In an **avulsion injury,** a skin flap is usually created with a distal base. The blood supply to the skin of the edge of the flap is frequently compromised, and this skin may die if the flap is simply sutured back in place. The blood supply is evaluated by the use of intravenous fluorescein (10 ml of a 10% solution in an adult) and a Wood's lamp, or by a tourniquet test, in which a tourniquet is applied to the arm for 10 min and then deflated. The return of circulation to the flap is observed. If any skin does not blanch or refill within 1 sec, consideration should be given to microvascular anastomoses of the veins or to cutting the avulsed flap skin at the line of demarcation and applying the detached skin as a free full-thickness skin graft.

e. Skin is usually sutured with 4-0 or 5-0 nylon. Deep dermal or subcutaneous absorbable sutures are not needed for hand wounds and are usually used only in arm or forearm wounds that are under some tension. Sutures in the hand are usually removed no sooner than 14 days after repair to avoid wound separation. Those in the arm and forearm are frequently removed before 10 days to avoid increased scarring from the stitch marks that may result if the sutures cut through the skin.

6. Specific injuries

a. Fingertip injuries are the most common hand injuries. If the tip has been amputated, the length should be maintained in many cases by use of a skin graft or flap if the bone is protruding. Replacement of the amputated tip is seldom successful and should be attempted only in a clean, sharp amputation in a child. Skin from the amputated tip, if not traumatized, may be used as a free skin graft.

b. If the **nailbed** is injured, the loose nail should be removed and the nail matrix repaired accurately with 6-0 or 7-0 catgut. The nail should be replaced as a splint to align the edges of the cut matrix. Deformity of the growing nail may result from adhesions of the eponychium and paronychium to the matrix and can be prevented by nail replacement or by packing for 10 days.

c. Nerve injuries should usually be repaired primarily. Digital nerve lacerations are repaired if the laceration is proximal to the DIP joint in a finger, or proximal to the base of the nail in the thumb, using magnification (loupe or microscope) in the operating room.

d. Tendons are repaired primarily except in special instances (e.g., human bite). Such repairs are also operating room procedures. Flexor tendons cut in "no-man's-land" (between the distal palmar crease and the middle of the middle phalanx) should be repaired by a hand surgeon. If one is not immediately available, the wound should be cleaned, the skin closed, and the patient referred as soon as possible for delayed tendon repair.

e. *Fingers or a hand or forearm that has been completely amputated or is still partly attached but devascularized should be considered for replantation or revascularization.* Patients with a thumb amputation or with multiple finger amputations are always candidates, and others should be discussed with the replantation surgeon. If the patient is a candidate, the stump or wound should be cleaned and a compression dressing applied. Supportive care is given, and the patient is transferred with the limb elevated. A tourniquet is used only if absolutely necessary to control bleeding initially and is removed as soon as the dressing is applied.

The amputated part is cleaned and placed in a sterile sponge, which is put in a sealed plastic bag. The bag is laid on a bed of ice. Replantation has been successful more than 24 hours after amputation if the amputated part has been cooled for most of this time.

The success of microvascular surgery obligates emergency service personnel to be aware of potential microsurgical cases and the replantation centers that are available.

f. Fractures must be reduced accurately and splinted for 3–4 wk, though occasional gentle motion with the finger or hand out of the splint helps to minimize joint stiffness. Unstable, unsatisfactorily reduced, or open fractures require open reduction, which is an operating room procedure.

g. A stable injured joint should be immobilized for 14 days, an unstable one for 21 days. Some unstable or irreducible joint injuries require surgical repair.

h. A **burned hand** is cleaned with bland soap and water and dressed with an occlusive (not pressure) dressing. Blisters can be left alone if unbroken. Immobilization in the safe position (see 7.b) is essential, for a hand left unsplinted will go into a badly deformed position. A burn deep enough to require grafting should be referred to a hand surgeon.

i. Human bites are frequently complicated by infection if not treated properly. It must always be suspected that a laceration over the dorsum of an MCP joint has been caused by a clenched fist hitting a tooth. The patient may be reluctant to admit to being in a fight, and the history of injury should be elicited with the patient's awareness of the complications that may result from not telling the truth. The laceration frequently involves the extensor tendon and the MCP joint, and infection can severely damage either or both. X-rays should be obtained. Debridement, irrigation, and broad-spectrum antibiotics are essential. Wound closure is considered only if the time between injury and treatment is less than 6 hr. If longer, the wound should be treated but left open and secondary closure carried out some days later if the wound is not infected.

j. Dog bites are much less likely than human bites to cause infection and can usually be closed primarily after thorough cleaning.

k. Wringer or roller injuries sometimes appear trivial but may actually be severe crushing or shearing injuries, depending on how far the extremity is pulled in, the distance between the rollers, and the time before the machine is turned off. Considerable swelling may gradually develop and cause ischemia and necrosis of the deep structures and ultimately a severely disabled extremity. The danger lies in **underestimating what appears to be a trivial injury.** Most patients, especially children, should be admitted to the hospital for observation, with the extremity in a resilient compressive (not pressure) dressing and elevated. Signs of vascular compromise may require fasciotomy of fingers, hand, or forearm.

l. A high-pressure **injection injury** caused by a grease or paint gun may cause severe damage and a useless finger that requires amputation. The injury may appear innocuous initially, but treatment requires immediate meticulous removal of the injected material in the operating room.

7. Dressings, splints, and elevation

a. Wounds of the wrist or proximal fingers, palm, or dorsum of the hand usually require a complete **hand dressing** initially. Dressing sponges are placed between the fingers and on the sides of the index and little fingers. The distal fingers are left exposed. A bulky group of sponges is placed between the thumb and index finger, with the thumb in an abducted and opposed position. The sponges are held in place with a Kling bandage, with the Kling brought back and forth between the fingers to keep the sponges in place. A stockinette with openings cut for the fingertips can be applied for observation.

b. Splinting may be necessary to protect the skin closure. The **safe position,** or position of function, is preferred. This is the position of the wrist and finger joints from which the joint motion regained after injury is in the most functional range. The wrist is extended 15 degrees, MCP joints are flexed 45 degrees, and the interphalangeal joints are slightly flexed 15 to 25 degrees. The thumb is abducted and rotated into an opposing position. After padding is applied over the forearm, a plaster splint of 15 thicknesses and 3 or 4 in. wide is applied to the dorsal aspect of the dressing and held in place with a Kling bandage. The hand and wrist must be held in position until the plaster hardens. If a tendon or nerve repair is to be protected, the position of the joints is adjusted appropriately.

c. Wounds of the fingers often require only a simple dressing. Splinting may promote healing and also prevent increased pain if the finger is accidentally hit. A foam-padded aluminum splint is taped to the finger with the joints slightly flexed. Tubegauze makes an attractive dressing and may be applied over the dressing or splint.

d. Elevation of the extremity minimizes swelling and discomfort. The patient is advised to keep the hand above the heart at all times and is shown how to keep the hand elevated at night by propping it against several pillows with the elbow on the bed.

IV. Infections

A. General principles

1. A hand infection may progress so rapidly that structures in the hand are destroyed in a few hours. Pressure caused by edema and pus in a closed space leads to ischemic necrosis of tendons, nerve, bones, and joints. The useless finger or hand that results may require amputation.

2. History

a. Heat, erythema, swelling, pain, and tenderness.

b. Ask about a preceding blister, minor laceration, or prick with a needle or thorn.

3. Examination

a. Swelling may be localized or generalized. Edema on the dorsum of the hand is common with deep infections of the palm or extensive infections of the fingers.

b. Discoloration.

c. Tenderness on palpation.

d. Local heat.

e. Pain on movement of adjacent joints.

f. Fluctuance, if the infection has progressed to an abscess.

g. Look for a recent minor cut or penetrating wound.

h. Lymphangitis with red streaks extending up the forearm.

i. Enlarged epitrochlear or axillary nodes.

j. Temperature elevation may be minimal; high temperature usually indicates lymphatic involvement.

4. Treatment

a. Immobilization to avoid spreading bacteria.

b. Elevation to minimize swelling and later joint stiffness.

c. Antibiotics.

d. Immediate drainage of pus if present. Obtain a smear, culture, and sensitiv ity test. The abscess cavity should be explored carefully to be sure that drainage is adequate and no foreign material is present.

e. A careful follow-up with frequent observation is necessary to be sure the infection is resolving.

f. Tetanus prophylaxis.

B. Management of early infections (cellulitis)

1. In an infection seen early, i.e. before pus has formed, there is a tender, red, swollen area in the hand but no fluctuance to indicate the presence of pus. Be alert to the possibility that pus may be present in a deep infection, but the overlying tissue may be so indurated that fluctuation may not be present. Frequent examination is needed, and incision is indicated at the first sign of fluctuation or if the induration does not resolve after several days of appropriate therapy.

2. Treatment consists of **immobilization** with a dry, bulky hand dressing and plaster splint in the safe position, elevation, and antibiotics.

3. **Hot, wet soaks are contraindicated.** Neither mosisture nor heat is needed, and frequent soaks prevent proper immobilization, which is most important.

C. Management of established infection (pus)

1. **Any pus present must be drained immediately.**

2. A small incision is made over the site of maximum fluctuation, or skin necrosis or skin thinning, the pus drained, and the cavity carefully probed. There is no routine incision for the drainage of any hand infection. The skin incision is then extended over the abscess cavity only as far as necessary. If an incision is made and pus is not identified, care must be taken to be sure an abscess is not missed. On the other hand, extending the incision into uninvolved tissue may spread the infection, be it an abscess or cellulitis.

3. A drain is usually left in the abscess cavity and is sutured to the skin to prevent its extrusion before the cavity has become much smaller.

4. Antibiotics should be given prior to the incision and drainage.

5. Adequate anesthesia and a bloodless field are essential in draining an abscess in order to allow satisfactory exploration of the abscess cavity. Most infections should be treated in the operating room. One confined to the distal finger may occasionally be drained in the emergency room with a digital block and a tourniquet. If there is any suspicion that the infection has spread proximally to the site to be used to inject the local anesthetic, a block should not be done here lest an abscess occur at this site as well. **The use of a surface anesthetic such as ethyl chloride spray is not adequate.**

6. Immobilization, elevation, and antibiotics are continued after drainage until the infection has significantly resolved. Gradually increasing motion is then begun. If there is any sign of recurrence, immobilization is reinstituted.

7. If the infection is not resolving several days after incision and drainage, reexploration, with adequate anesthesia and with a tourniquet, is indicated to look for undrained loculations of pus, necrotic debris including bone, or undetected foreign material.

D. Management of specific infections

1. A **felon (pulp abscess)** is pus in the pulp space of the volar aspect of the fingertip. It often follows a minor penetrating wound and should not be confused with an infected intradermal blister. Treatment of the latter is simple and requires only excision of the epidermis, but one must search carefully for a sinus tract that leads to a deeper abscess. A felon may impair blood supply and

is drained through an incision in a skin crease over the site of fluctuation, skin necrosis, or maximum tenderness.

2. Paronychia is infection in the skin at the side of the fingernail. It is most commonly caused by picking or chewing on a hangnail.

   a. If seen early, when there is no pus under the nail, the skin over the nail can be elevated for adequate drainage. Anesthesia is not often necessary.

   b. If seen late, when pus is present under the nail, the part of the nail that is not attached to the bed must be removed with a fairly strong, sharp-pointed scissors for adequate drainage. This requires a digital block.

3. Subcutaneous abscess of the finger usually follows a minor penetrating wound of the volar surface of the finger. The abscess usually points on the lateral surface of the finger. The incision is placed directly over the abscess, with care taken to avoid injuring the digital artery and nerve. A tourniquet is essential. To avoid spreading the infection around the tendons, the incision must not be made through the tendon sheath.

4. Acute tenosynovitis is infection inside the tendon sheath. The most common cause is a penetrating wound, and the history is important. Destruction of the tendons may occur early and result in a useless finger.

   a. The diagnostic signs are a finger held in slight flexion, uniform fusiform swelling, a significant increase in pain with full extension of the finger, and tenderness over the course of the flexor tendon on palpation.

   b. If the condition is seen early, treatment with immobilization, elevation, and antibiotics may prevent the development of pus and avoid the need for incision. The finger must be reexamined after 12 hr. If the pain, swelling, tenderness over the tendon sheath, and temperature are not decreased, immediate exploration is indicated.

   c. Incisions are made over the distal tendon sheath and the proximal sheath in the palm. If pus is noted inside the sheath, the sheath is opened and irrigated with antibiotic solution.

   d. A common error is mistaking a subcutaneous abscess for an acute tenosynovitis. The diagnostic signs may be similar, but the treatment is radically different. If a subcutaneous abscess is present, the incision must not be extended into the sheath.

   e. Infection of the thumb or little finger sheath may extend to the radial or ulnar bursa respectively. Extension above the wrist is very uncommon, and an incision should be made at the wrist only if there is significant tenderness there.

5. Palmar abscesses are usually located deep to the palmar fascia. They may occur in conjunction with a suppurative tenosynovitis.

   a. The hand is very swollen, with pitting edema on the dorsum. Skin color may be normal but is usually red or purple. The fingers are held immobile in a somewhat flexed position, and they can be extended without significant pain, in contrast to an acute tenosynovitis.

   b. Treatment requires careful exploration of the abscess cavity to ensure adequate drainage and limit the severe compromise of hand use that is likely to result. The swelling on the dorsum of the hand is rarely due to pus and should not be incised.

Suggested Reading

Bailey, D. A. *The Infected Hand*. London: H.K. Lewis, 1963.

Connolly, W. B., and Kilgore, E. S., Jr. *Hand Injuries and Infections*. London: Edward Arnold Publishers, 1979.

Flatt, A. E. *The Care of Minor Hand Injuries* (4th ed.). St. Louis: Mosby, 1979.

Weeks, P. M., and Wray, R. C. *Management of Acute Hand Injuries* (2nd ed.). St. Louis: Mosby, 1978.

Bites and Stings

I. **General principles.** The management of bites and stings involves the therapy of soft tissue wounds as well as the recognition of infectious risk of various bites. In addition, the possibility of an immediate or delayed hypersensitivity reaction must be considered.

II. **Bites**

A. **Human bites.** The management of human bites is complicated by the fact that the human mouth contains many more pathogenic organisms than most animals. The human oral cavity contains a mixed aerobic and anaerobic flora of both gram-positive and gram-negative organisms. The risk of tetanus from a human bite is real. The **principles of treatment** include the following:

1. A human bite wound should be cultured, thoroughly scrubbed with a bacteriostatic soap, and irrigated with saline. After cleaning, any damaged tissue should be debrided. Any vital structures that are severed should undergo secondary repair.

2. **Do not close any human bite wound.**

3. **Tetanus toxoid** should be administered when indicated (see Chap. 1, Sect. I. **D.1**).

4. **Antibiotics should be administered.** Penicillin is the drug of choice, since it covers both the aerobic and anaerobic flora of the human oral cavity quite well.

5. The injured portion should be **elevated** above the level of the right atrium, and, in the case of an extremity, the part should be dressed lightly.

6. Human bites should be inspected frequently; this usually requires **hospitalization.** Occasionally, an extremely reliable patient may be treated without hospitalization. However, the site of injury still must be inspected frequently.

7. Wounds with cellulitis or secondary infection seen late should be treated as outlined in 1–6. Hospitalization is mandatory. Intravenous antibiotic therapy and immobilization in the position of function are required.

B. **Animal bites.** Most animal bites are bites from domestic animals, particularly dogs. These bites differ from human bites in that the wound contains fewer bacteria, particularly fewer anaerobes, than a human bite.

1. **Local treatment** consists of thorough scrubbing with a bacteriostatic soap and water, debridement if necessary, and closure in most cases. A massively contaminated bite or wound with excessive tissue destruction should not be closed.

2. **Tetanus toxoid** should be administered.

3. **Antibiotics** are required only in the dirty wound with a significant amount of tissue destruction and contamination.

4. **Rabies prophylaxis** is indicated when a bite occurs from an animal not known to be healthy, including pets not properly vaccinated against rabies, as well as bites by animals that have escaped (condition unknown). Certainly, prophylaxis is indicated when an animal is suspected of being rabid because of lack of provocation of a bite, the species of the biting animal, type of exposure, and the presence of rabies in the region.

a. Rabies is known to be endemic in bats, foxes, skunks, and bobcats, but is rare in squirrels, rodents, and rabbits. Both **passive and active immunization** with human rabies immune globulin (RIG) and duck embryo vaccine (DEV) is indicated for all bite exposures in which rabies cannot be excluded and for all non-bite exposures if the animal is proved to have or is strongly suspected of having rabies. For non-bite exposures from escaped dogs or cats in a rabies endemic area, active immunization (DEV) alone may be used. Human rabies immune globulin, 20 IU/kg body weight, is given. The area of the wound is infiltrated with up to 50% of the solution, and the remainder is given intramuscularly in the buttocks. As this is a human immune globulin, serum sickness is not a problem. However, febrile responses and local pain can occur. Duck embryo vaccine is given in 23 doses: 1 dose is given daily for 21 days, with additional doses 10 and 20 days after the primary series is completed. Local reactions to DEV are common and do not contraindicate continuing treatment. For **non-bite exposures,** DEV alone is given in a daily dose for 14 days subcutaneously. **This is the only indication for administration of duck embryo vaccine without passive immunization.**

b. The key to administration of postexposure rabies prophylaxis is recognition or capture of the biting animal. If the animal is observed and remains healthy for a 10-day period, prophylaxis for a person bitten by that animal is not indicated. Remember that saliva of a rabid animal on an open wound (usually a bite) or on any mucous membrane constitutes exposure to rabies and requires prophylaxis.

C. Snakebites. A number of poisonous snakes are indigenous to the United States. Most are members of the family Crotalidae (rattlesnake, copperhead, water moccasin (cotton mouth), but some are members of the family Elapidae (coral snake). The mortality and morbidity from venomous snakebites remain high. At least one venomous snake species is indigenous to every state in the United States except Maine, Alaska, and Hawaii. Over 5000 poisonous snakebites occur each year. Most snakebites occur in the extremities, usually in young males. The venoms are neurotoxic as well as hematotoxic.

The **management** of snakebite includes both local and systemic considerations. The principles are as follows:

1. Retard absorption of venom by making an incision approximately 6–8 mm long and 3–6 mm deep over the bite and employing mechanical suction to remove as much venom as possible from the wound. **Cruciate incisions are not required and heal poorly.** Suction by mouth may be used if necessary; the venom is not absorbed through intact oral mucosa, and digestive juices will neutralize any swallowed venom. A tourniquet should be applied several inches above the bite to occlude venous and lymphatic return but not arterial inflow. The tourniquet should be left in place **without release** for up to 2 hr. Immobilization of the bitten extremity also slows spread of the venom. The extremity should be kept at heart level and not be heated or cooled.

2. Neutralize venom. Polyvalent snake antivenin should be given **intravenously,** not intramuscularly or locally. The amount of antivenin given varies with the severity of venenation. For minimal venenation (fang or tooth marks, severe pain, 2–12 cm of surrounding edema in the first 12 hr), 10 ml of antivenin should be given. For moderate venenation (12–25 cm of surrounding edema, erythema in the first 12 hr, and minimal signs of systemic involvement), 30–40 ml of antivenin should be given. For more severe involvement, 50 ml of antivenin should be given. Since sensitivity will occur, a test dose should be given first; the incidence of serum sickness in recipients of more than 20 ml of antivenin is appreciable. Serum sickness will occur approximately 7–10 days after antivenin administration.

3. Prevent or reduce the effects of the venom. Appropriate infusions of crystalloid and colloid solutions should be instituted when indicated to prevent shock.

A baseline hematocrit and blood coagulation studies should be obtained. Coagulopathy should be searched for; any evidence of coagulopathy or the presence of hemoglobinuria necessitates rapid treatment to prevent the ill effects of hemolysis and resultant renal failure.

4. **Prevention of complications.** Broad-spectrum antibiotics and tetanus prophylaxis are administered as indicated. Bites of the extremity are loosely bandaged in a position of function and kept at heart level or elevated slightly. All patients bitten by a coral snake shoud be admitted to a hospital for at least 48 hr, since the effects of venenation by this snake are slow to develop.

D. **Spider bites** produce a local reaction in humans; in sensitive persons, this may progress to a systemic reaction. Systemic and local treatment is then indicated. Two particular spider bites are of greater concern because of the severity of reaction to their venom.

1. **Brown recluse spider** *(Loxosceles reclusa)* is common in the southern and central United States; 1.0–1.5 cm long, light tan to dark brown in color, they have a characteristic dark, violin-shaped band over the dorsal portion of the body. The venom is necrotizing and hemolytic and results in progressive local ischemia. Several hours after the bite, a painful red area appears with a pale mottled cyanotic center that later blisters. Hemorrhage and induration with a surrounding halo of erythema occur. A central black eschar later develops and sloughs, leaving an open ulcer. Systemic symptoms of fever, chills, nausea, vomiting, weakness, arthralgias, and petechiae can occur. Rarely, hemoglobinuria occurs and can result in death. **Therapy** involves excision of the involved area, tetanus prophylaxis, and administration of broad-spectrum antibiotics. Excision of the area of necrosis must be complete in order to avoid a recurrence of this lesion. Skin grafting often is necessary.

2. **Black widow spider** *(Latrodectus mactans)* is endemic in the continental United States. Only the female of the species bites. The female may be distinguished by a shiny, black, globular body with a red hourglass mark over the ventral portion. The venom is neurotoxic; the victim may recall a small pricking sensation, followed by a dull pain. Local swelling always occurs. Severe chest pain may result after an upper extremity bite; abdominal pain and rigidity simulating peritonitis may follow a lower extremity bite. The abdomen usually is nontender, and signs resolve in approximately 24–48 hr. The mortality risk from a female black widow spider bite is 4–5%. In adults, **therapy** consists of narcotics for analgesia and muscle relaxants. In children under 6 and debilitated or aged adults or in cases of severe bites, antivenin may be given.

III. **Stings.** Arthropods of the order Hymenoptera (bees, wasps, hornets, yellow jackets, and ants) inflict more bites on humans than any other venomous group. Their venom is just as toxic as that of a rattlesnake. More people die yearly in the United States because of allergy to insect stings than from snakebites. Although less venom is injected in insect bites, severe allergic reactions can occur, which account for most fatalities. All these insects, except the bee, retain their stinger and can sting repeatedly. Stings of the head, face, and neck tend to cause the most serious effects. The reaction can be immediate, varying from local signs only to systemic anaphylaxis, or a delayed hypersensitivity reaction resembling serum sickness may occur 10–14 days after the person is stung.

A. **Local care.** A retained stinger should be removed, the wound washed with soap and water, and any necrotic tissue debrided.

B. **Toxic reactions.** In multiple bites, the amount of injected toxin may cause systemic symptoms, particularly fainting, vomiting, diarrhea, edema, muscle spasms, and convulsions. Supportive therapy with sedation, intravenous fluids, antibiotics, and antihistamines may be given as necessary. Calcium gluconate given intravenously or intramuscularly may counteract toxic muscle spasms or convulsions.

C. **Allergic reactions.** Give epinephrine (1:1000), 0.3–0.5 ml, subcutaneously. The dose should be reduced for children. Since this is a short-acting drug, the dose may have to be repeated at 20-min intervals. An antihistamine is also given immediately. Supportive therapy with intravenous fluids, vasopressors, and mechanical respiration may be required. Any patient with a known severe reaction to insect bites should undergo desensitization.

Cardiac Arrhythmias

I. General comments

A. Arrhythmias can be grouped into the following **three prognostic categories:**

1. Those that are usually benign and require no specific therapy (e.g., atrial premature contractions, first-degree heart block).

2. Those having no immediate hemodynamic consequences but often presaging more ominous rhythms (e.g., multiple ventricular extrasystoles).

3. Those causing immediate hemodynamic deterioration (severe bradyarrhythmias, severe tachyarrhythmias, and chaotic rhythms).

B. The implications of an arrhythmia influence the urgency and scope of therapy; **an accurate diagnosis** is therefore essential and always requires an electrocardiogram (ECG). An oscilloscopic monitor and direct recorder are usually acceptable, but multiple simultaneous leads may be required on occasion (see **III.H,** and Fig. 3-2). Consultation with a cardiologist is often wise, since the unsophisticated may mistake a dangerous rhythm for a benign one (e.g., mistake paroxysmal atrial tachycardia with 2:1 block for sinus tachycardia).

C. **Effective treatment** of arrhythmias entails one or more of the following:

1. Identification and, if possible, reversal of the cause.

2. Pharmacological therapy (discussed in **III** in conjunction with each arrhythmia).

3. Electrical cardioversion (discussed in **IV**).

II. Causes of arrhythmias

A. **Decreased or maldistributed myocardial oxygen supply** due to:

1. Intrinsic cardiac factors (coronary atherosclerosis, ventricular hypertrophy).

2. Extrinsic, usually acute noncardiac factors (inadequate respiratory function, hypotension).

B. **Areas of chronic ectopic impulse formation** or **abnormal impulse conduction** (reentry), usually due to chronic ischemic heart disease with fibrosis.

C. **Acid-base and electrolyte disorders.** Acidosis and hypokalemia increase cardiac irritability; hyperkalemia can cause cardiac standstill.

D. **Trauma** (e.g., myocardial contusion).

E. **Drugs** (e.g., excess digitalis, catecholamines, antiarrhythmics, antidepressants, or tranquilizers).

F. **Congenital factors** (e.g., mitral valve prolapse).

G. **Neurogenic reflex irritability** secondary to such thoracic procedures as pneumonectomy and endoscopy.

H. **Inflammation** or **neoplasm** of the pericardium or myocardium.

III. **Specific arrhythmias: diagnosis and treatment.** Table 3-1 lists the features of the arrhythmias seen most frequently and Table 3-2 the pharmacological features of commonly used cardiac drugs.

A. **Sinus bradycardia.** The **ECG** shows a normal sinus mechanism; the heart rate is less than 60/min. This arrhythmia is common in trained athletes. Otherwise, it is due to increased vagal tone, as with increased intracranial pressure, traction on abdominal viscera or the carotid artery during operation, or general anesthesia. It is usually transient.

If persistent and associated with hypotension, **treat** with 1 mg atropine IV (the dose needed for vagal blockade is much higher than that for operative premedication). If ineffective, repeat in 3–5 min. Isoproterenol or cardiac pacing, or both, are effective but rarely necessary. Isoproterenol is best used as a continuous IV infusion (1 mg/250 ml, 5% D/W, i.e., 4 μg/ml, beginning with 10–20 micro-drops/min, i.e., approximately 1–2 μg/min).

B. **Sinus tachycardia.** The **ECG** shows a normal sinus mechanism; the heart rate is 100–180/min (up to 200 in children). This arrhythmia must be differentiated from paroxysmal atrial tachycardia with 2:1 block and concealed alternate P waves. Sinus tachycardia accompanies stress, fever, hypoxia, hypovolemia, congestive heart failure (CHF), anemia, and hyperthyroidism.

Treat the underlying cause. If tachycardia persists and CHF is absent, use propranolol, 0.5 mg IV, with increments up to 2 mg over 10–15 min; or give 10–40 mg PO qid. Digitalis is occasionally effective by its vagal action but rarely so in this setting.

C. **Sick sinus syndrome.** The **ECG** shows sinus bradycardia with sinus pauses, wandering atrial pacemaker, and atrial premature beats; at other times, atrial tachyarrhythmias, atrioventricular (AV) dissociation, and junctional escape are observed. (See cardiology texts for complete discussions of the pathophysiology of this complex syndrome.) Syncope, dizziness, or both often result from bradycardias.

Treat by insertion of a permanent ventricular pacemaker. Atrial pacing may not be effective, since AV conduction abnormalities are common. Subsequently, maintenance digitalis and propranolol may also be necessary for the arrhythmic component.

D. **Atrial premature contractions.** The **ECG** shows a normal sinus mechanism with premature P waves of variable morphology, followed by a normal QRS complex and an incomplete compensatory pause. The QRS may be deformed by aberrant conduction. Although this arrhythmia is ordinarily benign, it may presage other atrial tachyarrhythmias.

If treatment is necessary, use quinidine sulfate, 200–400 mg q6h PO or IM. Procainamide is equally effective. Give 500 mg q4h PO or IV (no more than 100 mg/min should be given). Digitalis, or propranolol, or both, may be useful.

E. **Paroxysmal atrial tachycardia (PAT)** The ECG (Fig. 3-1) shows an atrial mechanism with a **1:1 ventricular response.** The heart rate is 140–240. PAT has a sudden onset and cessation with a regular ventricular response, but atrial activity may be obscured. The arrhythmia is usually due to a reentry mechanism. The QRS complex may be distorted at rapid rates by intraventricular conduction delays (Fig. 3-1). Wide QRS tachycardia must be distinguished from ventricular tachycardia; 1:1 AV conduction, triphasic QRS complexes in a right bundle branch block pattern, normal QRS frontal axis, and QRS duration less than 0.14 sec favor the diagnosis of supraventricular tachycardia with aberration. Atypical right bundle branch block (monophasic R or biphasic qR, QR, or RS in lead V1) with left axis deviation and AV dissociation is more suggestive of ventricular

Table 3-1. Features of Common Clinical Arrhythmias

Arrhythmia	Rate Atrial	Rate Ventricular[a]	Rhythm	QRS Morphology	Carotid Sinus Pressure
Sinus tachycardia	100–180	Same	Regular	Normal[b]	Slight ↓ HR or no effect
Paroxysmal atrial tachycardia	140–240	Same	Regular	Normal[b]	Abrupt return to normal sinus rhythm or no effect
Paroxysmal atrial tachycardia with block	140–240	Same or less	Regular or irregular	Normal[b]	↑ Atrioventricular (AV) block or no effect
Atrial flutter	250–350	75–350 (150)	Regular or irregular	Normal[b]	↑ AV block
Atrial fibrillation	>375	140–160	Irregular	Normal[b]	↑ AV block
Ventricular tachycardia	—	150–250 (180)	Regular or slightly irregular	Wide	No effect

[a]Rate in parentheses is most common rate.
[b]QRS may be wide due to aberrancy. See text.

Table 3-2. Pharmacology of Commonly Used Cardiac Drugs

Drug	Loading Dose	Average Maintenance Dose	Half-Life	Blood Level	Metabolic Pathway	Side Effects and Toxicity
Digoxin	0.75–1.0 mg	0.125–0.5 mg daily	36 hr	1–2 ng/ml	Kidney	Nausea, bigeminy, atrioventricular block, paroxysmal atrial tachycardia with block
Quinidine	2–4 mg/kg IM 3–6 mg/kg PO	200–400 q6h PO	4–6 hr	4–6 mg/L	Kidney	GI symptoms, vertigo, hypotension, ventricular arrhythmias, thrombocytopenia
Procainamide	1–2 mg/kg IV 15–20 mg/kg PO	1–5 mg/min IV 250–750 mg q3–4h PO	3–4 hr	5–10 mg/L	Kidney	GI symptoms, lupus syndrome, fever, myalgia, hypotension (I.V.)
Propranolol	0.05–0.15 mg/kg IV 15–20 mg/kg PO	10–80 mg q6h	4 hr	40–85 ng/mL	Kidney	Bradycardia, heart failure, bronchospasm, GI symptoms
Disopyramide	2–3 mg/kg PO	100–200 mg q6h	4–6 hr	2–4 mg/L	Kidney	Dry mouth, urinary retention, constipation, heart failure
Phenytoin	3–10 mg/kg IV 15–30 mg/kg PO	400 mg daily	22 hr	10–25 mg/L	Liver	Hypotension or respiratory arrest (I.V.) vertigo, ataxia, rash
Lidocaine	1–2 mg/kg IV	2–4 mg/min IV	10–15 min.	1.5–5 mg/L	Liver	Seizures, paresthesias, respiratory arrest
Bretylium	4–5 mg/kg IM or IV	Same as loading dose q6–8h	6–8 hr	0.4–0.6 mg/L	Kidney	Postural hypotension, angina, premature ventricular contractions, GI symptoms

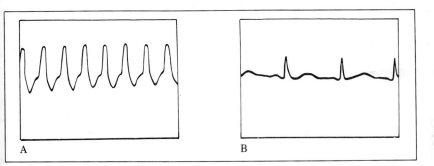

Figure 3-1. Paroxysmal atrial tachycardia (A) with aberrant conduction simulating ventricular tachycardia and (B) after conversion to sinus rhythm.

tachycardia. PAT is often found in patients with no other evidence of heart disease.

Treat in the following order: sedation (optional); carotid sinus pressure (CSP), which terminates the arrhythmia or has no effect at all; edrophonium (Tensilon), a parasympathomimetic, 10 mg IV; repeat CSP; repeat 10 mg edrophonium after 10–15 min; repeat CSP; phenylephrine, a vasopressor, 0.5–1.0 mg IV; rapid digitalization; propranolol, 0.5–2.0 mg IV by increments; cardioversion (see **IV**).

F. PAT with block. The **ECG** shows atrial tachycardia at 140–200/min, with a variable ventricular response and a prolonged P–R interval; premature ventricular contractions (PVCs) are common. P waves are often small, with a bizarre shape, and are easily confused with atrial flutter. An intra-atrial or esophageal electrode helps differentiate the two. Carotid sinus pressure may slow the ventricle and reveal P waves. The commonest cause of PAT is digitalis toxicity.

Treat by withholding digitalis, giving K+, and monitoring. Cardioversion is usually contraindicated in digitalis toxicity because it may elicit irreversible ventricular arrhythmias.

G. Atrial flutter and fibrillation. The **ECG** shows an atrial rate of 250–350/min (flutter) and 375–600/min (fibrillation). Atrial wave contours range from a regular sawtooth pattern (flutter) to virtually imperceptible contours (some cases of fibrillation). These arrhythmias are seen in rheumatic or coronary heart disease, following thoracotomy, in pericarditis (postsurgical or nonsurgical), hyperthyroidism, and pulmonary embolism. The ventricular rate varies with the degree of AV block. Rapid rates impair cardiac diastolic filling and cardiac output; loss of atrial systole has its major hemodynamic effects in patients with decreased left ventricular compliance.

1. In acute forms, unless severe hemodynamic deterioration mandates urgent electrical cardioversion, initiate **treatment** with rapid digitalization (1.5–2.0 mg digoxin in 24 hr) to increase AV block. Conversion often occurs from the vagal effects of digitalis. If it does not occur, begin quinidine sulfate, 400 mg q6h, or procainamide, 500 mg q4–6h. (Use these only after digitalization; they can increase AV conduction and the ventricular rate.) If ineffective, taper digitalis and cardiovert (see **IV**). Atrial flutter may require unusually high blood levels of digitalis, and initial electrical cardioversion may therefore be preferable. If tachycardia is a major problem and cardioversion is ineffective or undesirable, use propranolol to control the rate (0.5-mg increments IV).

2. In chronic forms, digitalis is usually needed for rate control. Conversion is often temporary unless the underlying cause is treated. Anticoagulation should be considered before conversion in patients with mitral valve disease, since

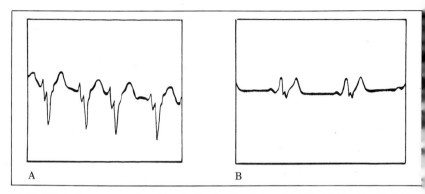

Figure 3-2. A. Irregular and rapid arrhythmia stimulates atrial fibrillation (lead V_4). B. Multiform P waves with inconsistent P-R intervals of multifocal atrial tachycardia (lead II).

atrial thrombi may embolize with restoration of atrial systole. Anticoagulation is mandatory in patients with a previous embolus.

H. Multifocal atrial tachycardia. The **ECG** shows a grossly irregular rhythm simulating atrial fibrillation; the ventricular rate is less than 100/min. P waves are visible, but with varying morphology and P–R intervals. Multiple ECG leads are often necessary to recognize the P waves (Fig. 3-2). This arrhythmia is usually seen with chronic lung disease and other hypoxic states. It rarely responds to drugs unless the hypoxic state is reversed.

I. Wolff-Parkinson-White (WPW) syndrome. The **ECG** shows a short P–R interval and a wide QRS complex, with slurred upstroke (delta wave). The symptoms are produced by paroxysmal tachycardias. An abnormal conduction pathway (Kent's bundle) between the atrium and ventricle allows circus movements to perpetuate supraventricular tachycardia with impulses traveling antegrade in the normal pathway and retrograde in Kent's bundle. Antegrade conduction through the normal conduction pathway results in normalization of the QRS complex during the tachycardia. Extremely rapid atrial rates (atrial flutter or fibrillation) may be accompanied by antegrade conduction through the bypass tract with more rapid ventricular rates than usual, since the abnormal conduction pathway lacks the conduction delay inherent in the normal pathway. Dangerously rapid ventricular rates can result (Fig. 3-3).

Treatment with digitalis and propranolol may disrupt the reentry by altering conduction in the AV node. Quinidine affects the bypass tract and is the preferable pharmacological treatment in the presence of atrial fibrillation. Digitalis is contraindicated in the presence of atrial fibrillation with WPW syndrome, since it has no effect on the abnormal pathway. Countershock is often necessary.

J. Junctional (nodal) rhythm. The **ECG** shows inverted or absent P waves. The QRS complex is regular but may be deformed by aberrant conduction. This arrhythmia occurs when the sinoatrial node is inhibited by vagal reflex, digitalis toxicity, or infarction, or when junctional automaticity is enhanced, as in inferior myocardial infarction. Specific **treatment** is rarely necessary; treat the underlying cause.

K. Ventricular extrasystoles (PVCs). The **ECG** shows premature QRS complexes of wide and abnormal configuration, with compensatory pauses. This arrhythmia is seen with ischemic heart disease, digitalis toxicity, hypokalemia, acid-base imbalance, stress, and mitral valve prolapse. Sporadic PVCs usually need no treatment.

Treat when frequent (more than six per minute), multifocal, on or near the

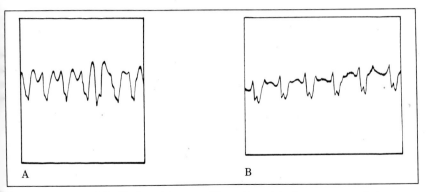

Figure 3-3. A. Atrial fibrillation with unusually rapid ventricular response and aberrancy (suspected WPW). B. Typical WPW pattern after conversion to normal sinus rhythm. Note delta wave, prolonged QRS, and short P–R interval.

wave, or in bursts of two to three or more. Lidocaine is the first choice: A 100-mg IV bolus is followed by a continuous infusion (2 gm/500 ml 5% D/W, i.e., 4 mg/ml) begun at 4 mg/min. Give an additional bolus of 100 mg in 30–40 min to maintain the blood level. If ineffective, add procainamide, 500 mg IV or PO q4h (not more than 100 mg/min or 1 gm/dose). Because of the risk of lupus syndrome with long-term procainamide therapy, quinidine, 200–400 mg q6h, is preferred for maintenance. Propranolol is occasionally useful for maintenance.

L. Ventricular tachycardia. The ECG shows abnormal QRS complexes at a rapid rate (150–250/min). The rhythm is often slightly irregular in contrast to atrial tachycardia with aberrant ventricular conduction (see **E**). The causes are the same as for PVCs. Ventricular tachycardia is an ominous rhythm that often heralds ventricular fibrillation.

Treat immediately with lidocaine as for PVCs (see **K**). Correct hypoxia and acid-base and electrolyte abnormalities. Procainamide, quinidine, disopyramide, and propranolol are useful. Immediate countershock is essential if the hemodynamic state deteriorates (see **IV**).

M. Ventricular fibrillation. The chaotic rapid sine-wave pattern seen on the **ECG** must be converted immediately by electrical countershock (see **IV**). If a defibrillator is unavailable or its arrival is delayed, a sharp blow to the precordium is effective on rare occasions. Simultaneously, give lidocaine, 100 mg IV, and consider infusion as in **K**. Correct acidosis with bicarbonate, since acidosis lowers the fibrillation threshold. For additional measures, see Chapter 4.

N. Heart block. The **ECG** shows impaired AV conduction of various degrees (see **1–3**). Heart block is caused by (1) increased vagal tone, (2) drugs that prolong AV nodal conduction (most often digitalis), or (3) injury to the AV node due to ischemia or surgery.

    1. First-degree block. The **ECG** shows a P–R interval of more than 0.2 sec. First-degree block causes no symptoms or disturbances of heart function, and no specific therapy is necessary.

    2. Second-degree block. The **ECG** shows one of three patterns:

        a. Wenckebach's phenomenon (Mobitz type I) consists of a progressive increase in the P–R interval with successive beats, until failure of conduction occurs for one beat. Conduction then resumes, and the cycle repeats.

        Since conduction delay is in the nodal region, **treat** initially with atropine. Also treat by withholding digitalis and correcting hypoxia, electrolyte and acid-base abnormalities, etc. ECG monitoring is essential.

b. **Mobitz type II block** consists of intermittent failure of impulse conduction from atrium to ventricle. Conduction delay is below the nodal region, and atropine is ineffective. Ventricular pacing is usually required.

c. **High-grade second-degree block** (2:1 or 3:1) Atropine is ineffective for the same reason as in Mobitz type II block, and ventricular pacing is usually required.

3. **Complete heart block.** The **ECG** shows complete dissociation between P waves and ventricular complexes. The idioventricular rate ranges from 30 to 60/min. Patients may be asymptomatic in the chronic phase but often are fatigued or dizzy or even have syncopal episodes (Adams-Stokes attacks) due to asystolic intervals. **Treatment** is insertion of a temporary or permanent cardiac pacemaker.

IV. Electrical cardioversion

A. **Supraventricular arrhythmias.** When indicated for specific arrhythmias (as discussed in **III**), cardioversion should be carried out with a synchronized direct-current instrument.

1. A reliable IV route must be established for drug administration, and equipment for ventilatory support must be at hand. Continuous ECG monitoring is mandatory. In the alert patient, sedation is essential. Premedication may include any common agent, such as pentobarbital, 100 mg. Amnesia and sedation are usually obtained with diazepam (Valium) IV. Increments of 5 ml are injected until the desired level of somnolence is reached.

2. For elective cardioversion of supraventricular arrhythmias, it is preferable to have one paddle posterior to the heart (i.e., just to the left of the spine) and one anterior, just to the right of the mid-sternum. If design of the available paddles prohibits this arrangement, both paddles are placed anteriorly, one on each side of the mid-sternum. Higher energies than usual may be needed with paddles placed in this way.

3. The paddles are well coated with electrode paste, the synchronizing switch is activated, and the instrument is fired. Actual discharge may be delayed for several beats until a synchronized discharge is possible. Initial energy settings are 25–50 watt-sec, with increments of 50 watt-sec as needed. If conversion occurs but is not maintained, higher energy levels have no advantage.

4. Intravenous lidocaine should be used to control ventricular irritability, and some advocate its use prophylactically (100 mg IV) before shock.

B. **Ventricular tachycardia and fibrillation** are acute, ominous arrhythmias, and the niceties of premedication, sedation, and synchronization of the shock have no place in their management. (Some cases of ventricular tachycardia may be subacute and reasonably well tolerated; these may be managed as in **A**. We refer here to the remainder.)

1. A 100-mg bolus of lidocaine is injected IV, and simultaneously, without delay for the medication, an unsynchronized shock of 100–400 watt-sec is administered, depending on the size of the patient.

2. Subsequent management has been described in **III.L** and **M** and includes rapid reversal of inciting causes, such as hypoxia, acidosis, and hypokalemia. A continuous lidocaine infusion should be initiated to prevent recurrence.

3. If frequent countershocks become necessary, reduced energy settings should be tried, since they may prove adequate and will be less traumatic.

Suggested Reading

Bigger, J. T.   Arrhythmias and antiarrhythmic drugs. *Adv. Intern. Med.* 18:251 1972.

Collinsworth, K. A., Kalman, S. M., and Harrison, D. C.   The clinical pharmacology of lidocaine as an antiarrhythmic drug. *Circulation* 50:1217, 1974.

Wellens H. J. J., Bar F., and Lie K. I.   The value of the electrocardiogram in the differential diagnosis of a tachycardia with a widened QRS complex. *Am. J. Med.* 64:27, 1978.

Winkle R. A., Glantz S. A., and Harrison D. C.   Pharmacologic therapy of ventricular arrhythmias. *Am. J. Cardiol.* 36:629, 1975.

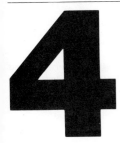

Cardiac Arrest

I. **Definition and general comments.** Cardiorespiratory arrest is the sudden cessation of effective circulation and respiration. In effect, there is failure of oxygenation (respiratory) and the transport system (circulation) that delivers oxygen to the peripheral tissues. Either one may be the primary event, but failure of the other quickly follows, and both must be restored for survival. In the interval between these events and the onset of irreversible cellular death, resuscitation may be performed with minimal sequelae. The extent of irreversible injury depends on the degree of preexisting cellular hypoxia; the brain, being almost totally dependent on aerobic metabolism, is the organ least able to withstand hypoxia. Following circulatory arrest, the pupils begin to dilate in 30–40 sec, respiration ceases within 60 sec because of medullary depression, and in the normothermic adult, serious brain damage may ensue within 3–5 min. If respiratory failure occurs first, the circulation may continue for a short period, with diminishing effect as hypoxic acidosis rapidly depresses myocardial contractility.

A. **Cardiac arrest** may be manifested as:

1. **Mechanical asystole,** which accounts for 80% of cardiac arrests occurring in the operating and recovery rooms and is usually related to inadequate ventilation.

2. **Ventricular fibrillation,** which accounts for 75% of cardiac arrests in intensive care units and is the most common form of arrest following myocardial infarction.

3. **Ineffective ventricular contraction,** which produces an inadequate cardiac output and may be caused by situations depressing contractility, e.g., acidosis, hypoxemia, drugs, arrhythmias, and acute coronary insufficiency.

B. **Respiratory arrest** may be manifested as:

1. **Cessation of effective mechanical breathing.**

2. **Ineffective gas exchange.**

II. **Etiology.** The mechanisms of sudden cardiac and respiratory arrest are multiple, complex, and interrelated.

A. **Usual causes of respiratory arrest**

1. Airway obstruction by a foreign body or by vomitus, blood, mucus, or laryngeal or bronchial spasm.

2. Central nervous system depression found in head trauma, stroke, hypercapnia, or overdosage of a barbiturate, narcotic, tranquilizer, or anesthetic agent.

3. Neuromuscular failure secondary to poliomyelitis, muscular dystrophy, myasthenia, or curarelike drug overdosage.

B. **Usual causes of either cardiac or respiratory arrest**

1. Flail chest.

2. Pneumothorax.

   3. Massive atelectasis.

   4. Acute pulmonary embolization.

   5. Alveolar-capillary block from congestive heart failure, overwhelming pneumonia, lung burn, gram-negative septicemia, or heavy metal poisoning.

   6. Carbon monoxide poisoning.

   All these causes result in ineffective gas exchange.

C. Usual causes of cardiac arrest

   1. Cardiogenic shock secondary to decreased coronary perfusion or congestive heart failure.

   2. Hypercapnia leading to respiratory acidosis, resulting in a depression in contractility.

   3. Hyperkalemia following anuria or excessive potassium replacement therapy in the presence of an oliguric state.

   4. Direct stimulation of the heart by an intracardiac catheter or electrode or during operative displacement or manipulation of the heart, usually resulting in ventricular fibrillation.

   5. Coronary occlusion by embolus, thrombus, or ligature, air bubbles, or contrast substances.

   6. Drug sensitivity or overdosage with cardiac glycosides, inotropic agents, anesthetic agents, and beta blockers.

   7. Hypothermia from exposure or rapid transfusion of large volumes of cold banked blood.

   8. Severe metabolic acidosis secondary to diabetes mellitus, inadequate extracorporeal circulation, pancreatic fistula, renal failure, or starvation.

   9. Electric shock.

   10. Hypocalcemia or hypercalcemia.

III. Diagnosis

A. Early signs

   1. Central nervous system. Restlessness, anxiety, disorientation, and combativeness. A previously cooperative patient who becomes difficult to manage postoperatively is much more likely to be hypoxemic than psychotic.

   2. Respiratory. Dyspnea, tachypnea, gasping, gurgling, laryngeal stridor, wheezing, pallor, and cyanosis.

   3. Cardiovascular. Mottling, cyanosis, peripheral venous distention, weak or irregular pulse, hypotension, and profuse sweating.

B. Late signs indicating that cardiorespiratory arrest is present include:

   1. Absence of a pulse in major arteries.

   2. Absence of audible or visible breathing or the presence of gasping respirations.

   3. Dilation of the pupils seen 1–2 min after complete arrest, indicating the beginning of anoxic damage to the brain.

   4. Sluggish, dark-colored bleeding at operative site.

   5. Flaccidity.

   6. Convulsions.

IV. Treatment. The aims of treatment are the earliest possible restoration of effective circulation and recognition and correction of the cause of the arrest. **Resuscitation**

alone is not sufficient. The grave threat of recurrent arrest can be averted only by correcting the physiological derangements that precipitated arrest and by appreciating and correcting the damage caused by the arrest itself.

A. During the resuscitative attempt, the patient is in a state of partially controlled shock, creating the situation for the following **functional derangements:**

  1. Ventilation-perfusion relationships may be altered by the creation of functional arteriovenous shunts that result in hypoxia despite ventilation with pure oxygen.

  2. Increased physiological dead-space may produce hypercapnia.

  3. Depressed cardiac output may reduce peripheral arterial flow by a factor of 30–50%.

  4. Tricuspid and mitral regurgitation may result from cardiac compression.

  5. Severe and progressive metabolic acidosis causes peripheral vasodilation, pooling of blood, and further impairment of circulation.

B. Steps in cardiorespiratory resuscitation. See Figure 4-1.

  1. Airway. Establishing a **patent airway** is the first most important step in successful resuscitation. Put one hand under the back of the shoulders and lift the head and neck slightly upward, thus hyperextending the head. Next, shift the tongue forward to open the airway by lifting the vertical rami of the mandible and visually inspect the airway. Foreign material in the mouth or pharynx may be manually removed and is often a cause of respiratory arrest in the feeble elderly patient.

  2. Breathing

   a. Adequate ventilation of the lungs is the crucial prerequisite to cardiac massage. If the patient does not spontaneously begin to breathe as the airway is opened, mouth-to-mouth ventilation is begun immediately.

   (1) Cover the patient's mouth tightly with your own and pinch the nose. Take a deep breath and blow until the patient's chest rises. Remove your mouth and allow passive expiration to occur. Repeat 12 times/min. The patient's chest must rise, the lungs must produce resistance as they inflate, and air must be felt to escape during expiration; otherwise, ventilation is not adequate. The exhaled air of the rescuer, who doubles his or her own ventilation, is about 18% oxygen and 2% carbon dioxide, an adequate composition for resuscitation.

   (2) In infants and children, both the nose and mouth can be covered by the resuscitator's mouth; care must be taken not to overinflate the lungs. The lungs are inflated 20–30 times/min in infants.

   b. A portable self-filling, nonrebreathing bag and tight-fitting mask, together with an oral airway, may be used as soon as they are available. Tracheal intubation minimizes the danger of regurgitation and aspiration but should not be attempted except by a skilled person and then not until the patient is well oxygenated by external ventilation.

  3. Cardiac resuscitation

   a. After four or five effective lung inflations, feel for the carotid pulse. If it is absent, place the patient on the floor unless a bed board is immediately at hand. Strike the sternum sharply with the fist; this may stimulate the heart to beat, especially in cardiac asystole. If a carotid pulse is not felt, begin external cardiac compression. Even in the operating room, external compression should be tried before thoracotomy is considered. Apply pressure with the heel of one hand covered by the second hand over the lower fourth of the sternum in the midline. Do not apply pressure over the xiphoid, since

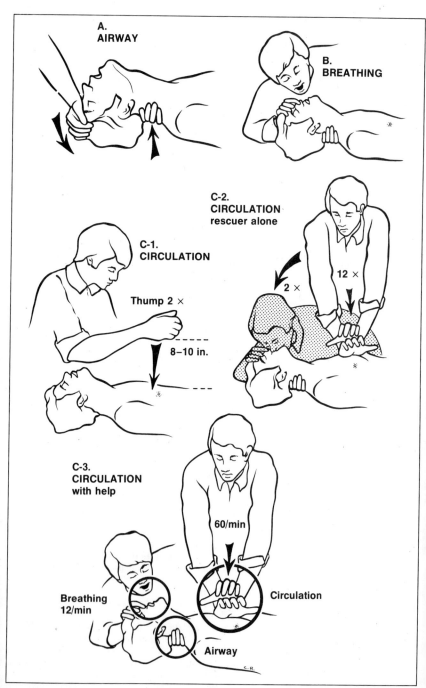

Figure 4-1. The essential steps in cardiopulmonary resuscitation are to establish an airway (A), restore breathing (B), and restore circulation (C-1–C-3).

laceration of the liver may result. Do not touch the chest wall with the fingers. Hold the elbows straight to minimize fatigue. Lean the weight of your torso toward the patient until the sternum in the adult is compressed 1.5–2.0 in.; extra pressure does not produce greater blood flow and may fracture the sternum. Compression time of 0.5 sec is followed by sudden release for an interval of 1 sec, accomplished by shifting your weight backward. Release of pressure should be complete, but the hands should remain in position in contact with the lower fourth of the sternum, lest the hands shift and the ribs or underlying viscera be injured. Compression should be at the rate of 60/min and should never be interrupted for more than 5 sec.

b. **In small children,** only the heel of one hand is used. **In infants,** encircle the chest with both hands and exert midsternal pressure with the thumbs; compression rate should be 100/min and displacement only ½–¾ in.

c. **In children and adults,** if only one rescuer is available, he or she should ventilate the patient twice, then compress the sternum 12 times at the rate of once per second. Carotid pulses should be checked repeatedly. The pupils are an effective means of judging results. Maintenance of pupillary constriction, following previous dilation, is evidence that oxygenated blood is reaching the brain.

4. Restoration of function and metabolic control

a. Start an IV infusion, preferably in a large vein, using an IV catheter.

b. For obese patients, or if the person performing external massage is of slight build, straddling the patient aids in effective sternal compression.

c. Inject sodium bicarbonate ($NaHCO_3$, 2 mEq/kg) and obtain arterial blood gas and pH values to guide further treatment.

d. Begin electrocardiographic monitoring; placement of lead II is sufficient.

e. If the electrocardiogram shows fibrillation, initiate external defibrillation. Apply two electrodes firmly on the chest wall. Start with an external direct-current stimulus of 200 watt-sec in an adult; if ineffective, progress to 400 watt-sec. If unsuccessful, resume massage and:

(1) Compress the chest several times immediately after defibrillation to prevent overdistention of the heart.

(2) Improve myocardial oxygenation by improving ventilation by endotracheal intubation.

(3) Warm the patient with hot water bags, heating pads, or a hyperthermia blanket if body temperature is below 34°C (93.2°F).

(4) Give intracardiac epinephrine, 1–2 ml of a 1 : 1000 solution diluted in 10 ml saline. If this fails, give intracardiac calcium chloride, 100–200 mg.

(5) Repeat $NaHCO_3$ administration unless the pH is normal. If irritable foci are present, administer lidocaine, 50 mg. Inotropic agents may not function in the presence of acidosis.

(6) Repeat defibrillation shocks after each therapeutic maneuver.

f. When fibrillation ceases or is converted, and the heart is beating too slowly or hypotension is present:

(1) Administer an IV infusion of epinephrine, 4 ml in 250 ml.

(2) Give atropine, 0.4–0.6 mg IV, for marked bradycardia with supraventricular rhythm. If effective repeat in 15 min.

(3) Give isoproterenol HCl (1 mg in 250 ml 5% D/W by IV infusion) to control bradycardia resulting from heart block. The rate of infusion is determined by the patient's response.

(4) Start external cardiac pacing by transvenous (cephalic or external jugular), transthoracic myocardial, or epicardial electrodes if complete or progressive heart block is present or if there is refractory bradycardia or myocardial irritability.

5. Closed or open cardiac resuscitation. External cardiac compression with a closed chest offers the best chance of successful resuscitation, even if the arrest occurs in the operating room. The following are the rare indications for open resuscitation:

a. The cause of arrest is within the chest, e.g., cardiac tamponade or a stab wound of the heart.

b. Only an internal defibrillator is available.

c. The chest is already open in the course of a thoracic operation.

d. There is tension pneumothorax or a flail chest.

e. The patient is very obese or barrel chested, so that external cardiac compression is ineffective.

f. The patient has undergone recent open-heart surgery.

V. Care following resuscitation. The underlying conditions leading to the cardiorespiratory arrest must be corrected or arrest will recur.

A. Transfer the patient immediately to an intensive care unit.

B. Maintain adequate ventilation. Use a mechanical respirator if necessary.

C. Monitor arterial pressure and the ECG constantly. If cardiogenic shock is present, pulmonary artery wedge pressure should be measured and use of an intra-aortic balloon-assist device should be considered.

D. Determine arterial blood gases, pH values, and serum electrolytes frequently to permit maintenance of normal values.

E. Use pharmacological agents, i.e., inotropic drugs, vasopressors, antiarrhythmic drugs, and diuretics, as indicated.

F. Corticosteroids given IV may be of assistance in reducing cerebral edema.

G. Anticipate subsequent episodes of arrest.

H. Look for trauma associated with arrest:

1. Pneumothorax.

2. Fractured ribs.

3. Hepatic and splenic injuries.

4. Intrathoracic or abdominal hemorrhage.

VI. Summary

A. Despite philosophical discussions of selection of patients for resuscitation, most surgical patients can be saved and deserve an all-out effort.

B. Confirm the diagnosis (apnea, pulselessness). Resuscitatory efforts starting 5 min or longer after the cardiac arrest are doomed to fail.

Suggested Reading

American Heart Association and National Academy of Sciences. National Research Council standards for cardiopulmonary resuscitation (CPR) and emergency cardiac care (ECC). *J.A.M.A.* 227 [Suppl. Feb. 18]:1, 1974.

Goldberg, A. H. Current concepts: Cardiopulmonary arrest. *N. Engl. J. Med.* 290:381, 1974.

Levitsky, S. New insights in cardiac trauma. *Surg. Clin. North Am.* 55:43, 1975.

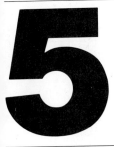

Acute Abdominal Pain

Pain, along with hemorrhage, represents a catastrophe of major proportions. Abdominal pain is among the most frightening of all, since the connotation to the patient experiencing it encompasses the entire gamut of catastrophes. Abdominal pain is the most common presenting complaint in patients with acute surgical disease of the abdomen (Table 5-1). It is incumbent on the surgeon first to decide what is the most likely diagnosis; second, to prove that diagnosis correct; and third, to undertake the specific treatment indicated for that diagnosis. In the course of investigating a patient with abdominal pain, it is extremely important that no analgesics or sedatives capable of masking the clinical findings be given until a decision is made as to the appropriate working diagnosis or until operation is obviously indicated.

I. **The history.** In acute surgical disease, perhaps more than in any other area of medicine, the history assumes overwhelming importance. The primary points that assist in making a diagnosis are:

A. **Localization of pain.** Certain viscera provide reasonably good localization of the pain they generate, whereas others afford little information in this regard. The stomach and duodenum, for example, reliably exhibit localized pain in the vicinity of the epigastrium, either to the right or the left of the midline. The pain in pancreatitis similarly is localized reasonably well in the upper abdomen (Table 5-2). The appendix classically causes pain in the right lower quadrant. The fallopian tube and ovary yield pain to the right or the left of the suprapubic area. Other organs, such as the small intestine, have poor pain localization; the pain may be perceived anywhere in the abdomen, although periumbilical pain is most common.

B. **Radiation and referral of pain.** Although a great deal is written about the diagnostic value of pain radiation, it may not be helpful and can be confusing. Biliary tract pain traditionally radiates around the right side of the back to the angle of the scapula, whereas pain of pancreatic origin commonly radiates directly through to the back. Appendiceal pain, for an entirely different reason, occasionally commences in the epigastrium and ultimately migrates to the right lower quadrant. Pain referred to remote areas can be highly suggestive of specific organ involvement, e.g., perihepatic inflammation referred to the right shoulder, and uterine and rectal disease to the low back.

C. **Quality of pain.** Acute abdominal pain is characterized in one of two ways: It is more or less **constant**, or it is **cramping (colicky).**

1. **Constant abdominal pain** frequently waxes and wanes, but is neither rhythmical nor cyclical and does not appear in successive waves, as is the case with abdominal cramps. Constant abdominal pain is usually caused by inflammatory or neoplastic involvement of a solid viscus.

2. **Cramping abdominal pain** is almost always caused by obstruction of a hollow viscus (e.g., intestinal obstruction, ureteral calculus, dysmenorrhea [blood clot obstructing the cervical os]) or by increased intraluminal pressure in a hollow viscus without obstruction (e.g., subsiding ileus after operation, or enteritis with hyperperistalsis and increased intraluminal fluid volume). Early arterial

Table 5-1. Differential Diagnosis of Acute Abdominal Pain by Location

Right upper quadrant
  Acute cholecystitis
  Perforated duodenal ulcer (forme fruste)
  Acute pancreatitis (bilateral pain)
  Acute hepatitis
  Acute congestive hepatomegaly
  Pneumonia with pleural reaction
  Acute pyelonephritis
  Angina pectoris
  Acute hepatitis
  Hepatic abscess

Left upper quadrant
  Ruptured spleen
  Perforated gastric or marginal ulcer
  Acute pancreatitis (bilateral pain)
  Ruptured aortic aneurysm
  Perforated colon (tumor, foreign body)
  Pneumonia with pleural reaction
  Acute pyelonephritis
  Acute myocardial infarction

Central (periumbilical)
  Intestinal obstruction
  Appendicitis
  Acute pancreatitis
  Mesenteric thrombosis
  Strangulated groin hernia
  Dissecting or rupturing aortic aneurysm
  Diverticulitis (small intestine or colon)
  Uremia

Right lower quadrant
  Appendicitis
  Acute salpingitis, tubo-ovarian abscess
  Ruptured ectopic pregnancy
  Twisted ovarian cyst
  Mesenteric adenitis
  Incarcerated, strangulated groin hernia
  Meckel's diverticulitis
  Cecal diverticulitis
  Regional ileitis
  Perforated cecum (tumor, foreign body)
  Psoas abscess
  Ureteral calculus

Left lower quadrant
  Sigmoid diverticulitis
  Acute salpingitis, tubo-ovarian abscess
  Ruptured ectopic pregnancy
  Twisted ovarian cyst
  Incarcerated, strangulated groin hernia
  Perforated descending colon (tumor, foreign body)
  Regional ileitis
  Psoas abscess
  Ureteral calculus

Table 5-2. Differential Diagnosis of Severe Epigastric Pain

Diagnostic Features	Perforated Peptic Ulcer	Acute Pancreatitis	Acute Cholecystitis
Onset	Sudden, sharp	Gradual	Gradual
Location	Epigastric → generalized rapidly	Epigastric → slowly spreading	Right upper quadrant only (early)
Radiation	Diffuse	Through to back	Around to back and angle of scapula
Vomiting	Absent to few times	Multiple episodes, persistent	Few to many times
Alcoholic intake	Variable	Usually heavy preceding attack	Occasional, not heavy
Previous attacks	Ulcer history (45%)	Frequently similar to current episode	Frequently similar to current episode
Dietary intolerance	Spices, alcohol	Fatty foods	Fatty foods, cabbage
Shock, prostration	Common early	Seen late	Unusual
Tenderness	Diffuse	Epigastric → diffuse	Right upper quadrant
Rebound tenderness	Early (first 4 hr)	Late (after 24 hr)	Rare
Rigidity	Boardlike	Moderate to severe	Unilateral rectus guarding
Peristaltic sounds	Absent	Hypoactive	Normal to hypoactive
Costovertebral angle tenderness	Bilateral	Left-sided	Right-sided
Position	Flat (supine)	Lying on side, hips flexed	Flat (supine) or on side
X-ray	Free air (70%), ileus	Ileus, sentinel loop, colon cutoff sign	Ileus, calculus in right upper quadrant (10%)
		Sonogram (B-mode) positive for pancreatic mass	Sonogram positive for stones in gallbladder
Laboratory	Moderate amylase elevation, elevated hematocrit, high leukocyte count	Marked amylase elevation, modest hematocrit elevation, low calcium and magnesium (after 5 days), glycosuria	Minimal amylase elevation, moderate rise in leukocyte count

insufficiency of the superior mesenteric artery may present with severe cramping pain, especially following ingestion of food or fluid. The pain becomes constant when progression to gangrene occurs.

D. Duration of pain. The duration of abdominal pain is of great significance. Acute appendicitis will not persist as a local process for more than 72–96 hr; acute cholecystitis may not persist for more than 36–48 hr before a complication ensues. As a rule, inflammation that is acute remains so for only 5 days or less. In contradistinction, regional enteritis may cause abdominal pain for several weeks, a neoplasm of the intestinal tract may cause pain for weeks or months, and metabolic disease (e.g., diabetes mellitus, porphyria) may cause abdominal pain in recurrent attacks over long periods of time.

E. Intensity of pain. Although not invariably the case, the most acute surgical entities usually cause the most intense or severe pain. A perforated peptic ulcer characteristically causes very severe pain resulting from the highly irritating nature of duodenal and gastric contents. On the other hand, the pain of acute pancreatitis is a result of retroperitoneal and intraperitoneal dissemination of enzyme-laden fluid that does not cause pain of as great intensity as is experienced in perforated ulcer. Colon perforation (diverticulitis, perforated carcinoma, trauma) is also marked by pain of moderate intensity at first, but the amount of pain increases with time until the findings become similar to those in perforated ulcer.

F. Nature of onset of pain. Some surgical diseases are characterized by a very sudden and abrupt onset, such as acute perforation of a hollow viscus (stomach, duodenum). The patient frequently likens this to being struck a severe blow. In patients with intestinal obstruction, appendicitis, or diverticulitis, the pain is much more likely to be gradual in onset. One can often differentiate the pain of pancreatitis, with its gradual onset, from the pain of perforated peptic ulcer, with its sudden, abrupt onset, by questioning the patient about the manner in which pain began.

G. Associated vomiting. In some diseases, vomiting is frequent and persistent, whereas in others it is infrequent or absent. Frequent vomiting at the onset of symptoms is seen in patients with irritation or inflammation of the pancreas and biliary tract. It is extremely unusual to observe patients with acute pancreatitis without vomiting, and it is relatively uncommon to see acute cholecystitis with no vomiting whatsoever. Among patients with intestinal obstruction and distention, those with colon obstruction are less likely to vomit. In patients with high small-intestine obstruction, vomiting is persistent and characteristic of the lesions causing the obstruction (e.g., carcinoma of the pancreas, stenosing duodenal ulcer). The character of the vomitus is of little help unless no bile is observed, suggesting a preampullary lesion, or, unless the vomitus is feculent in appearance and odor, indicating distal intestinal obstruction.

H. Other diagnostic points

1. The **age** of the patient is of considerable importance, since certain diseases are largely limited to certain age groups. Appendicitis is generally a disease of patients between 5 and 50 yr; intussusception is seen primarily under the age of 2; cholecystitis is unusual under the age of 20; and colon obstruction is uncommon under the age of 35.

2. The **position** the patient assumes to obtain relief from pain can also be extremely helpful in diagnosis. The victim of pancreatitis characteristically lies on his left side with the vertebral column, knees, and hips flexed. This position relaxes the psoas muscle, which is irritated and in spasm because of retroperitoneal inflammation. Patients with retrocecal appendicitis occasionally flex the right hip and knee to relax the right psoas muscle. The patient with diffuse peritonitis of any origin commonly prefers to lie in bed in an immobile

state; motion or position change is resisted because of the exquisite pain occasioned by movement of the parietal peritoneum.

3. Certain **drugs** are associated with acute surgical diseases. For example, if the patient is known to have been on corticosteroids, perforation of a peptic ulcer is likely; the chronic use of salicylates or other antirheumatic agents would lead to the same conclusion. A history of antacid ingestion suggests esophagitis, ulcer, or biliary-pancreatic disease. If the patient has ever used potassium chloride in tablet form, ulceration and subsequent stenosis of the small intestine may occur, with the acute abdominal pain based on intestinal obstruction due to a stricture.

4. It is helpful to know whether the patient has taken any **medication to relieve pain.** Vomiting (frequently digitally induced) that produces relief from pain is indicative of ulcer or high obstruction. Relief from pain with passage of flatus or after an enema could indicate incomplete left colon obstruction.

5. The **previous medical history** is of considerable importance. A history of similar episodes of pain in the past, and the diagnosis attached to such episodes, can be illuminating. Patients with acute appendicitis have had previous attacks in approximately 35% of instances. A history of perforation of a viscus, as with acute diverticulitis, can clarify the cause of left lower quadrant pain. In addition, the gynecological history in the female, specifically including the use of contraceptives, time of last menstrual period, nature of the last menstrual period, and potential exposure to communicable venereal disease may be essential information. A reasonably comprehensive gastrointestinal and urinary tract history in both male and female patients can shed considerable light on abdominal pain.

II. **The physical examination.** A careful physical examination is absolutely essential in the intelligent evaluation of a patient with acute abdominal pain. Thoroughness and a systematic approach are important; errors of omission far outnumber errors of commission. An examination pattern rigidly adhered to will pay handsome dividends in these patients.

A. **General considerations, vital signs**

1. The **appearance** of the patient will frequently give some general clues as to the severity of the illness. The detection of pallor, cyanosis, or simply facial features contorted by pain supports the supposition that a grave abdominal catastrophe has occurred.

2. **Tachycardia** is common in patients with profound illnesses, such as ruptured viscus, gangrenous intestinal obstruction, or diffuse peritonitis. The initial pulse rate has less value than serial observation of this sign. An unexplained rising pulse rate in a patient undergoing active but nonoperative treatment for acute abdominal pain is an ominous sign and usually means that an operation is required.

3. **Tachypnea** has somewhat the same connotation as tachycardia, although very rapid respiratory rates are observed in patients with peritonitis from pancreatitis, hemorrhagic shock, and similar lesions. The value of the respiratory rate as a physical finding is largely comparative; a respiratory rate that increases under management is alarming and may herald the need for an operation.

4. **Fever** is common in patients with acute abdominal disease, although the temperature is likely to be normal or only slightly elevated early in the course of the disease. It is essential that the temperature in patients on surgical services be obtained rectally. The initial temperature is not as valuable as the constant observation of this sign during the course of expectant management. As a rule, the temperature in patients with acute appendicitis, uncomplicated intestinal

obstruction, ruptured ectopic pregnancy, and other acute surgical emergencies is close to normal; the initial rectal temperature will rarely exceed 38.3°C (101°F). When perforation occurs or intestinal gangrene supervenes, the temperature will increase to 39.4–40.0°C (103–104°F) but will then fall if shock ensues. With an initial temperature over 39.4°C (103°F) it is far more likely that pulmonary or urinary tract infection rather than an intra-abdominal process is the cause of the fever. A temperature over 40.0°C (104°F) at any time means abscess, fulminant systemic infection, or infection involving the central nervous system, lung, or urinary tract.

B. Examination of the abdomen. The astute physical diagnostician is made, not born. Meticulous attention to small details will frequently spell the difference between diagnostic success and failure. The principles to be emphasized include the following:

1. **Always examine the area remote from the site of maximal pain first.** It is important to examine both sides of the abdomen with both hands; the examiner's right hand examines the left side of the patient's abdomen; his or her left hand examines the right side of the patient's abdomen. The assessment of rigidity can be enhanced by placing a pillow under the patient's knees and having the patient breathe gently, but deeply, through the mouth. The finding of unilateral rectus spasm is indicative of an acute inflammatory process beneath that rectus muscle, since the patient is unable voluntarily to contract one rectus to a greater degree than the other.

2. **True rigidity or intense bilateral guarding is suggestive of diffuse peritonitis.** This impression can be substantiated by the finding of rebound tenderness, in which gentle manual pressure elicits somewhat less tenderness than the sudden release of that pressure. It is important not to cause excessive or intense pain by injudicious eliciting of tenderness or rebound tenderness. Only one examiner should attempt to detect this finding. As a rule, such a finding requires operative treatment.

3. **Cutaneous hyperesthesia** can be demonstrated by stroking the skin with the fingernail or a needle. The patient is requested to tell the examiner if any area of skin stroking causes pain; this will indicate the spinal segment innervating the area of parietal peritoneum irritated by the acute inflammatory disease.

4. **Palpation of solid viscera** is important, but rarely diagnostic. Of greater value is the finding of referred tenderness, in which pressure at a distance from the inflamed viscus will cause acute tenderness over that viscus (Rovsing's sign in acute appendicitis). This suggests parietal peritoneal involvement by an inflammatory lesion. Also of importance is the physical finding of iliopsoas spasm (psoas sign), reflected in persistent flexion of the hip or by severe pain on passive hyperextension of the hip with the patient lying on the contralateral side, suggesting an inflammatory retroperitoneal lesion on the affected side. The psoas sign is seen, on the right side, in acute retrocecal appendicitis, in perinephric abscess, and in posterior perforation of a cecal carcinoma. Left-sided psoas spasm can be observed with perinephric abscess, perforated sigmoid diverticulitis, and perforated sigmoid carcinoma.

5. Of considerable importance is the assessment of the **frequency of peristaltic sounds.** In patients with diffuse peritonitis or intense localized inflammatory disease, the bowel sounds disappear or become markedly hypoactive. Normal activity in the fasting state is 10–20 sounds/min. With localized peritonitis, such as in appendicitis or diverticulitis, the intestinal sounds are somewhat hypoactive, but they usually are present. The bowel sounds are hyperactive in diffuse inflammatory disease of the intestinal tract, early intestinal obstruction, or subsiding paralytic ileus. It must be remembered that an acute inflammatory process anywhere in the body, severe metabolic disease (diabetic coma, uremia), or acute trauma can cause moderate to severe ileus with nearly total (but rarely complete) loss of peristaltic sounds.

6. The **pitch of intestinal peristaltic sounds** is difficult to describe and can only be learned by repeated auscultation of the abdomen. It is imperative that the house officer and student auscultate the abdomen with the same care with which auscultation of the chest is practiced. The pitch of bowel sounds is dependent on the tension of the wall of the intestinal tract and the length of the air-fluid interface in that particular section of intestine. Just as the pitch of a drum is raised by increasing the tension of the drum head, so the pitch of bowel sounds is raised by increased intraluminal tension. As paralytic ileus subsides, the large amount of air and fluid that has accumulated during the period of intestinal inactivity is subjected to ever-increasing pressure by the contracting smooth muscle; this situation is identical to that existing early in a mechanical intestinal obstruction while active peristalsis proximal to the obstruction continues. High-pitched bowel sounds are not always indicative of intestinal obstruction unless the other three prime findings of intestinal obstruction—distention, cramping abdominal pain, and obstipation—are observed.

7. **Abdominal distention** is best assessed by measuring the abdominal girth at the umbilicus and by viewing the lateral contour of the anterior surface of the abdomen in relation to an imaginary line between the symphysis pubis and the xiphoid. In patients without distention, the anterior abdominal border usually will be observed to lie below the xiphopubic line. When the patient lies flat in bed, the normal abdominal contour is scaphoid or flat even in the very obese patient. When the abdomen is moderately distended, lateral inspection will demonstrate the abdominal wall to be at or slightly above the xiphopubic line. As distention increases, the abdominal contour becomes grossly rounded, accompanied by increased tension of the abdominal wall and tightness of the skin.

8. In addition to determining the presence of distention, the examiner must decide whether the distention is gaseous or fluid by careful **percussion** of the abdomen. Distinguishing ascites from ileus or obstruction is a matter of determining the percussion note as well as the presence or absence of **shifting dullness.** The presence of fluid, with its dull note, may signify carcinomatous ascites, portal hypertension, congestive heart failure, hemoperitoneum, or inflammatory ascites. With tympany to percussion, the presence of mechanical or paralytic ileus is apparent; massive pneumoperitoneum will also produce this finding.

C. Rectovaginal examination

1. The rectovaginal (pelvic) examination is frequently done in a cursory fashion or is not attempted at all. This omission can be disastrous in the assessment of patients with acute abdominal pain. The **lower third of the abdomen** is hidden in the lower false and true pelvis by bone and soft tissue and **can be evaluated only by digital rectal or rectovaginal examination.** The presence of a pelvic abscess will be detected by finding severe tenderness and cul-de-sac fullness on digital examination. Fullness may be apparent in intestinal obstruction or paralytic ileus when it is caused by markedly distended and edematous loops of intestine impinging on pelvic structures.

2. Of great importance is the finding of a **unilateral mass or extreme tenderness on one side** of the pelvis, most frequently suggesting appendicitis or appendiceal abscess on the right or tubo-ovarian abscess on the left. It can be difficult to distinguish right-sided tubo-ovarian disease from appendiceal inflammatory disease, but **tenderness on manipulation of the cervix** will be extreme in patients with pelvic inflammatory disease. Ovarian cysts may cause severe abdominal pain and present as a unilateral mass ballotable between the vaginal examining fingers and the hand placed on the abdominal wall. This **bimanual examination** is helpful in delineating masses in the uterus, fallopian tubes, or ovaries. It should be remembered that rectal or rectovaginal examination is relatively unsatisfactory unless the bladder is empty; furthermore, the

simplest approach to cul-de-sac disease from a diagnostic standpoint is the rectovaginal route (digital examination, colpocentesis, culdoscopy). The use of the cervical smear to detect gonococcal disease of the genital tract is not particularly rewarding. Finding intracellular gram-negative diplococci is difficult and infrequent.

The patient should have been questioned about the use of an intrauterine device. These devices can be detected on physical examination by finding in the cervix a "tail" or bit of material used to retrieve them. In the presence of lower abdominal tenderness and an intrauterine contraceptive device, the frequency with which uterine infection and subsequent tubo-ovarian disease are seen is considerable. When the intrauterine device appears to be at fault, it should be removed, following appropriate consultation with the patient's gynecologist, in order to eradicate the possible infectious source. On the other hand, in the male patient, acute or chronic prostatic inflammation can be detected readily by the bogginess, extreme tenderness, and enlargement of the prostate on rectal examination.

3. If possible, the **female patient** should be examined on a firm table during this part of the evaluation. If the patient is too ill to be moved from her bed, a board or serving tray covered with a bath towel and placed under the sacrum will provide a firm surface for a reasonably satisfactory rectovaginal examination in bed. Little or nothing will be learned if the patient is examined on her side, since it is impossible to utilize bimanual examination, a key part of this examination, in this position. Twisted ovarian cysts, pedunculated uterine myomas, presacral tumors, and other ballotable or fixed pelvic masses are much easier to detect by bimanual examination.

III. Laboratory tests. The laboratory provides little help in the differential diagnosis of acute abdominal pain. Routine tests, such as a complete blood count, urinalysis with microscopic examination, blood urea nitrogen, creatinine, blood sugar, and serology, are usually done on admission.

A. Urinalysis. The presence of proteinuria and the finding of erythrocytes or leukocytes in the urine on a clean or catheterized specimen can be significant; pyonephrosis, perinephric abscess, retrocecal appendicitis, or retroperitoneal abscess from rupture of the duodenum, colon, or rectum can lead to these findings. Pancreatitis characteristically causes slight proteinuria (trace to 1+) because of the secondary inflammation induced by the proximity of the tail of the pancreas to the left kidney.

B. The leukocyte count and the differential count have no specific diagnostic significance except in children; the finding of leukopenia with lower abdominal pain is suggestive of acute viral infection (e.g., measles) rather than acute appendicitis. Patients with mesenteric adenitis as the cause of abdominal pain usually exhibit a leukocyte count between 6000 and 16,000, exactly the same range as in acute appendicitis. A shift of the differential count to the left suggests an acute inflammatory disease or abscess but does little to differentiate surgical from nonsurgical inflammatory conditions. Serial leukocyte counts in a patient with obscure or variable findings may be helpful in that a rising leukocyte count may be an indication for operation.

C. Serum, urine amylase. Obtaining amylase or lipase values (amylase is preferred because of the greater ease with which the test is performed) in patients with acute abdominal disease can provide evidence that the patient has acute pancreatitis. Levels over 400 Somogyi units/100 ml serum or over 700 Somogyi units in the urine are definitely suggestive of acute pancreatitis. Values over 700 Somogyi units in the serum and over 1200 Somogyi units in a single urine specimen are diagnostic of acute pancreatitis. Amylase also may be elevated in a number of acute abdominal diseases (e.g., intestinal obstruction, perforated peptic ulcer, mesenteric thrombosis) and following the administration of drugs such as morphine sulfate. However, the level does not approach the diagnostic values previously indicated for pancreatitis. On the other hand, it must be remembered that acute pancreatitis may occur with normal or minimally elevated amylase levels (see Table 5-2).

There has been a rash of enthusiasm for the diagnostic use of the ratio of the clearance of amylase to the clearance of creatinine; a ratio exceeding 5% is highly suggestive of acute pancreatitis. In our hands, this has not proved to be a successful test either for acute or traumatic pancreatitis, and it is not recommended. The "spot" or single-specimen urine amylase is helpful, but it is exceeded in diagnostic sensitivity by the 2-hr urine collection for amylase concentration or, if time permits, the 24-hr urine collection. Urine amylase excretion exceeding 50 units/hr is suggestive of acute pancreatitis, and values over 100 units/hr are diagnostic of acute pancreatitis.

IV. Other diagnostic approaches. Following a careful history and physical examination, the diagnosis may still be obscure, and further diagnostic tests may be indicated.

A. X-ray studies. Four x-rays of the abdomen and chest should be made during the initial period of evaluation of patients with acute abdominal disease.

1. Upright posteroanterior chest x-rays are utilized to exclude pulmonary parenchymal disease, to detect subphrenic free air suggesting perforation of the gastrointestinal (GI) tract, and to demonstrate air-filled viscera in the chest (traumatic diaphragmatic hernia), mediastinal abscess, or spontaneous perforation of the esophagus.

2. Flat x-rays of the abdomen can be used to delineate the pattern of gas in the intestinal tract, to differentiate gaseous from fluid distention, to detect fluid-filled loops of intestine, and to visualize abnormal soft tissue densities or calculi. Some 90% of urinary tract calculi contain sufficient calcium to be radiopaque and will be seen. Conversely, only 10% of biliary tract stones will be seen. Of great diagnostic value is the detection of air in the biliary tree, indicating biliary-intestinal fistula and possible gallstone ileus as the cause of small-intestine obstruction. Further, the psoas shadows can often be seen; if both are visible, retroperitoneal pus, blood, or intestinal content can be ruled out. When neither is visible, either extensive retroperitoneal contamination with one of the above has occurred, or, more commonly, the psoas shadows are simply obscured by fat or other soft tissue. If one psoas is seen and the other is not, most likely the disease process in the retroperitoneum is present on the side where the psoas shadow cannot be discerned. Bony abnormalities of the vertebra or pelvis may also be detected.

3. Upright x-rays of the abdomen are used to determine air-fluid levels, especially at different heights, in mechanical intestinal obstruction. In addition, masses or soft tissue densities and their relationship to air-filled loops of intestine may be helpful in arriving at the diagnosis.

4. Left lateral decubitus x-rays are taken after the patient has been lying on the left side for at least 10 min to allow any free air that may have escaped detection in the upright view of the chest to gravitate upward to the space between the right lobe of the liver and the parietal peritoneum. This can be best achieved by sending the patient to the radiology department lying on his left side on the cart. The first x-ray, the left lateral decubitus view, can then be taken with the patient on the cart. Furthermore, a long air-fluid level on the right side of the abdomen, representing the ascending colon air-fluid interface, will be seen in patients with colon obstruction or paralytic ileus.

B. Diagnostic abdominal paracentesis

1. Of great importance is the concept that a **negative, or "dry," abdominal paracentesis has no diagnostic significance;** in other words, if no fluid is obtained, the abdominal tap cannot be assumed to have yielded any information and should be ignored. It is common to fail to aspirate fluid even by several needle insertions into the peritoneal cavity, despite the presence of a considerable amount of fluid.

2. Paracentesis should not be employed until after abdominal roentgenograms have been obtained, since small amounts of air may be introduced inadvertently during needle paracentesis and lead to an erroneous x-ray diagnosis of perforation.

3. The technique commonly employed for simple abdominal paracentesis involves turning the patient on the left side for 5 min, allowing the fluid to gravitate into the left paracolic area, and then inserting a needle into the abdomen (with the patient still in the left ducubitus position), halfway between the umbilicus and the pubis at the left lateral edge of the rectus sheath. This puncture site will obviate laceration of the deep inferior epigastric artery. The urinary bladder should be emptied prior to insertion of the needle.

4. It is *important not to use local anesthesia of the peritoneum,* so that penetration will be perceived by the patient as a sharp pain, thus serving to identify the level of the peritoneum. Gentle suction should be applied to the needle with a sterile 10-ml syringe after it has been determined that the needle has entered the peritoneal cavity. The hub of the needle should not be moved about in an arc in an attempt to obtain fluid, since this will markedly increase the chances of causing serious injury to subjacent viscera.

5. If the left lower quadrant paracentesis is negative (no fluid is obtained), the right side should be aspirated in the same fashion. It is not desirable to use the upper quadrants, as damage to the liver, spleen, or stomach may occur.

6. The preferred technique in abdominal trauma—and a very sensitive and useful technique in patients with subtle acute abdominal findings—is the **lavage paracentesis.** This procedure is done by placing a catheter into the peritoneal cavity in the lower abdominal midline, 2 cm below the umbilicus (see Fig. 25-20). The catheter may be introduced percutaneously, or with a tiny stab wound made by a scalpel through the skin only, and should be of the arterial catheter variety, that is, a metal central trocar with a peripheral sheath, the central trocar being removed as soon as the peritoneum has been entered. Probably a safer procedure is to introduce the catheter under direct vision, making a small incision under local anesthesia, and utilizing either the catheter described or a standard peritoneal dialysis catheter. Under either circumstance, the catheter should be directed toward the pelvis. If the procedure is done under direct vision, the peritoneum and fascia are closed around the catheter with a single absorbable purse-string suture, so that there is no leakage of irrigation fluid. When the catheter has been placed, 500 ml of sterile saline solution buffered with 30 ml 7.5% sodium bicarbonate should be allowed to enter the peritoneal cavity over a 10- to 15-min period. The fluid can then be aspirated and examined as indicated in **8**. In children, the placement of the catheter is somewhat difficult, but if a cooperative older child is encountered, the use of 10 ml/kg of body weight can be satisfactory. Larger volumes of saline, or, alternatively, Ringer's lactate, in adults or children tend to increase abdominal discomfort and may have an adverse effect on diaphragmatic excursion. The use of a smaller volume of fluid then requires that the numbers of cells be calculated as in **8**.

7. A logical plan is to utilize simple needle aspiration first and, if no fluid is obtained, to proceed to catheter irrigation.

8. **Study of paracentesis fluid** should consist of measurement of pH, a test for bile with Smith's reagent or other appropriate material, laboratory evaluation of amylase content, and microscopic examination of the fluid for leukocytes or erythrocytes. The presence of blood, large numbers of polymorphonuclear cells, bile, or the detection of an acid pH of the fluid usually represents a solid indication for exploratory laparotomy. If significant numbers of red cells or

polymorphonuclear cells are found, a cell count is indicated. With a 500-ml volume infusate, red cell counts in the vicinity of $100,000/ml^3$ of fluid or more should be an indication for operation. With regard to polymorphonuclear cells, a count of $500-700/ml^3$ or more represents a similar finding. The protein concentration of undiluted peritoneal fluid is important. If the concentration is 3 gm/100 ml or less, the fluid is a transudate, most probably from congestive heart failure, portal hypertension, or other mechanical causes. With concentrations in excess of 3 gm/100 ml, the fluid is the result of an exudative process, inflammation or neoplastic involvement of the peritoneum being the most likely.

9. An alternative to abdominal paracentesis in the female is **colpocentesis.** During this procedure, the patient must be in stirrups on a gynecological examining table. A spinal needle with a short bevel, usually 17- or 18-gauge, customarily is employed. With a vaginal speculum in place, the needle is introduced posterior to the cervix and directed straight cephalad. The needle should never be introduced more than half of its length in order to avoid perforation of intestine in or above the cul-de-sac. The technique is useful in patients thought to have a pelvic abscess or other pelvic disease. In a seriously ill patient, it is more troublesome and more difficult to perform than simple abdominal paracentesis.

C. **Special x-ray studies.** Under certain circumstances, the use of contrast material in the GI tract or the injection of dye into the arterial tree may yield significant information.

   1. **Contrast material by mouth.** Two types of medium can be given by mouth: diatrizoate (Gastrografin) and barium. The former is a water-soluble dye that is helpful in elucidating the size of the intestine and the presence of obstruction in the upper GI tract. It has little value in detecting mucosal lesions; for these, barium is the more satisfactory contrast medium. Barium may be harmful when given by mouth to a patient with significant gaseous intestinal distention. Use of oral barium should be limited to patients with acute abdominal disease in whom no perforation of the GI tract is judged to be present and in whom the abdomen is scaphoid or flat.

   2. **Barium enema.** This is usually indicated to differentiate small-intestinal from large-intestinal obstruction. *A barium enema should not be utilized under any circumstances* in patients with diffuse abdominal tenderness, frank peritonitis, or other signs of a perforated viscus. The examination should always be done with great care in patients with acute abdominal pain, under the direct supervision of the radiologist, and barium flow should be stopped immediately if there is either aggravation of the abdominal pain or fluoroscopic evidence of barium extravasation during the procedure.

   3. **Injection or exploration of stab wounds.** There has been some enthusiasm for detecting peritoneal penetration by sewing a catheter into the subcutaneous area of the wound of the abdomen, injecting dye, and obtaining a lateral abdominal x-ray to determine whether the dye is within the peritoneal cavity. This has not proved to be particularly effective or desirable, since penetration of the peritoneum does not require operation in small stab wounds of the abdomen unless the wound results in findings of peritoneal irritation or other signs suggesting injury to the viscera. In gunshot wounds, operation without the use of this diagnostic technique is ordinarily indicated.

   Exploration of stab wounds under local anesthesia has recently become popular. This would be undertaken only if there were insufficient abdominal findings to suggest the need for abdominal laparotomy, but the wound itself could be opened to its depths to ascertain the presence or absence of peritoneal damage. This has been suggested as an emergency room procedure and might allow the patient's discharge from the emergency room if the operator were certain that the peritoneum was intact as determined by the exploration. Such a procedure requires considerable experience, not to mention a cooperative patient. Under any circumstances, the immediate discharge of the patient without further observation is to be discouraged.

4. **Ultrasound (B-mode sonography).** Sophisticated instruments utilizing the Doppler principle of ultrasound detection have been developed and are helpful in detecting masses in the abdomen and in determining whether those masses are solid or fluid-filled. When a mass is palpated, it is sometimes helpful to subject the abdomen to ultrasound study, so that the precise nature of the mass may be ascertained. Abscesses, twisted cysts, and encapsulated hematomas are identified as fluid-filled, whereas solid tumors or other solid lesions are identified as such. Abdominal aneurysm can be definitely delineated, as to both presence and size. Localization of an intra-abdominal abscess is simplified considerably in patients with signs of sepsis and vague abdominal findings. This is particularly helpful in the postoperative period, provided the abdominal incision does not interfere with the application of the sonographic probe. Ultrasound has proved to be extremely valuable in the pancreatobiliary system, with great accuracy in detection of an enlarged gallbladder, the presence of calculi in the gallbladder or common bile duct, and the presence of an enlarged pancreas or pancreatic pseudocyst. Renal masses, as well, can be identified and even characterized by the use of the sonogram.

5. **Angiography** has become increasingly valuable in determining the site of GI bleeding. A Seldinger catheter is inserted by the femoral or brachial route, and cannulation of the celiac or mesenteric arteries may be done. The same technique is applied to patients who have experienced abdominal trauma, in whom rupture of the spleen or liver is suspected. The injured kidney is precisely evaluated by this technique. Flush aortography, in which individual vessel cannulation is not attempted, is helpful in diagnosis of splenic or renal rupture, but is of no benefit in patients with rupture of the liver. Acute pancreatic lesions cannot be assessed with angiography. The angiogram can be particularly useful with the selective technique, when a catheter is inserted into a specific vessel for purposes of diagnosing obstruction or narrowing of that vessel, as in acute intestinal ischemia.

6. **Computerized tomography (CT)** has achieved an increasing role in the diagnosis of the acute abdomen with the advent of the newer-generation, rapid scanners. These instruments are capable of obtaining cuts at 4.8-sec intervals, so that a section of the abdomen can be completely visualized in less than 30–40 min. In very obese patients, the accuracy far exceeds that of sonography, since fat is an excellent contrast medium, with a very low number in the computer utilized by the CT scanner. Unfortunately, the cost of this procedure and the lack of general availability of the instrument have so far restricted its use.

D. **Radionuclide scanning.** Infectious processes can be localized reasonably well if ^{67}Ga scanning is done 24 and 48 hr after intravenous administration of 1.0 to 2.5 mc of ^{67}Ga citrate. Tumors (especially lymphomas) and chronic inflammatory lesions also concentrate ^{67}Ga. Liver and spleen scanning in trauma patients with ^{99m}Tc-sulfur colloid is extremely helpful, primarily if gamma camera scanning is available. Renal scans are performed with ^{197}Hg chlormerodrin; an accurate scan can be completed within 1 hr of injection.

A new scanning technique, the HIDA/PIPIDA isotope for the visualization of the hepatobiliary system, has recently become popular; this is a ^{99m}Tc isotope, secreted into the hepatobiliary system. When ^{99m}Tc is administered intravenously, the presence of jaundice is not particularly significant in interfering with the scan, and visualization of the common bile duct with failure to visualize the gallbladder is presumptive evidence of obstruction of the cystic duct, namely, acute cholecystitis. The scan can be obtained in 1–2 hr with reasonable certainty of accuracy.

Suggested Reading

Gelin, L. E., Nyhus, L. M., and Condon, R. E. *Abdominal Pain: A Guide to Rapid Diagnosis.* Philadelphia: Lippincott, 1969.

Requarth, W. *Diagnosis of Acute Abdominal Pain.* Chicago: Year Book, 1958.

Silen, W. *Cope's Early Diagnosis of the Acute Abdomen* (15th ed.). New York: Oxford University Press, 1980.

Suarez, C. A., Block, F., Bernstein, D., Serafini, A., Rodman, G., Jr., and Zeppa, R. The role of HIDA/PIPIDA scanning in diagnosing cystic duct obstruction. *Ann. Surg.* 191:391, 1980.

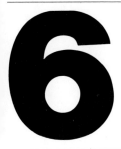

Upper Gastrointestinal Hemorrhage

I. General comments. The evolution of gastrointestinal **endoscopy** and **angiography** as diagnostic techniques has been immensely helpful to all who manage patients with upper gastrointestinal (GI) tract hemorrhage. The further therapeutic refinements of endoscopy (transendoscopic coagulation of bleeding points) and angiography (selective infusion of vasopressors, selective embolization of bleeding points) continue to raise our expectations that emergency operations will become less and less necessary. Until then, however, knowledge of the precise bleeding point simplifies the management of the patient, ensures that the most appropriate procedure will be done, and relieves the great anxiety that affects almost all those caring for such patients.

A. Definitions

1. **Massive GI hemorrhage** is the rapid loss of at least 1 liter of blood, or acute blood loss of any volume that is sufficient to cause hypovolemia.

2. **Hypovolemia** is an acute or chronic deficit in circulating blood volume and is manifested by rapid pulse and lowered systolic blood pressure (<100 mm Hg) and central venous pressure or by more subtle findings (postural changes in pulse and blood pressure).

3. **Upper GI hemorrhage** refers to bleeding from the esophagus, stomach, or duodenum. **Lower GI hemorrhage** refers to bleeding distal to the ligament of Treitz. Massive GI hemorrhage occurs most frequently from the upper GI tract.

4. **Hematemesis** means vomiting of bright red blood. **Melanemesis** (coffee-ground emesis) means vomiting of altered brown or black blood. Either indicates that the source of bleeding is above the ligament of Treitz, usually in the esophagus, stomach, or duodenum.

5. **Melena** refers to the passage of black blood per rectum. (**Hematochezia** means passage of bright red blood per rectum.) The color of blood passed in the stool gives no clue to the source of hemorrhage and the intestinal transit time. As blood passes through the GI tract, the action of bacteria and digestive juices changes the character of the blood from bright red to black and tarry, a process requiring some hours. Blood in the GI tract also may act as a cathartic, producing rapid transit. If transit is sufficiently rapid, blood shed in the stomach or duodenum may be passed unaltered per rectum. While melena is more characteristic of upper than of lower GI bleeding, it can occur with bleeding from a distal lower GI lesion. Conversely, hematochezia is more characteristic of mucosal lesions of the rectum and rectosigmoid but is not uncommon with upper GI hemorrhage.

B. Causes of hematemesis.
With the exception of very rare lesions, the causes of hematemesis are, in approximate order of frequency, as follows:

1. Duodenal ulcer.

2. Gastritis (acute, chronic, corrosive, infectious, stress).

3. Gastric ulcer.

4. Esophageal varices (portal hypertension).

5. Esophagitis or esophageal ulcer.

6. Gastric carcinoma.

7. Swallowed blood (epistaxis, hemoptysis).

8. Esophageal trauma (foreign body).

9. Esophageal carcinoma.

10. Aortoduodenal fistula.

11. Carcinoma of ampulla of Vater.

12. Hematobilia.

13. Blood coagulation dyscrasia (congenital or acquired).

14. Postemetic laceration (Mallory-Weiss syndrome).

15. Benign gastric tumor (e.g., hemangioma, leiomyoma).

16. Multiple telangiectasia.

17. Pseudoxanthoma elasticum.

A duodenal or gastric ulcer or gastritis is the cause of 85% of cases of upper GI hemorrhage.

II. Immediate management

A. Every patient with massive GI hemorrhage **must be admitted to a hospital** for further care. **Most patients with upper GI hemorrhage** (85%) **stop bleeding** either just before or just after admission to the hospital. Patients in whom bleeding continues or recurs after admission are unusual and probably need intra-arterial infusion therapy or operative control of the bleeding. Of course, many patients develop this complication during hospitalization after admission for burns or to intensive care units for such complications as shock, gastric distention, respiratory embarrassment, and sepsis. The diagnostic approach is similar; the therapeutic approach may be different.

B. Resuscitation and diagnostic maneuvers are used simultaneously. Hypovolemic shock must be corrected before this dual approach.

C. The **two prime objectives** of initial therapy are

1. **To replace the volume of lost blood** to stabilize the patient's condition.

2. **To determine the source** and approximate volume of the hemorrhage and whether or not bleeding is continuing.

D. The volume of blood lost is best estimated by the physical findings. The history is apt to be exaggerated in this regard. Estimating the volume of blood loss from the response of the blood pressure and pulse to a change from a supine to a sitting position is outlined in Table 9-2.

E. A rapid **physical examination** should be conducted, with particular attention to evidences of diseases that are associated with GI bleeding. Look for melanin spots, telangiectasia, hemangiomas, and the stigmata of cirrhosis. An enlarged liver or spleen, spider nevi, collateral circulation over the abdomen and chest, and loss of body hair are all indications of portal hypertension. Point tenderness in the epigastrium suggests duodenal or gastric ulcer.

F. **Place a large-bore central venous pressure (CVP) catheter** in one arm and a second IV catheter in the other arm. **Secure all IV catheters against inadvertent dislodgment** should the patient retch or be transferred to another area of the hospital. The Swan-Ganz balloon-tip catheter may be required to gauge the adequacy of fluid resuscitation in selected patients with heart or chronic pulmonary disease.

G. Type and cross-match whole blood, draw blood for a complete blood count and platelets, prothrombin time (PT) and partial thromboplastin time (PTT), serum electrolytes, sugar, and creatinine and for at least one additional tube. At least 6 units are required in the blood bank initially; notify the blood bank personnel that more blood may be required and determine whether the patient has a rare blood type—conservative treatment may not be possible if enough blood is not available.

H. Treat hypovolemic shock as the first priority. Give blood or plasma expanders as rapidly as possible, pumping them in if necessary. Once shock is reversed, transfusion should continue at a reasonably rapid rate to replace blood until (1) blood pressure and pulse are normal and stable, (2) an effective circulating blood volume has been restored, and (3) the hematocrit level is about 35%. Follow the precepts of shock therapy outlined in Chapter 1.

I. The following **laboratory examinations** may be helpful.

   1. Hematocrit. Serial determinations will be helpful in establishing the response to therapy and ongoing hemorrhage. Remember that initial hydration of the bleeding patient will dilute the remaining red cells, and that each transfused unit of packed cells will increase the hematocrit by two to three points. Conversely, the hematocrit falls by about three points for every 500 ml of blood lost.

   2. PT and PTT may reveal abnormal liver function, drug effects (sodium warfarin [Coumadin] or heparin), or coagulopathy.

   3. Comparison of platelet count fibrinogen and fibrin split products helps distinguish coagulopathy from dilutional decreases in serum clotting factors.

   4. Sodium sulfobromophthalein has been used to detect abnormal liver function in patients with possible esophageal varices. The test may be unreliable in patients with recent hypovolemia, must be performed with care to avoid local tissue damage, can cause a hypotensive reaction, and probably should not be done.

   5. An **electrocardiogram** may reveal recent myocardial infarction, drug effects, or electrolyte abnormalities (hypocalcemia), which can occur as a result of massive hemorrhage or transfusion.

J. A **careful history** should be obtained after replacement of lost blood volume has begun. **The history usually provides the best clues to the source of bleeding.** Because the patient may be frightened or even be incoherent, an effort must be made to obtain information from and corroborate the history with relatives or friends. Inquire particularly regarding symptoms of duodenal or gastric ulcer, alcoholism, and hepatitis. Make specific inquiries about medications or "blood thinners" and drug allergies.

K. Physicians who have treated the patient previously should be contacted. Old x-rays and records should be obtained for review, although they rarely arrive in time to be of much help in making the initial decisions regarding therapy.

L. The **"vigorous diagnostic approach"** should be followed in all patients with a major upper GI tract hemorrhage in order to provide or confirm a diagnosis.

   1. Lavage the stomach with iced saline solution via an Ewald tube; remove all old blood and clots. Lavage is continued until the returns are clear.

   2. As soon as the patient's condition is stable, perform **upper GI endoscopy:** esophagoscopy, gastroscopy, and duodenoscopy. A definitive diagnosis should follow.

   3. If after these studies the diagnosis is still in question and the patient continues to bleed, **selective angiography** of the visceral arteries (superior mesenteric, gastroduodenal, splenic, and left gastric) with injection of contrast material should be performed. Depending on the specific source of the hemorrhage, the catheters may be left in place for 2–6 days for injection of vasopressin.

4. If these diagnostic techniques are not available, an **upper GI series** with barium is performed; the esophagus must be carefully surveyed for varices or ulceration. Barium studies are not definitive, however, because varices or ulcers seen need not be bleeding, and additional pathological conditions such as gastritis will be missed.

M. The record must contain a "hemorrhage data sheet" that shows the exact quantities and types of fluids infused, serial hematocrit, electrolyte determinations, urine output, CVP, and serial vital sign determinations.

III. Therapeutic approach

A. Bleeding stops

1. Place a **nasogastric tube** on suction to provide a means of early warning of recurrent upper GI bleeding. **Antacids** should be instilled into the stomach. The pH of the gastric aspirate should be monitored frequently and kept above 6.0. Alternatively, intravenous cimetidine in a dose sufficient to maintain a similar pH may be used.

2. After the volume of estimated blood loss has been rapidly replaced, transfusions should stop, but IV maintenance fluids are continued. The recording of blood pressure and pulse at frequent intervals is continued. These data, together with the character of the nasogastric suction output, the presence or absence of borborygmi or hyperactive bowel sounds by auscultation, and the direction of change in the hematocrit, will allow early recognition of recurrent bleeding.

3. After it is certain that bleeding has stopped, the nasogastric tube may be removed. **Antacids** should be given hourly; milk and cream, despite their popularity, are not efficient antacids. The patient should be kept at bed rest or on restricted activity, and small doses of **sedatives** should be administered around the clock for the first few days. No anticholinergics should be given to patients soon after a major GI hemorrhage. A caffeine-free and alcohol-free general diet can be ordered. Depending on the source of the hemorrhage, a definitive operation on an elective basis may be indicated.

B. Bleeding continues: use of vasopressin

1. Assuming that the patient is hemodynamically stable and can be maintained on modest blood replacement (less than 1500 ml/24 hr), an attempt should be made to control the hemorrhage by the use of intravenous vasopressin. This technique particularly applies to hemorrhage from varices, gastritis, or stress ulceration; it is less effective for bleeding from chronic duodenal or chronic gastric ulcer. This method of treatment for ulcer should be reserved for high-risk patients who would be poor candidates for operation.

2. The **rationale for intravenous vasopressin** is best shown in the patient with elevated portal venous pressure. Vasopressin infusion **reduces portal pressure and flow by constricting splanchnic arterioles.** The use of vasopressin to control bleeding is a temporizing measure, since most patients rebleed when therapy is discontinued. The overall mortality associated with variceal bleeding has not been altered by use of this drug. Furthermore, numerous side effects may occur during vasopressin infusion: bradycardia (vagal effect?); elevation of blood pressure with narrowing of pulse pressure; cardiac arrhythmia; cardiac arrest; angina pectoris; myocardial infarction; cerebral, intestinal, or limb ischemia; and water intoxication. About one third of patients may be expected to have one or more such side effects.

3. Dose and route of administration

a. Intravenous infusion has approximately the same effect as intra-arterial infusion; earlier hopes that the intra-arterial route would be more advantageous have not been realized. The biological half-life of vasopressin (15–30 min) explains the comparable effects of the venous and arterial routes.

b. Preparation of vasopressin solution. Mix 20 units of vasopressin (Pitressin 20 units/vial) and 100 ml 5% D/W. Infuse with a continuous infusion pump set to deliver 1 ml/min (0.2 units vasopressin).

c. Begin infusion of vasopressin at 0.2 units/min using a continuous infusion pump. Routine electrocardiographic monitoring and serial hemodynamic measurements are advisable (cardiac output, wedged pulmonary capillary pressure, mixed venous oxygen tension). If adverse reactions are observed, discontinue infusion. Treatment is then directed toward the symptom, e.g., atropine for bradycardia, nitroglycerine for angina. If bleeding continues despite several hours of infusion, it is probably pointless (and possibly hazardous) to continue vasopressin therapy.

d. We no longer recommend high-dose vasopressin infusion (over 0.4 units/min IV).

C. Special problems in therapy

1. The single most difficult problem is the **decision to discontinue nonoperative therapy** (e.g., ice-water lavage or vasopressin infusion). The following few **guidelines** as to when to operate on the patient may help:

   a. Older patients tolerate continuing hemorrhage and prolonged resuscitation poorly. Although not a fixed rule, 24 hr should be sufficient time to control bleeding fully. Older patients who have persistent or recurrent bleeding should be operated on sooner than young patients with the same problem.

   b. Patients over 50 yr of age who have a history of chronic duodenal ulcer and present with massive bleeding require an operation.

   c. Operative therapy is often necessary in patients who bleed massively from a gastric ulcer.

   d. Immediate operative therapy is mandatory under the following circumstances:

      (1) When perforation and hemorrhage coexist.

      (2) When blood pressure and pulse are not normal and stable after rapid transfusion of 2500 ml of blood.

      (3) When, following initial stabilization, more than 1500 ml of blood must be transfused in less than 24 hr to maintain a normal pulse and blood pressure.

      (4) When bleeding, even of small amounts, continues for more than 24 hr from onset. In young, vigorous patients, persistence of bleeding for up to 48 hr may be tolerated in selected patients.

      (5) Having initially stopped, bleeding recurs while the patient is hospitalized and receiving nonoperative treatment.

      (6) There is a shortage of compatible blood.

      (7) The patient has a lesion that will invariably bleed again (e.g., aortoduodenal fistula).

2. **Esophageal varices and balloon tamponade.** If the intravenous vasopressin technique is not effective, a triple-lumen (Sengstaken-Blakemore) tube is both a diagnostic and therapeutic tool. The stomach first must be lavaged free of old blood. With a triple-lumen tube, the gastric aspirate can be isolated effectively from the esophagus. Balloon tamponade is a temporary, not a definitive, treat-

ment; half these patients will bleed again when the balloon is deflated. Great care in the use of tamponade technique is essential. Rupture of the gastric balloon, with asphyxiation, or rupture of the esophagus, may occur. Constant bedside attention by intensive care unit personnel is mandatory during periods of balloon inflation.

3. **Portosystemic shunts**

   a. Portosystemic shunts are **indicated** in the treatment of selected patients with variceal hemorrhage who do not respond to medical therapy means, or who have survived a major hemorrhage from esophageal varices. Such patients ideally have a normal or slightly elevated bilirubin, near-normal serum albumin levels, and absence of encephalopathy and ascites. Patients with extreme abnormalities of liver function are not candidates for a portosystemic shunt, since they will not survive the procedure.

   b. Types of shunts

      (1) End (of portal vein) **to side** (of vena cava). All blood from the portal circulation is diverted from the liver. This shunt is *not* performed if the liver is normal, or if hepatofugal flow has been established. This shunt is performed if other varieties cannot be constructed.

      (2) Side (of portal vein) **to side** (of vena cava). This is the ideal shunt for patients with ascites or with hepatofugal venous flow.

      (3) Distal splenorenal. This shunt allows continued perfusion of the liver and is the most physiological shunt. It is not recommended if ascites is present, or if hepatofugal flow is established.

   c. Preoperative study of venous vascular anatomy and flow and wedged hepatic vein pressures is recommended.

4. **Sclerotherapy of bleeding varices.** An alternative to portosystemic shunt is transendoscopic injection of esophageal varices with a sclerosing solution (e.g., sodium morrhuate). Encouraging early reports warrant further investigations of this promising technique.

Suggested Reading

Donahue, P. E., and Nyhus, L. M. Massive Upper Gastrointestinal Hemorrhage. In L. M. Nyhus and C. Wastell (eds.), *Surgery of the Stomach and Duodenum* (3rd ed.). Boston: Little, Brown, 1977.

Fiddian-Green, R. G., and Turcotte, J. G., (eds.). *Gastrointestinal Hemorrhage.* New York: Grune & Stratton, 1980.

Johnson, W. C., Widrich, W. C., Ansell, J. E., Robbins, A. H., and Nabseth, D. C. Control of bleeding varices by vasopressin: A prospective randomized study. *Ann. Surg.* 186:369, 1977.

Welch, C. E., and Hedberg, S. Gastrointestinal hemorrhage. General considerations of diagnosis and therapy. *Adv. Surg.* 7:95, 1973.

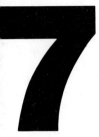

I. General comments

A. Normal motility

1. **Electrical activity** of bowel smooth muscle is characterized by slow waves and spike discharges.

2. **Slow waves** (pacesetter potentials, basic electrical rhythm, control activity) are omnipresent, aborally propagated, and regularly recurring low-amplitude depolarizations of the smooth muscle membrane. They permit contractile potentials (spike discharges) only just before or at the peak of partial depolarization; thus, they govern the maximal contraction frequency of the bowel. Slow waves are intrinsically generated and vary in frequency along the alimentary tract: about 12/min in the human duodenum; 8/min in the ileum; 3/min in the right and transverse colon; and 6–11/min in the rectosigmoid colon.

3. **Spike discharges** (contractile potentials, response activity) occur singly or in short bursts, are of variable amplitude, are superimposed on a slow-wave depolarization, and produce the several types of muscle contractions. The percentage of slow waves carrying spike discharges can range from 0 to 100%. Spike discharges are readily stimulated or inhibited by external and intraluminal mechanical and chemical factors, drugs, hormones, fasting, and feeding.

4. **Small-bowel muscular contractions** are of two types:

   a. **Ring contractions,** about 1 cm in length, displace fluid both ways. The frequency of ring contractions decreases along the length of the bowel; as a consequence, fluid is propelled caudad. Segmentation or ring contractions chiefly result in mixing of intestinal contents. These contractions occur at random and independently at multiple points in the intestine and have sufficient force to produce intraluminal pressures up to 8–12 mm Hg.

   b. **Peristaltic contractions** occur about 1/min; they are ring contractions that are propagated caudad over bowel segments about 4–6 cm in length. Although peristaltic contractions occur regularly with feeding, they also occur cyclically in bursts during fasting.

   c. Migrating myoelectrical complexes occur during fasting. They are peristaltic sweeps that begin proximally in the duodenum or jejunum and progress distally over long segments, often to the distal ileum.

5. The **ileocecal junction** is a 1- to 2-cm muscle segment that is tonically contracted for long periods, probably to prevent retrograde flow of colonic contents. It opens occasionally in response to propulsive contractions of the terminal ileum.

6. **Proximal colon muscular contractions** are of two types:

   a. **Rhythmic contractions** are asymmetrical mixing waves that tend to induce flow, usually toward the cecum (orad). Animal studies have shown that they are phase-locked, with slow-wave potentials about 67% of the time in the ascending colon and 90% in the transverse colon.

b. **Peristaltic contractions** occur with a "migrating spike burst" that is prolonged over several slow-wave cycles and slowly moves caudad over long distances. These actions are infrequent and begin at variable points along the transverse and descending colon.

7. **Distal colon muscular contractions** are similar. Standing rhythmic contractions are symmetrical, and their segmentation pattern produces little net directional flow. Peristaltic contractions develop intermittently from migrating spike bursts, often originating at the hepatic flexure and sweeping distally.

8. The **rectum** acts largely as a reservoir. Peristaltic contraction is its principal motility pattern, which is probably under complete neural and largely voluntary control.

9. Extrinsic neural activity is just a portion of the spectrum of peristaltic stimuli. Parasympathetic cholinergic nerves are generally considered excitatory and sympathetic adrenergic nerves inhibitory, at least in the small intestine. Preganglionic sympathectomy (e.g., epidural anesthesia) is followed transiently by some increase in peristaltic activity. Parasympathectomy (truncal vagotomy) usually has little effect on bowel motility. It is occasionally associated with episodic or persistent diarrhea for reasons that are unclear.

B. Incidence of bowel obstruction

1. An estimated 20% of hospital general surgical emergency admissions are for operative or nonoperative management of intestinal obstruction. This disease occurs at all ages. Among infants, 10% of deaths are caused by bowel obstruction, most frequently related to congenital malformation or hernia.

2. The **incidence** of obstruction rises progressively with age throughout adulthood; adhesions and groin hernias are the predominant causes of obstruction. There is a sharp increase in incidence after age 50 and again after age 70 as bowel neoplasms and colonic diverticulitis become more prevalent. Four common causes (**adhesions, hernia, tumor, diverticulitis**) in adults produce 80% of cases of intestinal obstruction.

C. Types of bowel obstruction

1. Obstruction means that **bowel content cannot pass normally** to the rectum due to an interposed extrinsic or intrinsic block in either the small or large bowel. Bowel obstruction may be complete or incomplete and may or may not involve compromise of vascular supply. In patients with mechanical obstruction, the site of obstruction is in the small bowel in 70–80% and in the colon in the remainder. This ratio diminishes somewhat with increasing age.

2. **Simple mechanical obstruction** is the result of occlusion of the bowel lumen without compromise of vascular supply. The source may be extrinsic (adhesions, hernia), intramural (tumor, hematoma), or intraluminal (polyp, fecal impaction). **Obturation obstruction** refers to intraluminal obstruction anywhere along the gastrointestinal tract by foreign body (gallstone, bezoar). **Closed-loop obstruction** involves obstruction at two levels such that content in the intervening loop of bowel cannot progress distally or reflux backward, i.e., the loop is closed in both directions.

3. **Strangulation obstruction** is an advanced stage of mechanical obstruction usually due to bowel protrusion through a constricting ring of tissue or to torsion of the bowel on its vascular pedicle. In both cases, venous occlusion develops, followed by arterial insufficiency, with consequent gangrene of the bowel wall.

4. **Paralytic (adynamic, neurogenic) ileus** is a functional obstruction due to ineffective or nonpropulsive peristalsis. Motor activity, though diminished, is never completely absent. No vascular compromise is involved. The causes are numerous (Table 7-1); paralytic ileus simulates mechanical intestinal obstruction and may be difficult to differentiate from it.

Table 7-1. Some Causes of Paralytic Ileus

Intra-abdominal
    Inflammation, infection: appendicitis, cholecystitis, pancreatitis, etc.
    Peritonitis: bacterial (perforated bowel), chemical (bile, pancreatic juice, acid gastric juice)
    Wound dehiscence
    Mesenteric embolus: arterial
    Mesenteric thrombosis:* venous, arterial
    Mesenteric ischemia:* shock, heart failure, vasopressors
    Blunt trauma*
    Distended bladder
    Gastric dilation
    Hirschsprung's (aganglionic) megacolon
    Postcoarctation syndrome: mesenteric arteritis
Retroperitoneal
    Infection: pyelonephritis, abscess
    Ureteral stone or obstruction
    Vertebral fracture: lumbar, thoracic
    Pelvic fracture
    Central nervous system: trauma, tumor
    Hematoma: trauma, anticoagulants, hemophilia
    Tumor: primary (sarcoma, lymphoma) or metastatic
    Strangulation of spermatic cord, testicular torsion
Systemic
    Potassium depletion
    Sodium depletion
    Drugs: ganglionic blockers, anticholinergics
    Emphysema
    Uremia
    Diabetic ketosis, neuropathy
    Lead poisoning
    Porphyria
    Septicemia
    Pneumonia, especially lower lobes
    Pulmonary embolus
    Empyema
    Meningitis

*Gangrene may be present with these lesions.

5. **Intestinal vascular occlusive disease** is neither a primary mechanical nor a functional obstruction of bowel but usually presents clinically with paralytic ileus. The possibility of vascular compromise of the bowel should be entertained whenever an older patient appears to have ileus or mechanical obstruction.

II. Simple mechanical small-bowel obstruction

A. Causes

1. In **adults who have previously had an abdominal operation,** 90% of mechanical obstructions are a result of **adhesions.** The cause of adhesions remains unproved, but it is most likely related to operative ischemic injury or postoperative inflammation of the peritoneal serosa. Adhesive obstruction can occur in patients who have not had a previous abdominal operation.

2. In **adults who previously have not been operated on,** an **external hernia** is the most common cause of obstruction.

3. In **infants,** segmental intestinal **atresia** and **imperforate anus** are the most frequent causes of obstruction.

4. Some of the myriad other causes of mechanical obstruction are listed in Table 7-2.

Table 7-2. Some Causes of Intestinal Obstruction

Mechanical-extrinsic

Adhesions:* postoperative, peritonitis, enteritis, abscess, carcinoma

Hernia:* external or internal

Carcinomatosis

Volvulus:* spontaneous, resulting from adhesions, congenital defect

Intra-abdominal mass: tumor, abscess, cyst duplication

Malrotation

Annular pancreas

Meckel's diverticulum

Congenital bands

Arteriomesenteric compression (superior mesenteric artery syndrome)

Mechanical-intramural and intraluminal

Carcinoma

Stricture or stenosis: congenital, trauma, regional enteritis, radiation, tuberculosis, lymphopathia, endometriosis

Hematoma: trauma, anticoagulants, hemophilia

Diverticulitis

Intussusception (lymphoid tissue in children, cancer in adults)

Stoma/ostomy: stricture, edema, ulcer

Polyp

Congenital atresia or diaphragm

Imperforate anus

Meconium

Gallstone ileus

Bezoars, foreign bodies

Fecal impaction

*Gangrene may be present with these lesions.

B. Pathophysiology

1. The disturbed physiology engendered by mechanical small-bowel obstruction is manifested as reactive hyperperistalsis, luminal distention by gas and fluid, increased bacterial growth, variable mural transudation of vascular volume and bacterial toxins, and contraction of extracellular functional volume, leading to hypovolemic shock.

2. **Hyperperistalsis** is a result of reactive intrinsic motor activity of the bowel both proximal and distal to the point of obstruction; a hyperactive bowel is evacuated, after which the patient passes no flatus or feces if the obstruction is complete. After 24–48 hr, edema and muscle exhaustion supervene; the clinical picture now resembles paralytic ileus.

3. **Intestinal gas** accumulates proximal to the obstruction and is the major cause of bowel distention. The gas is largely swallowed air; minor volume contributions are made by bacterial fermentation, digestion of some foods, and diffusion from blood gases.

4. **Fluid** accumulating proximal to the obstruction is derived chiefly from normal secretions. In addition to decreased insorption (lumen into blood) of water, sodium, and potassium, experimental studies also have documented increased exsorption (blood into lumen) of water and electrolytes after 24–60 hr of obstruction. The fluid is isotonic, with concentrations of potassium progressively higher than normal as the site of the obstruction becomes more distal.

5. The fluid contained in the bowel forms a "third space," which is functionally lost to the body. The small bowel may partially decompress itself by regurgitation into the stomach, resulting in vomiting. These processes lead to **contraction of extracellular (interstitial and plasma) volume,** which produces hypovolemic shock unless the functionally lost fluids are replaced parenterally. Shock compounds the problems of obstruction, since decreased arterial perfusion to already distended bowel results.

6. **Alkalosis** typically develops with pyloric or high jejunal obstruction in which copious vomiting produces external loss of acid gastric juice and chloride. Metabolic **acidosis** accompanies distal small-bowel obstruction, due to predominant loss (third space) of sodium-containing fluids.

7. Normal resting intraluminal pressure in the small bowel is about 2–4 mm Hg. In simple small-bowel obstruction, **sustained increased intraluminal pressures** of 10–14 mm Hg are usual; with vigorous peristalsis, they may increase temporarily to 30–60 mm Hg. The intestinal vascular supply is oriented so that most vessels travel transversely within the bowel wall, thereby minimizing the effects of peristalsis. It is the sustained intraluminal pressures in obstruction that alter or damage the bowel wall. Pressures above 30 mm Hg cause lymphatic and capillary stasis; pressures above 60 mm Hg cause venous congestion; and pressures above 100 mm Hg cause arterial occlusion. If intraluminal pressure is sustained just above 20 mm Hg for 10–20 hr, vascular congestion develops; if sustained for more than 28 hr, the bowel wall may lose viability. Regurgitation of bowel content usually prevents this hazardous development unless **a closed-loop obstruction** is present. In the latter case, focal gangrene and perforation occur before the small bowel literally bursts; the bursting pressure of the normal human small bowel is 170–280 mm Hg, a pressure unlikely to be achieved in any form of obstruction.

8. Abdominal distention reduces effective **pulmonary ventilation** by elevating the diaphragm and reducing the effectiveness of abdominal respiratory movements. This effect is particularly important in elderly patients with compromised pulmonary function.

9. Raised intraluminal pressure and bowel distention increase mural capillary

permeability and retard lymphatic drainage, both of which produce **edema** of the bowel wall. Submucosal edema alters the normal barrier function of the bowel and permits transudation of fluid, bacteria, and bacterial toxins into the peritoneal cavity. It also interferes with muscle contraction, so that ileus may persist for a time even after relief of the obstruction.

10. **Bacterial growth** is promoted by stasis; after a few hours of obstruction, the small bowel must be regarded as filled with fluid feces. The high concentrations of bacteria and their ability to transmigrate to the abdominal cavity are associated with an increased incidence of preoperative peritonitis and postoperative abscesses and wound infection, particularly if bowel resection or decompressive enterotomy is necessary during operation.

C. Clinical complex and diagnosis

1. The clinical signs and symptoms of obstruction in **adults** are summarized in Tables 7-3 and 7-4.

2. In **infants,** obstruction should be suspected when any of these cardinal signs are present: (a) failure to evacuate meconium within 12 hr of birth, (b) green or bilious vomitus, or (c) abdominal distention.

3. **Colic** (cramps) coinciding with rushing peristalsis and sometimes with loud borborygmi is the classic pattern of pain in small-bowel obstruction. Visible peristalsis is frequent in children and also is seen in adults with a thin body habitus. Later in the course of untreated obstruction, when the bowel has "decompensated" and is too distended and edematous to contract effectively, colic is diminished or absent and is replaced by dull, nonlocalized but persistent discomfort.

4. **If pain is localized, steady, and intense, particularly with percussion tenderness, suspect strangulation.**

5. **Obstipation** is present early in complete obstruction, as soon as the initial reaction of hyperperistalsis has evacuated the distal bowel. Continued passage of small amounts of feces (often diarrheal) or flatus suggests that the obstruction is intermittent or incomplete.

6. **Distention** usually is present and is most prominent with distal small-bowel obstruction. It is absent early in the course of obstruction, may be minimal with closed-loop obstruction, and is infrequent and limited to the upper abdomen in high small-bowel obstruction.

7. **Vomiting** begins early and is bilious and persistent in high small-bowel obstruction. Vomiting appears later with more distal obstruction; it is initially

Table 7-3. X-ray Signs in Intestinal Obstruction

Sign	Paralytic Ileus	Mechanical Obstruction
Gas in stomach	+++	+
Gas in bowel	+++	+
	Scattered in both large and small bowel	Only proximal to obstruction
Fluid in bowel	+	+++
Ladder pattern supine	++	+
Ladder pattern upright	+	++
Air-fluid interfaces at opposite ends of a bowel loop (upright film)	All tend to be at about same level across midabdomen; U-loops seen	Tend to be at different levels; J-loops seen

Table 7-4. Clinical Features in Intestinal Obstruction

Type of Obstruction	Pain	Distention	Vomiting	Bowel Sounds	Tenderness	Temperature°C (°F)
Simple mechanical						
High small bowel	++ Cramps, mid- to upper abdominal	+	+++ Early, bilious, persistent	Increased	Minimal, diffuse	<37.7 (<100)
Low small bowel	+++ Cramps, midabdominal	+++ Early	++ Later, feculent	Increased, rushes	Minimal, diffuse	<37.7 (<100)
Colon	+++ Cramps, mid- to lower abdominal	+++ Later	+ Very late, feculent	Usually increased	Minimal, diffuse	<37.7 (<100)
Strangulation	+++ Continuous, may localize, severe	++	+++ Persistent	Variable, usually decreased	Marked, localized	50% > 37.7 (>100)
Paralytic ileus	+ Diffuse, mild	++++ Very early	+	Decreased	Minimal, diffuse	None
Vascular ileus	++++ Continuous, midabdominal and midback, may be severe	+++ Early	+++	Decreased or absent	Marked, diffuse or localized	Usually >37.7 (>100)

bilious but later feculent. The early appearance of vomiting in low small-bowel obstruction suggests strangulation.

8. **Fever** is never caused by fluid loss in obstruction. If the temperature is above 37.7°C (100°F), suspect strangulation or perforation.

9. **Leukocytosis** is not usually prominent in simple obstruction. A high or low leukocyte count may indicate perforation or strangulation.

10. Serum **amylase** levels may be elevated, particularly if there is vomiting, but more often than not, the amylase is normal.

11. Clinical signs of **saline depletion** (furrowed tongue, increasing hematocrit, oliguria, hypotension) and **water depletion** (thirst, dry axillae, increasing serum sodium) are present to some degree in every patient (see Chap. 9). Fluid losses may account for all the systemic effects in many patients with obstruction.

12. Supine anteroposterior (AP) **x-rays** of the abdomen show distended bowel proximal to the obstruction and absence of gas distally. Multiple air-fluid levels are noted on upright or lateral decubitus views (see Table 7-3). Gas in the small bowel may be a normal finding in young children. Radiographic evidence of bowel-wall edema is not a reliable indicator of duration of obstruction. A **barium enema** may help to rule out colon obstruction. This examination must be conducted entirely under fluoroscopic control to prevent passage of barium proximal to a colon obstruction. Barium lodged proximal to a partial obstruction of the colon may become inspissated and convert the partial obstruction to a complete obstruction. A **barium meal** can be useful if the diagnosis of small-bowel obstruction is in reasonable doubt. Barium administered PO will not cause further obstruction or perforation if colon obstruction has first been ruled out by barium enema.

D. Treatment

1. The **three steps** in the treatment of simple mechanical obstruction are (a) nasogastric suction, (b) correction of fluid imbalances, and (c) removal of the cause of obstruction, usually by operation.

2. **Nasogastric suction** using an 18 Fr tube removes fluid regurgitated into the stomach, prevents further accumulation of swallowed air, may partially decompress the bowel, and reduces the risk of aspiration.

3. **IV fluid therapy** (see Chap. 9) should be prompt and aimed at restoration of major deficits.

   a. If marked deficits are apparent, a central venous line is advisable and will be helpful in administering and monitoring the responses to large volumes of fluid therapy before and after operation.

   b. All patients need crystalloid solutions with potassium; estimated plasma volume deficits should be replaced with plasma substitutes. *A history of heart disease should never deter administration of saline solution.*

   c. Major fluid deficits and imbalances should be repaired before operation is undertaken. Correction is appraised by obtaining a normal blood pressure and heart rate, a satisfactory urine output and central venous pressure, and improved or corrected serum electrolyte concentrations. Rehydration should be accomplished within a maximum of 8 hr in nearly all patients.

4. **Antibiotics** in experimental animals reduce mortality from obstruction associated with strangulation. In patients without strangulation, the evidence for benefit is less clear. However, bowel ischemia cannot be excluded preoperatively in any patient; bacterial diapedesis into the peritoneal cavity may be ongoing, and bowel resection or enterotomy with possible contamination may be necessary during operation. **Broad-spectrum antibiotics** should be ad-

ministered systemically before operation (see Chap. 14) and should be continued postoperatively if indicated by the operative findings.

5. **Urinary catheterization** is performed in patients with prolonged obstruction or marked fluid imbalance. Notation of the initial amount of urine in the bladder and its specific gravity is helpful, and the catheter provides an accurate means of monitoring the response to fluid resuscitation.

6. *No cleansing enemas of any kind should be used in cases of small-bowel obstruction.* Enemas confuse the x-ray picture by introducing gas into the bowel distal to the obstruction.

7. **Nonoperative treatment with a long intestinal suction tube** is applicable as alternative management only in special circumstances. One must then be extremely alert to fluid management and the patient's progress. It is often helpful to use nasogastric tube suction simultaneously. The long tube, once past the pylorus, is connected to intermittent suction, and the nasogastric tube is then changed to gravity drainage for gastric air decompression. It is also expedient to accomplish pyloric traversal by the long tube in the radiology suite by manipulation under image fluoroscopy. However, if the tube in the duodenum fails to progress aborad over the next 2 hr, it should be abandoned. The special situations in which long-tube management is applicable include:

   a. An incomplete obstruction that is progressively improving.

   b. Obstruction occurring in the immediate postoperative period.

   c. Initial decompression that promptly converts a complete to an incomplete obstruction.

   d. The "frozen abdomen," i.e., patients with a history of many previous operations for relief of obstruction resulting from adhesions, particularly if they appear incomplete.

   e. Obstruction known to be related to abdominal carcinomatosis or radiation enteritis (these rarely strangulate).

8. **Operative treatment** should be conducted through a midline incision, with careful lysis of abdominal-wall adhesions as they are encountered. It is helpful to search first for the cecum and distal ileum, then follow the small bowel proximally until dilated bowel is encountered. The **objective of operative treatment** is release, removal, or repair of the cause of the obstruction. Diseased or necrotic small bowel must be resected; a primary anastomosis is preferable to exteriorization. Decompression of obstructed bowel should be accomplished with a Baker or Leonard tube passed orally. If decompressive enterotomy is necessary, it should be performed aseptically with an 18-gauge needle connected to suction and inserted through a small purse-string suture in the intestinal wall. It is not necessary to lyse intestinal adhesions obviously unrelated to the obstruction. Bypass of the obstruction is acceptable only when definitive treatment is neither safe nor feasible; it may produce a blind-loop syndrome.

9. Operative treatment of **recurrent adhesive obstruction** may require more than complete enterolysis, particularly when accompanied by massive dilation and ileus. A Baker tube is inserted through a gastrotomy or high jejunotomy, its distal balloon inflated and then the tube progressively maneuvered through the entire small bowel into the cecum. The enterostomy is secured to the abdominal wall, and the bowel is permitted to lie in the abdomen without angulation or kinking. The cecal balloon is deflated on the first day, and the tube is removed after 12–14 days, permitting time for adhesion formation without obstruction.

10. **Mortality** in operative treatment for nonstrangulated small-bowel obstruction

varies from 0–5% and is influenced both by the patient's general condition and the cause of obstruction (particularly malignancy). In patients with adhesive obstruction, recurrence after operative treatment is 10%.

III. Simple mechanical obstruction of the colon

A. Causes

1. **Carcinoma** is the commonest cause of colon obstruction. Most obstructing lesions lie between the splenic flexure and the rectum.

2. Other frequent causes include **volvulus** (sigmoid, cecum) and colonic **diverticulitis,** with or without acute abscess formation.

3. Particularly in older patients, **fecal impaction** and idiopathic **adynamic ileus** may closely simulate colon obstruction.

B. Pathophysiology

1. The disturbed physiology of colon obstruction is similar to that of small-bowel obstruction but develops more slowly.

2. **Accumulation of gas** is very marked. Swallowed air still contributes the major volume, but methane, hydrogen sulfide, and other products of bacterial fermentation provide about one fourth of the gas volume in colon obstruction.

3. **Accumulation of fluid** in the obstructed colon also is marked, resulting largely from failure of normal water absorption in the right colon. Both fluid and gas collection regurgitate and progressively distend the distal small bowel if the ileocecal valve is incompetent (in 50–60% of patients) and eventually can lead to feculent vomiting. Otherwise, with ileocecal valve competence, the most distensible colon segment, the cecum, enlarges; if the cecum is distended to more than 10 cm in diameter in the presence of obstruction, perforation may occur.

4. Fluid losses into the luminal third space have the same consequences as in small-bowel obstruction, namely, **contraction of the extracellular fluid volume,** progressing to hypovolemic shock.

5. The intraluminal pressure in unobstructed colon is 2–4 mm Hg. In complete mechanical colon obstruction, with reflux past an incompetent ileocecal valve, the **sustained intraluminal pressure** is usually 10–25 mm Hg. A higher pressure of 70–95 mm Hg is needed to force open a competent ileocecal valve; if the valve does not yield, closed-loop obstruction is present. Because the bursting pressure of the normal colon is about 95–110 mm Hg, which is considerably lower than the bursting pressure of the small bowel, dangerous intraluminal pressures can develop rapidly. With high but equal pressures through the colon, increased surface tension and threat of primary rupture will follow the law of Laplace (tension = pressure × diameter × 3.14); this relationship also explains why the greatest distention occurs in the segment with the widest initial radius, usually the cecum. Moreover, elevated intraluminal pressures, particularly if sustained over a number of hours, compromise lymphatic and capillary circulation and may lead to serosal tears, patches of ischemic gangrene, and perforation.

C. Clinical complex and diagnosis

1. Clinical **signs and symptoms** are similar to those of low small-bowel obstruction but develop more slowly.

2. Abdominal **distention,** once it develops, is more prominent than in small-bowel obstruction. Alternating diarrhea and constipation may have preceded frank obstruction. A discrete carcinomatous mass or a tender diverticular abscess may be discernible early. Segmental volvulus usually is associated with more diffuse distention than in small-bowel obstruction and is more apparent on abdominal x-rays.

3. **Vomiting** also occurs late, sometimes only after regurgitation of colonic content back to the stomach, and usually is feculent.

4. **Hyperperistalsis** accompanies **colic,** which progresses to eventual exhaustion, resulting in ileus.

5. On supine or upright AP **x-rays** of the abdomen, the cecum distended beyond 10 cm or the transverse colon distended beyond 8 cm should be viewed as in imminent danger of rupture.

6. In cases of questionable or early colonic obstruction, a **barium enema,** performed after proctoscopy and with the surgeon in attendance, may be helpful in delineating both the site and nature of the obstructive lesion. It must be carefully executed so as to prevent either passage of barium proximal to the obstruction or perforation at the obstructing site.

D. Treatment

1. Treatment of **complete colon obstruction** (other than a sigmoid volvulus) **always involves an early operation.** There is no place for prolonged nonoperative tube suction therapy.

2. The principles of **preoperative preparation** for colon obstruction are similar to those for small-bowel obstruction. The timing of intervention will demand more urgency in patients in whom colonic rupture is threatening.

   a. A **nasogastric tube** should be passed in all patients and put on suction.

   b. **Vigorous IV fluid therapy** (see Chap. 9) should prepare the patient for operation as quickly as possible.

   c. **Proctoscopy** must be performed; a barium enema may be indicated (see **C.6**). Regular enemas for the purpose of evacuating the bowel are not indicated; they only confuse the x-ray picture.

   d. **Broad-spectrum antibiotics** should be administered systemically and, if indicated, continued after the operation. Although oral antibiotic bowel preparation (see Chap. 14) is always preferable if the colon is to be resected electively, it is not applicable in the acute preoperative preparation of patients with obstruction.

3. Since **most obstructing colon lesions** are in the descending or sigmoid colon, standard operative principles for colon obstruction apply to this usual location. A decompressive proximal loop colostomy, if used, should be placed as close as possible to the obstruction but must not compromise future definitive resection.

4. **Resection of necrotic bowel** is mandatory. Adequate abdominal exploration must be made to ensure that all obstructed bowel not resected is viable. If resection is necessary, or if a noninflammatory descending or sigmoid colon obstruction is present and the patient can tolerate an extended procedure, colonic resection with end colostomy and distal mucous fistula exteriorization is advisable. Primary anastomosis of unprepared bowel or in the presence of peritonitis should be avoided.

5. **Diverticular abscess with obstruction** poses some additional operative considerations. Emergency proximal transverse colostomy with abscess drainage leaves a column of stool in the left colon that may continue to contaminate the abdominal cavity during the early postoperative days; election of a sigmoid loop colostomy may be preferable for this reason. Alternatively, when exteriorization of a sigmoid diverticular mass is technically feasible, it may be resected with creation of an end colostomy and distal mucus fistula.

6. **Sigmoid volvulus** usually can be reduced by careful entry of a sigmoidoscope (see Fig. 25-22) or a rectal tube into the twisted loop. Be prepared for a sudden, copious passage of flatus and feces. The 60-cm flexible sigmoidoscope can be

used; its advantages are that it may reduce a higher sigmoid volvulus, air can be more readily evacuated from the reduced loop, and the mucosa can be inspected for viability. If sigmoidoscopic reduction is successful, a rectal tube is left in place, secured to the perianal skin, and the patient then may be prepared for elective resection of the redundant loop. Failure of sigmoidoscopic reduction often means that strangulation of the twisted loop has occurred. If reduction is not successful, or if volvulus promptly recurs, sigmoid resection should be carried out at once.

7. **Cecal volvulus** always should be managed by operation. Gangrenous cecum requires resection. If it is not gangrenous, after reduction, cecopexy by broad fixation of the mobile cecum with sutures to the abdominal wall is preferable to cecostomy. Unprepared bowel is not entered, and postoperative infections and persistent fistulas are avoided.

8. **Other ascending colon obstructions** usually are resected as a right hemicolectomy with a primary ileotransverse colon anastomosis. In the presence of peritonitis, a temporary ileostomy and distal mucus fistula are preferable to anastamosis.

9. The **mortality** of procedures for colon obstruction relates to the cause of obstruction and the age of the patient. The overall operative mortality for neoplastic colon obstruction is 10–15%. The operative mortality figure for obstructing diverticulitis is about 1% but varies upward with increasing age and associated complications. The mortality for a successfully deflated sigmoid volvulus is 15%; when followed by elective resection, there is an additional mortality of 8–15%, whereas emergency sigmoid resection for this disease carries a 45–50% mortality. Old age is the major factor influencing these mortality figures. Despite a generally younger age group, the operative mortality for cecal volvulus is about 10%, largely because of delays in diagnosis until gangrenous bowel has supervened.

IV. Strangulation obstruction

A. Causes

1. Strangulation involves the small bowel more often than the colon and is simply an **advanced stage of mechanical obstruction** in which vascular compromise due to constriction by a hernial ring or torsion of the bowel on its vascular pedicle has produced or is producing gangrene. Usually, the type of obstruction is a closed loop.

2. The two most common causes are **adhesions** with internal herniation and incarceration of bowel in an **external hernia.** Cecal and sigmoid volvulus are other causes.

3. Two forms of mechanical obstruction that are particularly unlikely to lead to strangulation are those associated with abdominal carcinomatosis and radiation enteritis.

B. Pathophysiology

1. The disordered physiology seen in strangulation obstruction is superimposed on that of mechanical obstruction.

2. **Bacteria** multiply rapidly in the lumen of obstructed bowel but they and their toxins do not transmigrate into the peritoneal cavity until marked distension or vascular occlusion has produced ischemic mural changes and effectively removed the mucosal barrier. This progression also leads to **plasma and blood loss** into bowel lumen and the peritoneal cavity, functionally displaced as a third space.

3. The primary cause of toxicity and shock in strangulation obstruction is related to the presence of coliform **endotoxins** in the intestinal fluid that traverse the bowel wall and are readily absorbed from the peritoneal cavity. These

endotoxins have primary deleterious effects on both the pulmonary and peripheral vasculature. Exotoxins, principally clostridial alpha-toxin, also enter the bloodstream and can produce septic shock.

4. Endotoxemia and sepsis are more rapid and more pronounced with long segments of strangulated bowel.

5. Protection against the lethal effects of strangulation has been obtained experimentally in animals by all of the following:

    a. Preventing access to the body of the contents of the strangulated loop by placing it in a plastic bag.

    b. Pretreating the intestinal lumen with antibiotics. Confirmation of the importance of bacteria in producing the lethal effects of strangulation is provided by the fact that strangulation in germ-free animals is not fatal.

    c. Simultaneous IV and intraperitoneal instillation of broad-spectrum antibiotics increases animal survival despite leaving ischemic bowel in place.

6. With strangulation obstruction, the shock state that develops and deepens is **mixed septic and hypovolemic shock.**

C. Clinical complex and diagnosis

1. Clinical **signs and symptoms** in strangulation obstruction are initially those of the underlying mechanical obstruction (colic, distention, vomiting), but there is rapid progression and early deterioration in the clinical state.

2. Early **differentiation of simple obstruction from strangulation obstruction** is often difficult. Cramps may be replaced by severe, constant pain. Localized abdominal **tenderness** is prominent; a palpable abdominal **mass** or irreducible and tender external hernia may be present. **Vomiting** occurs early and tends to be severe and persistent. **Tachycardia** and **leukocytosis** usually are present and, less frequently, **fever.** It is important to remember that these classic signs are less prominent or may be absent in the elderly patient. Furthermore, no one sign is of more value than another in distinguishing strangulation from simple obstruction.

3. Determinations of serum phosphate, lactic dehydrogenase, and alkaline phosphatase may show elevations, particularly with ischemic bowel, but they are not specific and reliable. Serum amylase and blood ammonia may both be elevated but are even less reliable in confirming the presence of strangulation.

4. **X-rays** of the abdomen do not reliably differentiate strangulation obstruction from simple obstruction. Other than the strangulated segment of a colonic volvulus, most strangulated loops do not become filled with gas. A radiographic abnormality peculiar to strangulated small-bowel obstruction in some cases is a bubbly appearance of fecal debris in the ascending colon.

D. Treatment

1. Strangulation obstruction is a **surgical emergency.**

2. **Preoperative treatment** involves vigorous and rapid IV fluid resuscitation, whole blood transfusion as necessary, nasogastric tube suction, and IV administration of large doses of broad-spectrum antibiotics.

3. **Inadequate blood replacement** is a prime cause of death in patients with strangulation. The short interval spent preparing the patient preoperatively with transfusion is rewarded with a lowered operative mortality.

4. Several **operative principles** deserve emphasis and are unique to this particular type of obstruction:

    a. All necrotic bowel must be resected.

    b. A twisted vascular pedicle with gangrenous bowel is first isolated and its vessels ligated prior to untwisting the pedicle. This avoids sudden release of bacteria and toxins into the portal circulation, which can produce a prompt severe metabolic acidosis and endotoxemia.

c. In the presence of peritonitis and an initially precarious clinical state, the simplest possible operative procedure should be carried out. Primary anastomosis after resection should be done only in small-bowel strangulation; temporary exteriorization of bowel ends almost always is more prudent in colonic strangulation and in some cases of small-bowel strangulation.

d. Occasionally, bowel viability is questionable, and the bowel has no motility. The involved bowel can be wrapped in moist packs for 10–15 min and reevaluated; if there is no improvement, it should be resected.

e. Peritoneal bacterial contamination must be presumed in these patients. After resection or exteriorization, intraoperative irrigation of the peritoneal cavity with large volumes of saline and a final rinse of antibiotic-saline solution is advisable to debride and dilute any remaining bacteria-laden exudate. The following is our antibiotic solution formula: kanamycin, 500 mg.; bacitracin, 50,000 units; normal saline, qs to 500 ml.

5. Operative mortality in strangulation obstruction is dependent on the extent of gangrenous bowel; 35% is an overall figure. This risk is decreased with early operation and the free use of broad-spectrum antibiotics. The morbidity in operations for this condition ranges from 20 to 60%; wound infection and pulmonary and urinary complications are the most common sequelae.

V. Paralytic ileus

A. Causes

1. Ileus is **ineffective or nonpropulsive bowel motility.** The intrinsic myogenic contractility of the bowel wall is unimpaired, but an imbalance develops in coordination by parasympathetic and sympathetic nerves. The apparent mechanism is reflex splanchnic-sympathetic inhibitory overstimulation. Alternatively, bowel distention with intramural edema leading to intrinsic paralysis is seen in the exhaustive stage of mechanical obstruction and in some postoperative situations.

2. A metabolic cause of paralytic ileus is intracellular hypokalemia, developed in a variety of conditions, in which acetylcholine synthesis and its neuromuscular effects are impaired.

3. Other causes of paralytic ileus are listed in Table 7-1.

B. Pathophysiology

1. Nonpropulsive bowel motility may involve the small bowel and colon, together or separately.

2. Gas derived from swallowed air accumulates in the involved segments of bowel, producing marked, early distention.

3. Fluid also accumulates in the involved bowel because of failure of normal absorptive mechanisms. While significant volumes of fluid may be sequestered in such a third space, the potential loss of extracellular fluid volume is not as great as in mechanical obstruction. Peculiarly, very little fluid collects in the distended segment in colonic ileus.

4. The accumulation of gas and fluid causes only a small rise in intraluminal pressure. Lymphatic drainage may be slightly compromised, so that some edema may accumulate in the bowel wall, but much less than in patients with mechanical obstruction. Colonic ileus is peculiar in this regard: segmental colonic distention may be considerable, although little bowel-wall edema develops. The distended cecum may threaten to rupture at diameters greater than 10 cm, literally splitting the longitudinal teniae coli, despite the relatively low pressure in the lumen.

C. Clinical complex and diagnosis

1. **Progressive abdominal distention** usually develops over 2–3 days. The abdomen may be tense and tympanitic.

2. **Anorexia** and **nausea** are common. Vomiting occurs as a result of ingestion of food or fluid but frequently does not occur if the patient does not eat or drink.

3. **Obstipation** is rarely complete, and small amounts of flatus may be passed throughout the period of ileus.

4. **Pain** is dull, diffuse, and related to the degree of distention. Colic sometimes is present early in paralytic ileus and reappears as the ileus clears and progressive peristalsis is resumed, but is never as prominent a part of the clinical history as in mechanical obstruction.

5. Peristalsis is depressed but does not completely disappear; bowel sounds may be infrequent. High-pitched and tinkling sounds are characteristic of paralytic ileus; the quality of bowel sounds is not a reliable criterion in differentiating paralytic ileus from mechanical obstruction.

6. Laboratory studies usually reflect only dehydration and are not particularly helpful in differentiating paralytic ileus from mechanical obstruction.

7. Abdominal flat and upright **x-rays** typically demonstrate multiple, dilated, fluid-filled small-bowel loops with some gas present throughout the colon. In colonic ileus, massive distention of colon segments is apparent, usually with an abrupt cutoff, but with some gas in the distal colon.

8. A **barium enema** may be indicated in cases of colonic ileus; it will show no obstruction distal to the dilated colon segment and should be terminated promptly as barium enters the dilated segment.

D. Treatment

1. Therapy first should be directed to the underlying cause of the ileus.

2. **Treatment of the ileus** itself involves:

   a. Provision of IV fluids and correction of any imbalances.

   b. Prevention of further distention by passage of a nasogastric tube. A long intestinal tube usually will not leave the stomach, so that long-tube therapy is not effective in paralytic ileus.

3. The best adjunctive therapy would appear to be observation and the passage of time. A number of pharmacological adjuncts have been used, directed toward reduction of splanchnic-sympathetic inhibition and parasympathetic motility stimulation. These agents are still undergoing clinical study and cannot be recommended for routine use at the present time.

4. Treatment of **colonic ileus** deserves special mention because of the threat of right-colon or cecal rupture. Such patients should initially be treated nonoperatively; frequent examination of the abdomen and serial abdominal x-rays every 12–24 hr serve to detect progressive distention and the threat of rupture. Laparotomy should be undertaken with failure to improve over a maximum of 72 hr, together with a cecal diameter greater than 10 cm or the development of right lower quadrant tenderness or spasm. A cecostomy can be performed, but right hemicolectomy and exteriorization should be undertaken if extensive necrosis or longitudinal splitting of the teniae coli has extended up the ascending colon.

5. The **mortality** of small-bowel ileus that is not treated surgically is minimal and

related much more to the underlying cause than to the ileus per se. Conversely, the overall mortality of colonic ileus in 25%; in patients who require surgical decompression, it is 40%.

VI. Acute intestinal vascular occlusion

A. Causes

1. Mesenteric vascular occlusion produces a functional obstruction to the normal flow of bowel content (e.g., ileus) rather than a mechanical obstruction.

2. A common cause of intestinal infarction is **nonocclusive ischemia,** which occurs in 30–50% of patients. Hypovolemia is a prominent factor, and reduced mesenteric blood flow is superimposed on mesenteric atherosclerosis. Many of these patients have heart disease, and a precipitating event usually produces the acute perfusion defect: an arrhythmia, an infectious process, an operation, or excess postprandial splanchnic flow requirement.

3. An equally common cause is **superior mesenteric arterial thrombosis,** which also occurs amid extensive aortic and mesenteric atherosclerosis, commonly at the origin of the superior mesenteric artery. It may be preceded by intermittent symptoms of ischemia but may not have an apparent precipitating cause.

4. A **superior mesenteric arterial embolus** produces acute infarction in 15% of patients. The thrombus usually arises from an intramural ulcerated plaque; less often after a myocardial infarction or from a dilated, fibrillating atrium associated with rheumatic heart disease. The embolus can lodge anywhere in the mesenteric arterial tree but most commonly lodges in the middle colic artery.

5. Acute **mesenteric venous thrombosis** is the least common cause, occurring in 10% of affected patients. It may be associated with polycythemia or another hypercoagulable state, carcinoma and tumor compression, sepsis, direct injury, or the use of contraceptive pills, but most often is spontaneous and agnogenic.

6. **Ischemic colitis** frequently is acute but seldom progresses to the stage of gangrenous bowel. The inferior rather than the superior mesenteric arterial tree is involved. The cause is mesenteric atherosclerosis; ischemic colitis may follow operative ligation of the inferior mesenteric artery.

B. Pathophysiology

1. The histological consequence of arterial or venous occlusion is the same: **hemorrhagic necrosis.** Hemorrhage occurs in the submucosa; the mucosa is ulcerated; the process may progress to transmural gangrene and bowel perforation. Bloody suffusion of the bowel wall and mesentery is more marked with venous thrombosis. If perfusion is restored, the changes may relent, or bowel-wall scarring and stricture formation may follow.

2. Initial hyperperistalsis is followed by marked bowel distention and disordered motility, then usually by decreased distensibility of the compromised segment.

3. Mucosal barrier disruption leads to bacterial and toxin transmigration into the peritoneal cavity, plasma volume losses into the intestinal lumen and abdominal cavity, peritonitis, dehydration, and, eventually, to septic-hypovolemic shock.

C. Clinical complex and diagnosis

1. A wide spectrum of signs and symptoms develop that are more a reflection of the extent of ischemic damage than of the cause or location of the ischemia.

2. **Pain** is the outstanding symptom and is present in almost all patients. Although it may be colicky and periumbilical at onset, it soon becomes severe, continuous, and diffuse. Numerous associated symptoms and signs may be

present, but they usually are so unimpressive that the most characteristic picture of bowel ischemia initially is a **lack of significant abnormalities even when pain is unbearable.**

3. **Abdominal distention** may develop early and eventually becomes prominent in the majority of patients.

4. **Gastrointestinal bleeding** (usually melena with diarrhea) occurs often but seldom is gross unless colonic ischemia is present.

5. Peritonitis with diffuse direct and percussion **tenderness** supervenes, as do severe **dehydration** and **shock.**

6. **Laboratory determinations** consistently show an elevated hematocrit and white blood count, reflecting dehydration, ischemia, and sepsis. Elevations in liver enzymes, blood urea nitrogen, amylase, phosphate, and intestinal alkaline phosphatase have been recorded in many patients but not reliably enough to be diagnostic.

7. Plain abdominal x-rays usually are equally nonspecific and demonstrate only **paralytic ileus.** Eventually, intestinal intramural gas or gas in the portal venous circulation may be seen, indicating a late stage with gangrenous bowel.

8. **Proctoscopy** with rectal biopsy may be diagnostic if ischemia arises from the inferior mesenteric circulation. A barium enema may delineate the nature and severity of colonic ischemia, typically showing the "thumb printing" of submucosal edema and hemorrhage, but it should be performed most carefully. Barium studies in small-bowel ischemia are not helpful in the acute stage.

9. **Arteriography** is the most important diagnostic step and should be conducted **very early** when gut ischemia is suspected. The examination begins with an aortic flush to demonstrate aortic atherosclerosis and the patency of the superior and inferior mesenteric arterial orifices. Thereafter, selective arterial catheterization is performed to determine the patency of proximal and distal smaller vessels, evidence of spasm, degree of acute or chronic arterial collaterals, extravasation of dye into the bowel lumen, and delay or inability to opacify the portal venous system. **Arteriography must precede** gastrointestinal barium studies.

10. A final diagnostic maneuver when mesenteric infarction is suspected is a **peritoneal tap.** Insertion of a peritoneal catheter carefully through the lower midline will reveal malodorous serosanguinous fluid if bowel gangrene is present. A Gram stain, culture, white cell count, and amylase determination should be obtained.

D. Treatment

1. Several vascular occlusive diseases are **surgical emergencies.** In these patients, arteriography is not delayed until hemodynamic stability is obtained. Laparotomy for suspected acutely gangrenous bowel must be undertaken promptly.

2. The usual preoperative measures for the management of intestinal obstruction are initiated and include vigorous crystalloid and plasma fluid resuscitation, nasogastric suction, urinary and central venous catheterization, and IV administration of broad-spectrum antibiotics.

3. The operative management of **acute arterial thrombosis** is immediate thromboendarterectomy or arterial bypass with a venous or prosthetic graft. Bowel resection should be limited; intraluminal inspection of resected bowel margins for mucosal hemorrhage and Doppler ultrasonography of mesenteric vessels at resection edges are useful adjunctive measures in assessing the need for addi-

tional resection. Often, a second-look operation and reassessment at 12–48 hr should be planned. The mortality is particularly high, probably over 60% with this disease, largely because the patients have diffuse systemic atherosclerosis.

4. The operative management of **acute arterial embolus** is immediate embolectomy without bowel resection. An appraisal of bowel viability and a decision to reoperate for a second look are made at the initial operation. Bowel with progressive ischemia, or gangrene, must be resected. The operative mortality depends on the promptness of diagnosis but with early surgical correction should be below 30%.

5. Operative management of **nonocclusive mesenteric ischemia** should be delayed for 8–12 hr, unless peritonitis is present, while volume resuscitation and hemodynamic stability is obtained. When the selective mesenteric arteriogram demonstrates vasoconstriction without occlusion, the arterial catheter can be left in place for vasodilator infusion. Most clinical experience has been obtained with papaverine: a test dose of 45 mg is given over 15 min, a positive vasodilatory response is seen on a repeat arteriogram, and therapeutic infusion is continued at 30–60 mg/hr for 8–16 hr. This permits a therapeutic interval for stabilization; but operation should be undertaken regardless of the response to early treatment to assure absence of segmental bowel infarction and to preclude overlooking other acute inflammatory processes. The mortality of this disease is high, due both to failure of diagnosis and to the postoperative effects of the underlying systemic disease. Survival through the acute period carries a good late prognosis, though resection of scarred and strictured bowel may be required several weeks later.

6. Operative management of **acute mesenteric venous thrombosis** is immediate laparotomy with resection of the involved bowel and its mesentery. The extent of bowel involvement can easily be determined intraoperatively. Venous thrombectomy is usually impractical because of small-vein involvement. Heparin anticoagulation or administration of dextran should begin preoperatively; anticoagulants are continued for several months after operation. Prompt diagnosis and treatment of this disease have reduced its mortality to 20%, although the recurrence rate remains at 25%.

7. A final caution regarding the **postoperative nutritional prognosis** should be emphasized in the operative management of all diseases involving gangrenous bowel. In a patient with a massive bowel infarction, resection of up to 75% of the small bowel is tolerable if the ileocecal valve remains; a total colectomy with ileoproctostomy also is well tolerated. But beyond these extremes in resection, despite survival through the early postoperative interval, the patient will always be a nutritional cripple, dependent on parenteral alimentation.

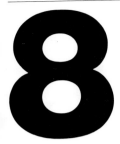

Preoperative and Postoperative Care

Routine Orders

Written orders afford the surgeon a means of communicating with other members of the surgical team—nurses, physical therapists, technicians. As much care should be taken with the formulation of orders as with the preparation of any legal document.

I. **Admission orders: elective.** Writing and reviewing orders in a routine manner will prevent important therapeutic measures from being overlooked. The same sequence should be followed for each patient each day, whether preoperatively or postoperatively.

    A. **Admit to.** Give room number, ward, intensive care unit, etc., and responsible attending physician or service.

    B. **Diagnosis and condition.** A record of the patient's diagnosis on admission will provide a basis for the hospital staff to integrate the orders that follow with their own experience in formulating plans for the overall management of an individual patient.

    C. **General measures** include **activity allowed, diet,** and **fluid restrictions** if any.

        1. Maximal activity within the limits of the patient's condition should be encouraged. Inactivity leads to complications such as venous thromboembolism, atelectasis, pneumonia, and muscle atrophy.

        2. Consideration of an appropriate diet will take into account the patient's **dentition;** those without teeth should be given a mechanical soft diet. Patients with an **oral tumor** or **obstructing esophageal lesion** may tolerate only a liquid diet. A fat-free diet for patients with **biliary tract disease** and a bland diet for **peptic ulcer patients** are almost routine. A low-salt diet is appropriate for **hypertensive or cardiac patients** with a history of congestive heart failure. Diabetic diets are encouraged for **diabetic patients,** although hospital inactivity often will result in lower caloric requirements. Little emphasis should be placed on weight-reduction diets for surgical patients, since their anticipated hospital stay will be too brief to result in any real benefit. Better results may be obtained by consultation with a dietician prior to discharge.

        Chronic illness may cause loss of weight and appetite. Such patients need frequent small feedings of high-caloric food with supplements such as milk shakes. If the appetite is so poor that the patient refuses food, a small tube should be passed through the nose into the stomach and liquified high-calorie foods dripped in continuously (see Chap. 10). In some cases, IV hyperalimentation may be necessary to supplement oral intake to ensure that the patient is in positive nitrogen balance (see Chap. 10).

        The water-soluble B and C vitamins are especially indicated in the debilitated patient prior to operation. B vitamins are essential in intermediary metabolism of carbohydrates. Vitamin C (ascorbic acid) aids in wound healing.

There are no great body stores of B or C vitamins, and they need to be provided daily. Vitamin K is indicated preoperatively in jaundiced patients with prolonged prothrombin time.

D. General observations include vital signs (temperature, pulse, respirations, and blood pressure), neurological status checks, weighing, intake and output, and urine sugar and acetone levels. Measurements should be taken as frequently as necessary; otherwise healthy patients need not have vital signs checked more than once daily. If fever is present, recording temperatures more often than every 4 hr is of no value.

E. Precautions and preventive measures. Detail here any allergy, isolation technique, seizure precautions, skin, eye, and mouth care, frequent turning, restraints, etc. Remember that many elderly patients, those at any age who smoke cigarettes, and patients with chronic bronchitis or emphysema are at increased risk for general anesthesia. Postural drainage, mucolytic agents, and when indicated by positive sputum cultures, appropriate antibiotics, should be ordered to help improve pulmonary function prior to the operation (see Chap. 12).

F. Equipment needed at the bedside and care of tubes, drains, etc. Anticipate a need for Gomco suction, wall suction devices, oxygen, electrocardiograph or other monitoring devices, respirators, etc.

G. Medications

   1. IV fluids should be considered first. Fluid orders must be revised at least daily to conform to patient requirements (see Chap. 9).

   2. The use of **analgesics** should be given careful consideration. Particularly in patients admitted with acute surgical illness, pain may be an important diagnostic clue. As a general rule: **No medication should be given for relief of pain until a diagnosis has been established and a decision made whether or not to operate.**

   3. The use of appropriate antibiotics, cardiac drugs, diuretics, etc., including the patient's current medications, must be considered. Although routine prn orders to ensure adequate sleep and to alleviate constipation and headache may be criticized, individualized orders for these common problems may save you or your colleague a telephone call late at night.

H. Laboratory testing. Routine preoperative laboratory testing, if not already done, should be promptly ordered on admission. Minimal tests needed for elective major surgery are a complete blood count (CBC), sickle cell preparation (in black patients), serum electrolytes, blood urea nitrogen (BUN) or creatinine, glucose, total protein, albumin, calcium, prothrombin time, partial thromboplastin time, platelet count, serology, chest x-ray, electrocardiogram (ECG), and urinalysis. Add a liver profile and amylase level for patients with biliary disease or malignancy and pulmonary function studies for heavy smokers and all thoracic surgery patients. When ordering contrast studies, consider the need for thyroid function tests before administering any iodinated material. Angiography should be performed before barium is given. Consider doing an intravenous pyelogram (IVP) before lower gastrointestinal x-rays, and oral cholecystogram before upper gastrointestinal studies if indicated.

I. Conditions for which a physician should be notified. This information will not only alert the hospital staff to potential problems, but will also alleviate any indecision about when to call a physician if the patient is doing poorly.

II. EMERGENCY ADMISSION FOR URGENT OPERATION. These patients are extremely ill, with possibly life-threatening problems. The diagnosis may or may not be obvious.

A. Diet. Any patient who is a candidate for an emergency operation should have nothing by mouth (NPO); this includes water and oral drugs.

B. **Medications.** The special problem in this group of patients is usually pain. Since pain may be the only clue to diagnosis and the only symptom that can be followed to determine whether the patient's condition is getting better or worse, it should not be masked by giving narcotics or other anodynes. Again, **no medication should be given for relief of pain until a diagnosis has been established and a decision has been made whether or not to operate.**

C. **Fluid therapy.** Almost all the patients in this group will require IV fluid therapy to correct dehydration and electrolyte imbalance (see Chap. 9).

D. **Antibiotics** should be given preoperatively to septic patients or when surgery involving a hollow viscus is contemplated (see Chap. 14).

III. **Elective operation.** Preoperative orders are written 1 day prior to operation.

A. **Proposed procedure and anesthetic.** This will enable the nursing staff and ancillary personnel to begin preoperative teaching and orientation, answer questions, etc.

B. **Consent.** A signed consent form should be obtained by the surgeon on the day before operation.

C. **Blood components to be cross-matched.** Knowledge of what is required will allow the hospital staff to assist in getting proper specimens to the blood bank.

D. **Shower and preparation of the operative site.** Ideally, an antiseptic soap (Hibiclens or Betadine) has been used for at least 1 wk prior to admission; regardless, a complete bath should be taken the night before the operation, and the patient should also have a shampoo. Skin is shaved the morning of the operation, or depilatory cream is used.

E. **Nasogastric tube, Foley catheter, and IV fluids.** Overnight nasogastric suction may be indicated prior to gastric operations. IV fluids may need to be administered to patients after mechanical bowel preparation for colonic operations or who are otherwise dehydrated. A Foley catheter may be desirable if the urine output is uncertain or lower tract obstruction is present.

F. **NPO after midnight.** Allow 6–8 hr for emptying of the stomach before operation to minimize the hazards of vomiting and aspiration. Infants may be fed clear fluid 4 hr prior to induction of anesthesia to minimize dehydration.

G. All **oral medications** that must be taken by the patient during the few hours immediately prior to operation should be changed to parenteral (IM or IV) administration.

H. **Premedication.** These orders are usually written by the anesthesiologist. However, when local anesthesia is used, the surgeon is responsible. A combination of drugs usually is used, the particular combination and dose depending on the size and condition of the patient. A healthy young adult patient weighing 150 lb or more may require IM administration of meperidine (Demerol), 100 mg; secobarbital (Seconal), 100 mg; promethazine (Phenergan), 25 mg, or diazepam (Valium), 10 mg; and atropine, 0.4 mg, a half hour before an operation under local anesthesia. Premedication should make the patient very drowsy. Reduce these doses to meperidine, 50 mg; secobarbital, 75 mg; promethazine, 25 mg, or diazepam, 10 mg; and atropine, 0.4 mg, for an adult patient weighing less than 150 lb. Reduce doses of all drugs except atropine by half after age 50. Eliminate all narcotics and sedatives in any patient with chronic respiratory or liver disease. Eliminate barbiturates in patients over age 60 and narcotics in patients over age 65. A 70-year-old, 125-lb patient may need only 0.4 mg of atropine.

Patients with a history of suppressive doses of corticosteroids (prednisone or equivalent) should be covered with hydrocortisone as hemisuccinate, 100 mg IM, at 12 midnight, on call to the operating room, with administration continued postoperatively in tapering doses. Administration of digitalis preparations should be stopped 1 day prior to cardiac procedures but continued up to and through most other procedures in patients with a definite indication for their use. Propranolol for hypertension may be tapered prior to operation but should be continued in full doses for angina pectoris.

I. Enema. The evening before operation, order an enema to empty the distal colon. On induction of general anesthesia, a patient may relax the sphincter and defecate on the operating table if the distal colon and rectum are not empty.

J. Voiding on call to the operating room will avoid embarrassment in the operating suite and obviate undue bladder distention under anesthesia.

IV. Postoperative orders. Orders for the postoperative patient follow the same general outline as those for admission. All orders must be rewritten, since no preoperative order is carried over. Orders are revised at least daily to reflect changes in the patient's condition and progress toward recovery.

A. Operation performed and type of anesthesia. The same rationale applies here as for detailing the admitting diagnosis.

B. Activity. Most patients having a general anesthetic and abdominal operation will be at bed rest during the afternoon after operation. Beginning in the evening—or certainly by the next morning—they should be up walking with assistance. Connection of tubes for IV fluids, nasogastric suction, catheters, etc., may complicate, but do not contraindicate, ambulation.

C. Vital signs will generally be taken frequently during the early postoperative period, then gradually less often. Temperature should be measured at least qid to detect postoperative fever.

D. A daily record of **intake** and **output** and of **body weight** should be kept to help decide the volume and type of fluid replacement required.

E. Care of tubes and drains. See pages 154–161.

F. Medications. IV fluid orders will need revision frequently as requirements change. Serum electrolytes, intake and output record, and body weight will reflect deficiencies or excesses. Narcotics will often be required initially: adequate doses encourage deeper breathing, cough, and movement, but administration of large doses may lead to hypoventilation, hypercapnea, atelectasis, and hypoxia. Small doses of morphine (5–7 mg) or meperidine (50–75 mg) given frequently (q2–3h) are more effective than higher doses given less often.

G. Vomiting. Nasogastric intubation and suction should be used in patients who **vomit repetitively** after an abdominal operation. Antiemetics such as prochlorperazine (Compazine) are effective in controlling short-term postanesthetic nausea. Remember that the patient who has gastric distention secondary to a plugged nasogastric tube also will vomit; antiemetic drugs will not correct this problem. Be sure of the cause of the vomiting before you treat.

H. Turn, cough, and hyperventilate. A "stir-up" regimen should be ordered every few hours in the early postoperative period. It prevents splinting of one side of the chest resulting from lying continually in one position, helps to prevent accumulation of secretions, and reduces the tendency to atelectasis. Incentive spirometry given hourly is of value in preserving functional residual volume and preventing atelectasis. The management of patients with compromised respiratory function is discussed in Chapter 12.

I. Laboratory tests. Postoperative laboratory tests should include a CBC and electrolytes, a chest x-ray after thoracotomy or after placement of central venous lines or endotracheal tubes, and a daily urinalysis while an indwelling urinary catheter is present. Other functions that were altered by the disease process should be monitored postoperatively.

J. Conditions for which a physician should be notified. Again, it is essential that the surgeon communicate his or her concern regarding changes in the patient.

The house officer's duties are frequently simplified by requesting notification of laboratory results, urine output, fever, etc.

V. Discharge orders. Ideally, these are written 24 hr in advance to allow the hospital staff adequate time to prepare for discharge. They include:

A. Date and time of discharge.

B. Discharge diagnosis.

C. Date and time of return visit.

D. Discharge medications, dosages, and amounts to be dispensed.

Preoperative and Postoperative Management of the Cardiac, Pulmonary, and Renal Systems

---

I. Cardiac system

A. Evaluation of cardiac status

1. History

a. Inquire about dyspnea, exercise tolerance, paroxysmal nocturnal dyspnea, orthopnea, peripheral edema, irregular heart beat, and chest pain.

b. Document significant past illnesses, such as congenital heart disease, rheumatic fever, myocardial infarction, atherosclerotic cerebrovascular and peripheral vascular disease, diabetes mellitus, hypertension, and autoimmune disease. Inquire about the need for a cardiac pacemaker, previous cardiac surgery, and the past or present use of diuretics, digitalis, coronary vasodilators, antihypertensives, and antiarrhythmics.

2. Physical examination. Record the heart rate and rhythm; measure blood pressure in more than one extremity. Note cyanosis, clubbing, petechiae, neck vein distention, hepatojugular reflux, and peripheral edema. Listen to the lungs for rales or wheezes. Inspect and palpate the precordium for the cardiac apex, thrusts, and thrills. Percussion of cardiac dullness reflects heart size. Auscultation permits evaluation of the first and second heart sounds, extra sounds and gallops, and murmurs. Note the quality and timing of peripheral pulses.

3. Chest x-rays. Anteroposterior chest x-rays demonstrate cardiac enlargement, pulmonary vessel distention, and pulmonary infiltrates. Lateral and oblique views permit diagnosis of individual chamber enlargement.

4. An **electrocardiogram (ECG)** detects arrhythmias, conduction defects, chamber enlargement, and myocardial ischemia. Changes due to imbalance of potassium and calcium ions may be apparent. The value of formal **stress electrocardiography** is debated; false-positive and false-negative tests are not unusual. However, nearly one half of patients who have no or only atypical cardiac symptoms, but who have an abnormal stress test, have significant coronary artery disease.

5. Blood tests. Concentrations of **hemoglobin, sodium, potassium,** and **calcium** may pertain to cardiac abnormality. **Arterial blood gas** and **pH** studies indicate the adequacy of oxygenation. Measurement of arterial and mixed venous O_2 concentrations with known O_2 intake allows estimation of right-to-left shunt. An arteriovenous O_2 content difference of greater than 5 vol % indicates a low cardiac output. Elevations of **serum glutamic-oxaloacetic transaminase (SGOT), lactic dehydrogenase (LDH)** (isoenzymes I and II), **creatine phosphokinase (CPK)** (isoenzyme MB), support a diagnosis of myocardial infarction.

6. **Hemodynamic studies. Pulse rate** and cuff **blood pressure** are helpful indicators of cardiac function. Monitoring arterial pressure with an intra-arterial line provides more accurate data and permits waveform analysis. **Central venous pressure (CVP)** and **pulmonary artery wedge pressure (PAWP)** are indicators of cardiac preload. The CVP reflects right ventricualr function; PAWP reflects left ventricular performance. In most patients, left heart function correlates well with right heart function. A CVP that exceeds PAWP by more than 5 cm H_2O indicates pulmonary artery hypertension; a PAWP exceeding CVP by more than 5 cm H_2O indicates isolated left ventricular failure. For patients with cardiac or pulmonary disease, monitoring of PAWP by a Swan-Ganz catheter provides the best indicator of left ventricular preload. **Cardiac output** can be measured at the bedside by thermodilution with an appropriate Swan-Ganz catheter.

7. **Other studies. Vectorcardiography** and **phonocardiography** provide little information of direct value to the surgical patient. **Echocardiography** may define the status of valvular disease, may detect pericardial effusion or restriction, and may measure myocardial contractile dynamics. The use of **nuclide scans** and **dynamic studies** to detect myocardial infarction and to evaluate myocardial contraction is being defined. **Cardiac catheterization** with **coronary angiography** remains the most definitive cardiac diagnostic study.

B. **Preoperative evaluation and preparation. Relative cardiac contraindications to** operation are recent myocardial infarction, uncontrolled congestive heart failure (CHF), unstable angina pectoris, intractable cardiac arrhythmias and conduction defects, and uncontrolled hypertension. Preoperative evaluation is directed to detecting and treating these conditions.

1. **Myocardial infarction. (MI)** The **excess cardiac mortality** of major operations is 25% within 3 wk of MI, 10% within 3 mo, and 5% within 6 mo. There is no excess cardiac mortality in asymptomatic patients 1 yr after MI. Only emergent and urgent operations are indicated within 3 mo; only semiurgent procedures are indicated within 6 mo. Elective operations should be postponed 6–12 mo following MI.

2. **CHF.** Treatable causes of CHF include myocardial ischemia and its sequelae, valvular disease, bacterial endocarditis, sepsis, arrhythmias, hyperthyroidism, and hypertension. These conditions should be looked for and treated appropriately. Minimal CHF in a patient with heart disease is treated first with restriction of fluid (2 liters/day) and Na (2 gm/day) and with diuretics; hydrochlorothiazide (50–100 mg/day) or furosemide (40–80 mg/day) are used most commonly. If these measures are insufficient, digitalis (digoxin, 0.125–0.5 mg/day) is indicated. *There is no place for prophylactic digitalis therapy prior to operation.* Treatment of severe CHF is discussed in **C.3.**

3. **Angina pectoris.** Anginal chest pain of any degree may reflect severe coronary artery disease. Severe disease is associated with these signs: sweating and nausea during the attack; poor response to coronary vasodilators; lack of relief by rest; increasing frequency of attacks; prolongation of pain; and ECG evidence of ischemia during the attack.

a. In the perioperative period, coronary vasodilators may be administered sublingually or as a paste. Although propranolol exerts a negative inotropic effect, it also protects the myocardium from ischemia. Indications for perioperative cessation or continuation of this drug are being defined; in general, the drug should not be stopped.

b. Patients with mild, stable angina may undergo minor elective procedures safely. Patients with severe angina or premature ventricular contractions (PVCs), those with atherosclerotic peripheral vascular disease, and those requiring major intra-abdominal or intrathoracic procedures should first undergo complete cardiac evaluation.

c. Especially risky coronary artery lesions include occlusion of the left main coronary artery, lesions high in the left anterior descending artery, and lesions in multiple vessels. Completely elective procedures should be postponed in patients with such lesions. Elective but necessary procedures may necessitate preliminary or coincident coronary artery bypass. Patients needing urgent or emergent procedures require intense perioperative management; temporary circulatory support by intra-aortic balloon counterpulsation may be necessary.

4. Arrhythmias and conduction defects. Treatment of arrhythmias is discussed in Chapter 3. Excessive operative risk is associated with more than five PVCs/min, coupled PVCs, ventricular tachycardia, PVCs occurring in the QRST complex, and a history of previous cardiac arrest. The need for elective surgery must be balanced against the nature of the arrhythmia and its response to treatment.

Patients with second- and third-degree heart block, bifascicular block, and some bradyarrhythmias require peroperative placement of a temporary cardiac pacemaker. Arrhythmogenic conditions, such as digitalis toxicity and hyperthyroidism (atrial fibrillation), must be excluded preoperatively and treated if present.

5. Hypertension. Blood pressure preferably should be returned to normal prior to elective surgery. However, if the diastolic pressure can be stabilized at 110 mm Hg or less, an operation should be safe. Diastolic pressure exceeding 110 mm Hg, or hypertension causing cardiac, neurological, renal, and ocular complications, must be stabilized prior to elective surgery. Pheochromocytoma particularly must be diagnosed and treated prior to elective operation. The acute management of hypertension is discussed in Section **C.3.b.(1).** It may or may not be desirable to discontinue antihypertensive medications preoperatively. Side effects of antihypertensive medications include K+ depletion and depletion of adrenergic amines from nerve endings. The anesthesiologist must be aware of all medications taken by the patient.

C. Operative and postoperative management

1. Patients with significant cardiac disease require close intraoperative and postoperative monitoring of the ECG, arterial pressure, PAWP, CVP, cardiac output, urine output, arterial blood gases and pH, hematocrit, potassium, and calcium. Monitoring requires that the patient be treated in an intensive care unit for the first 72 hr postoperatively.

2. Most **postoperative MIs** occur on the second or third postoperative days; serial ECGs for 3 days are in order for patients with known coronary artery disease. Chest pain may be difficult to evaluate in the postoperative period; an MI may become apparent only because of hypotension. Cardiac enzymes are difficult to interpret; the CPK should be nearly normal by the third postoperative day. Treatment of postoperative MI entails continued support and monitoring. Arrhythmias and cardiac failure are treated as they occur.

3. Cardiac failure frequently presents as hypotension or oliguria, usually due to hypovolemia in the postoperative patient. If hypotension or oliguria persist after administering fluids IV, complete evaluation of the patient is necessary. Factors affecting cardiac function are ventricular preload, afterload, myocardial contractility, and heart rate.

a. Preload. Insufficient preload (hemorrhage or gastrointestinal [GI] or "third space" fluid loss) lowers cardiac output, as does excessive preload (overinfusion of IV fluids). Measurement of CVP or, preferably, PAWP is necessary to guide fluid management. A PAWP of 10–12 cm H_2O is an ideal goal; pushing the PAWP to 15–18 cm H_2O may improve cardiac output without causing pulmonary edema. **Preload is increased** by infusing physiological saline solution. **Preload is decreased** by diuresis with furosemide (5–250 mg IV). In the absence of renal function, plasmapheresis or dialysis may be needed to decrease preload.

b. Afterload. Maintenance of cardiac output against an elevated systemic blood pressure requires an increased expenditure of work by a failing heart. In addition, peripheral vasoconstriction resulting from hypotension may impair peripheral perfusion sufficiently to produce acidosis and to release factors that further impair cardiac function.

   (1) When cardiac failure results from a **hypertensive crisis,** blood pressure can be reduced with nitroprusside (1 mg/ml by IV infusion), trimethaphan (1 mg/ml by IV infusion), diazoxide (300-mg IV bolus), alpha methyldopa (250–500 mg IV), or hydralazine (5–40 mg IV or IM). Hypertensive crisis due to pheochromocytoma can be treated with phentolamine (5–10 mg by IV injection, or 0.5 mg/min by IV infusion). Infusion of vasoconstrictors (norepinephrine, methoxamine) may be necessary if pressure falls too far following excision of the tumor or after phentolamine administration.

   (2) Cardiac failure unresponsive to other measures may respond to **afterload reduction.** Dopamine, a positive inotropic drug, has a vasodilator action at doses less than 20 μg/kg/min. If administration of dopamine proves unsuccessful, a nitroprusside infusion in addition to dopamine may be tried **cautiously.** This treatment should not be administered if PAWP is less than 18 cm H_2O, or if systolic blood pressure is less than 90 mm Hg.

c. Myocardial contractility. Maximal myocardial performance requires correction of hypoxia and acidosis. Adequate plasma and tissue levels of potassium and calcium must be maintained; administer calcium ($CaCl_2$) cautiously to patients receiving digitalis. Drugs with a positive inotropic effect include dopamine (begin infusion at 2–5 μg/kg/min), isoproterenol (begin infusion at 2–5 μg/min), and digitalis. In the absence of excessive tachycardia, the former drugs are preferred in acute situations.

d. Heart rate. The performance of the heart is most efficient at a rate of 100–120/min. Dopamine and isoproterenol may be used to increase heart rate and digitalis and propranolol, to slow it. Digitalis should never be administered when digitalis toxicity is present. The treatment of tachycardias and bradycardia is discussed in Chapter 3.

e. Mechanical assist. Intra-aortic balloon counterpulsation may be used to support the patient with intractable cardiac failure.

4. Cardiac tamponade. Pericardial restriction due to constrictive pericarditis or pericardial effusion is suggested by a decreased cardiac output with a high CVP. Jugular veins are distended, and a paradoxical pulse may be present. Echocardiography may assist in making the diagnosis. Treatment consists of pericardiocentesis or pericardectomy.

II. Pulmonary system

A. Evaluation of respiratory status

1. History. Inquire about dyspnea at rest or following minor exertion, cough, sputum production, wheezing, chest pain, and hemoptysis. Document a past history of pneumonitis, tuberculosis, fungal infection, recent upper respiratory infection, chronic lung disease, and asthma. Determine the degree of tobacco and alcohol use and previous occupational exposures to coal dust, asbestos, and silica dusts. Establish a medication history; the use of corticosteroids is especially pertinent.

2. Physical examination. Note the systemic blood pressure, pulse rate, and pulse irregularity. Look for cyanosis and clubbing of the nails. Determine the mental status. Observe the respiratory rate and respiratory effort. Examine the head and neck to rule out upper respiratory infection. Observe the chest configuration, and measure chest expansion with inspiration. Evaluate fremitus and chest tenderness by palpation. Percuss the chest to detect dullness and hyperresonance and to determine inspiratory diaphragm excursion. Auscultate the chest to hear rales, rhonchi, wheezes, and decreased breath sounds.

3. **Chest. x-rays** may demonstrate pulmonary infiltrate, granuloma, atelectasis, hyperlucency, pneumothorax, abnormalities of pulmonary vasculature, or a mass. A normal x-ray does not rule out pulmonary disease.

4. **Sputum examination.** Production of more than 30 ml of sputum/day is a sign of chronic or acute lung disease. Yellow, green, or brown sputum suggests active infection. Microscopic examination of a gram-stained specimen of infected sputum demonstrates neutrophils and organisms; acid-fast staining reveals mycobacteria. Sputum culture is indicated to identify specific organisms and to determine antibiotic sensitivities. Transtracheal aspiration yields the most representative specimen, particularly in postoperative patients.

5. **Arterial blood gases** are determined to evaluate respiratory gas exchange.

   a. **PaO_2.** The arterial partial pressure of oxygen is an indicator of how well oxygen is taken up by the blood in its passage through the lungs. PaO_2 is affected by the FIO_2, right-to-left shunting, and diffusion capacity across the alveolar-capillary membrane. Normally, PaO_2 is 70 mm Hg or greater. A PaO_2 of 60 mm Hg indicates mild respiratory failure; a PaO_2 of 50 mm Hg or less indicates severe pulmonary disease.

   b. The **oxygen saturation (O_2 Sat)** indicates the percentage of hemoglobin-binding capacity actually combined with oxygen. O_2 Sat is affected by the blood pH, red cell 2,3-DPG concentration, presence of abnormal hemoglobin molecules, and presence of competing substances such as carbon monoxide. Normally, O_2 Sat is 93% or more. An O_2 Sat of 90% indicates mild respiratory failure; an O_2 Sat of 84% or less indicates the presence of severe pulmonary disease.

   c. **$PaCO_2$.** The arterial partial pressure of CO_2 is an indicator of the adequacy of ventilation. Carbon dioxide diffuses across the alveolar-capillary membrane so readily that the $PaCO_2$ is not usually affected by shunting or by diffusion capacity. Normally, $PaCO_2$ is 38–43 mm Hg. A $PaCO_2$ of 48 mm Hg indicates mild impairment of ventilation; a $PaCO_2$ of 55 mm Hg or greater indicates severe impairment of ventilation.

   d. **Arterial blood pH (pHa)** is determined by both metabolic and respiratory factors. Normally, the pHa is 7.38–7.42.

   e. **Qs/Qt.** Right-to-left shunting may be accounted for by cardiac anomalies or by perfusion through pulmonary vessels not associated with ventilated alveoli. When FIO_2 is 1.0, Qs/Qt is derived from the equation:

   $$Qs/Qt = (CcO_2 - CaO_2) \div (CcO_2 - C\overline{v}O_2)$$

   where CaO_2 is O_2 content of arterial blood; $C\overline{v}O_2$ is O_2 content of mixed venous blood; and CcO_2 is the maximum possible O_2 content of arterial blood and is defined by the equation:

   $$CcO_2 = (1.39 \times \{Hb\} \times \%O_2 \text{ Sat}) + (0.003 \times PaO_2)$$

   where % O_2Sat is considered to be 100%; $PaO_2 = FIO_2 \times (PB - 47 \text{ mm Hg} - PaCO_2)$ PB is barometric pressure; and 47 mm Hg represents alveolar partial pressure of H_2O. A Qs/Qt of 15% or more indicates a significant ventilation-perfusion defect in the absence of a cardiac anomaly.

6. **Spirometry** The following are clinically useful measurements:

   a. The **vital capacity (VC)** is the maximum volume expired after a maximum inspiration. VC is decreased in restrictive disease but is usually normal in obstructive disease. A VC 50% or less of predicted indicates severe disease.

   b. The **forced expiratory volume (FEV)** is the maximum volume expired as forcibly as possible after a maximum inspiration. FEV equals VC in restrictive disease but is less than VC in severe obstructive disease.

   c. **FEV_1/FEV.** The percentage of FEV expired in 1 sec (FEV_1) exceeds 70% in restrictive disease but is less than 70% in obstructive disease. FEV_1/FEV is less than 40% in severe disease.

   d. **FEF25–75.** The maximum midexpiratory flow rate (mean FEF during the middle half of FVC) is usually normal in restrictive disease but is reduced in obstructive disease. An FEF25–75 less than 50% of predicted indicates severe disease.

7. **Nuclide scans.** A ventilation-perfusion scan may be used to predict the effect of pulmonary resection in the compromised patient. If the resected lung is not involved in gas exchange, its removal will not be detrimental and may improve lung function.

B. Preoperative evaluation and preparation

1. **Asymptomatic patients** can be expected to tolerate operation well. If a patient can climb two flights of stairs without difficulty, further evaluation of respiratory status prior to an abdominal operation is unnecessary.

2. **Factors predisposing** to postoperative pulmonary complications are long-term cigarette smoking, chronic obstructive lung disease, upper abdominal and thoracic procedures, acute respiratory infections, and restrictive disorders, such as obesity, neuromuscular and skeletal disease, and pulmonary fibrosis. Patients with one or more of these factors require special attention to preoperative preparation, and most of them should undergo complete spirometric and blood gas evaluation. Truly elective procedures are postponed until preparation produces maximum benefit. Then, function is reassessed, and pulmonary risk is weighed against the course of the surgical disease.

3. *No patient should be denied operation for emergent and urgent conditions because of lung disease.* The risk should be recognized, and management must be optimum.

4. All patients should **stop smoking** 2 wk prior to elective surgery.

5. Overweight patients should **lose weight,** trying to achieve ideal body weight.

6. All patients should receive **preoperative instruction** in coughing, deep breathing and the use of the incentive spirometer and other devices to be used postoperatively.

7. **Promote physical strength** by avoiding constant bed confinement preoperatively; adequate nutritional support is essential.

8. Treat **respiratory infection** prior to elective surgery. Viral infections resolve with symptomatic treatment; bacterial infections are treated with appropriate antibiotics. Ampicillin or tetracycline commonly are the first-line drugs in chronic obstructive lung disease patients.

9. Whenever possible, **outpatient** preoperative preparation should be achieved to avoid superinfection with hospital-acquired antibiotic-resistant organisms.

10. **Liquefy sputum** with adequate hydration, humidified air (steam, vaporizer, or ultrasonic nebulizer), and expectorants (glyceryl guaiacolate, potassium iodide).

11. Postural drainage and chest percussion help to clear secretions of patients producing large amounts of sputum.

12. Bronchodilators are helpful to patients with chronic obstructive lung disease. Patients with bronchospasm or asthma may benefit from the administration of bronchodilators by aerosol or intermittent positive-pressure breathing (IPPB). Corticosteroids may be necessary for patients with severe asthma and certain pulmonary fibrotic disorders.

C. Operative and postoperative management

1. Intraoperative respiratory management is largely in the hands of the anesthesiologist. Nevertheless, the surgeon should note the color of the blood and, when operating in the abdomen, be sure both diaphragms are moving.

2. The postoperative effects of major procedures done under general anesthesia include decreased total lung capacity, vital capacity, functional residual volume, and compliance. Aggressive postoperative care minimizes these effects.

    a. Administering low doses of **analgesics** at frequent intervals promotes improved respiration by controlling pain without oversedation.

    b. Frequent **change of position** (side to side, sitting) and early ambulation are beneficial.

    c. Changing the **volume of ventilation** prevents atelectasis. Maneuvers promoting deep inspiration (incentive spirometry) are more effective than IPPB.

    d. Continued effort to liquefy secretions is necessary.

    e. **Oxygen administration** should be added only when necessary. Administration of 100% oxygen promotes atelectasis by the nitrogen washout effect and may result in oxygen toxicity. Administration of oxygen to patients with chronic hypercapnia may depress respiratory drive.

3. Consider planned **ventilator support** (intermittent mandatory ventilation) over the first postoperative night for those with moderate to severe preexisting pulmonary disease, the weak and elderly, and those with acutely acquired respiratory impairment. Monitor arterial blood gases and fluid therapy closely; administration of both insufficient and excessive fluid impairs respiratory function. Respiratory failure and ventilator support are discussed in Chapter 12.

4. Patients with bronchospasm may benefit from bronchodilator therapy.

5. Massive atelectasis may require bronchoscopy for directed suctioning. Bronchoscopy results in an immediate reduction of PaO_2; this reduction must be anticipated.

III. Renal system

A. Evaluation of renal status

    1. History. Inquire about frequency and volume of urine, dysuria, nocturia, poor stream, incontinence, and hematuria. Note past history of renal disease, calculi, diabetes mellitus, hypertension, gout, oxalosis, cystinuria, atherosclerosis, and heart disease. Establish the use of diuretics and potential nephrotoxins.

    2. Physical examination is relatively unimportant in evaluating renal status. Note evidence of edema and dehydration. Acidosis may result in hyperventilation. Pericardial effusion may produce a friction rub.

    3. Urinalysis

        a. Specific gravity. Random urine samples usually have a specific gravity of 1.012–1.015. A higher specific gravity reflects dehydration or the presence of solutes, such as x-ray contrast media, glucose (each 1 gm of glucose/100 ml of urine increases specific gravity by 0.003), or mannitol. Dilute urine (specific gravity < 1.007) reflects overhydration, diuretic therapy, water intoxication, or diabetes insipidus. A fixed specific gravity of 1.010–1.014 (isosthenuria) signifies a lack of renal tubular concentrating ability and occurs in renal parenchymal disease, congenital tubular defects, and acute tubular necrosis.

b. **pH.** The normal range is 4.3–8.0, reflecting diet and acid-base balance. Aciduria may result from metabolic or respiratory acidosis, potassium depletion (paradoxical aciduria of metabolic alkalosis), starvation, or fever. Alkaline urine results from metabolic or respiratory alkalosis, certain urinary infections, and carbonic anhydrase–inhibiting diuretics.

c. **Protein.** Transitory proteinuria results from fever, cold exposure, strenuous exercise, and acute stress. Persistent proteinuria signifies renal disease. Proteinuria is the earliest sign of aminoglycoside toxicity. Proteinuria should be quantitated in a 24-hr urine collection (normal is < 250 mg/24 hr).

d. **Glucose.** Glucosuria usually signifies diabetes mellitus but may result from benign renal glucosuria, renal tubular disorders, pregnancy, and glucose infusion. Ascorbic acid, cephalosporins, salicylates, paraldehyde, and chloral hydrate alter reactions measuring reducing agents.

e. **Ketones.** Ketonuria occurs in diabetic ketoacidosis, excessive vomiting, starvation, cachexia, and following strenuous exercise and cold exposure.

f. **Bilirubin and urobilinogen.** Normally, urine contains no unconjugated bilirubin. Some urobilinogen, reabsorbed from the gut, is excreted by the kidneys (0.5–1.4 mg/24 hr). Urobilinogen excretion is increased in liver disease and hemolysis.

g. **Occult blood.** The dipstick test for occult blood is positive (abnormal) with more than 10 red blood cells/high-power field (RBC/hpf) in a spun urine sediment. Myoglobinuria and hemoglobinuria also cause a positive reaction.

h. **Urine sediment.** Examination of the spun sediment may reveal a few RBCs and white blood cells (WBCs)(<5/hpf), tubular cells, and occasional (0–1) hyaline casts/low-power field; more than this is abnormal. Tubular cells and tubular cell casts are seen with aminoglycoside toxicity and acute tubular necrosis. Bacteria are not seen in the sediment of a clean voided specimen until the concentration of bacteria exceeds 10^5/ml.

4. **BUN** concentration varies with dietary nitrogen consumption, hepatic urea production, and endogenous protein catabolism. It is increased by dehydration, gastrointestinal (GI) hemorrhage, hemolysis, corticosteroid therapy, and the tissue breakdown of trauma, shock, or sepsis.

5. **Creatinine.** The serum creatinine concentration reflects glomerular filtration. Creatinine production is related to muscle mass and, in a given individual, remains nearly constant unless muscle destruction occurs.

6. **Creatinine clearance (Clcr)** is a more exact indicator of glomerular filtration and is determined by the equation:

Clcr = (U [cr] × V) ÷ P[cr]

where U[cr] = urine creatinine concentration (mg/100 ml), P[cr] = serum creatinine concentration (mg/100 ml), and V = urine volume (ml/min). (There are 1440 min/24 hr and 120 min/2 hr.) Normal creatinine clearance is 125 ± 25 ml/min/1.73 m^2. A minimal clearance of 10 ml is necessary to maintain life without dialysis. Serum creatinine level may remain normal until the clearance is reduced by more than half.

7. **Urine concentration test.** The osmolality or specific gravity of a first-voided, morning urine specimen is a simple indicator of tubular function; specific gravity above 1.025 or osmolality more than 750 mOsm/liter implies normal function.

8. **Urine sodium concentration** is another indicator of tubular function. With dehydration, hypovolemia, low sodium intake, and following trauma, the concentration should be under 5 mEq/liter; in these circumstances, a urine sodium level of over 40 mEq/liter indicates tubular dysfunction. The validity of this test is impaired in the elderly and in patients receiving diuretics and sodium infusions. An abnormally elevated urine sodium concentration raises the possibility of hypoadrenalism.

9. **Free water clearance.** Disordered tubular function is usually the first abnormality detected in acute tubular necrosis or drug (e.g., aminoglycoside) toxicity. Free water clearance, the best test for tubular dysfunction, is abnormal up to 3 days prior to an apparent decrease in creatinine clearance or elevation of BUN or creatinine. Free water clearance is determined by the formula:

$$ClH_2O = \text{total urine output} - \text{osmolal clearance}$$

where $ClOsm = [UOsm \times V \text{ (ml/hr)}] \div POsm$. Normally, free water clearance is -25 ml/hr or **less**. With renal failure, free water clearance approaches 0 or becomes positive. The test should be performed prior to diuretic administration.

10. **An ultrasound scan** is particularly helpful in demonstrating hydronephrosis or absence of a kidney and in guiding renal needle biopsy.

11. A **radioisotope scan** gives an indication of renal blood flow, concentrating ability, and urinary obstruction.

12. **IVP.** Contrast studies may reveal renal structural abnormalities, calculus disease, or urinary tract obstruction. Infusion studies with tomography may visualize moderately to severely diseased kidneys.

13. **Arteriography** and **renal biopsy** are useful in selected cases.

B. **Preoperative evaluation and preparation.** Anephric patients, if managed carefully, tolerate operations well. Preoperative preparation should maximize renal function and is important in preventing postoperative failure.

1. **Urinary tract infection** should be treated preoperatively with appropriate antibiotics as determined by urine culture and sensitivity tests.

2. **Obstructive lesions** of the urinary tract should be removed or corrected prior to other major operations.

3. **Dehydration, hypovolemia, and electrolyte imbalance** should be corrected and adequate urine volume assured preoperatively.

4. **Metabolic acidosis,** even though compensated, should be corrected with sodium bicarbonate.

5. **Anemia** is evaluated preoperatively. A hemoglobin of 9 gm/100 ml and a hematocrit of 25% are satisfactory levels for patients with chronic renal insufficiency.

6. **Coagulation defects** in chronic renal disease patients should be identified and corrected.

7. If preoperative **hemodialysis** is required, it should be planned for the day prior to operation. The next hemodialysis, with its attendant anticoagulation and fluid shifts, can then be delayed until the second or third postoperative day.

C. Operative and postoperative management

1. The diseased kidney is unable to concentrate urine and must excrete a urine volume greater than normal to excrete metabolic end products but may be unable to excrete water and electrolytes. There is a slim margin between further renal insufficiency from underhydration and CHF due to excess salt and water. Effective management requires monitoring of body weight, intake, and output, serum electrolytes, pH, CVP, and PAWP. Measuring urine electrolyte concentrations and all measurable losses guides appropriate IV fluid therapy. Urine output and specific gravity do not reflect the state of hydration reliably.

2. Administration of an **osmotic diuretic** (e.g., mannitol) may have a protective effect on renal tubular function. Consider mannitol therapy if intraoperative hypotension is anticipated or actually occurs, if indicators of renal function (creatinine, Clcr, and ClH$_2$O) deteriorate, or if a transfusion reaction occurs. Care must be taken to prevent hypovolemia following mannitol therapy.

3. **Nephrotoxic drugs** must be administered carefully and in reduced doses to patients with impaired renal function; these agents include aminoglycoside antibiotics, cephaloridine, colistin, polymyxin B, and amphotericin B. Spot checks for urine protein are useful to detect early aminoglycoside toxicity. Drugs to avoid because of other side effects include tetracycline, nitrofurantoin, methenamine mandelate, phenylbutazone, ethacrynic acid, spironolactone, triamterene, chlorpropamide, phenformin, and probenecid. Other drugs requiring major dose modification include phenobarbital, quinidine, procainamide, methotrexate, tolbutamide, allopurinol, and digoxin.

4. **Postoperative anuria and oliguria.** A postoperative urine output of less than 25 ml/hr requires immediate evaluation. Oliguria suggests either prerenal or renal parenchymal failure; total anuria suggests vascular obstruction, cortical necrosis, or urinary tract obstruction. Acute renal failure is discussed in Chapter 11.

Anesthesia and Anesthetic Premedication

I. Local versus general anesthesia

A. The pharmacodynamic action of all anesthetic agents depresses the central nervous system (CNS) and other systems. In debilitated patients this poses a significant risk; local anesthesia often is preferable if careful attention is paid to the total dose of local anesthetic used and intravascular injection is avoided. Remember that local anesthetics also produce CNS and cardiovascular depression by intravascular injection, rapid absorption from highly vascular tissue, or rapid infiltration.

B. Inadeqate local anesthesia, on the other hand, often has to be supplemented by depressant analgesics, producing respiratory and circulatory depression. If a general anesthetic then becomes necessary to maintain respiration and circulation, the patient (and surgeon) would have been better served by the use of a well-planned general anesthetic in the first place.

C. The multitude of anesthetic agents and methods available today permits the use of general anesthesia in the vast majority of patients.

II. Choice of anesthesia

A. The patient's age, previous anesthetic experience, complicating diseases, drugs being administered for these diseases, the operation to be performed, the habits of the surgeon, and the position required for the operation must be considered in choosing anesthetic agents and technique.

B. On the basis of past experience a patient may have formulated preferences that differ from those of the anesthesiologist. A clear explanation of the reasons for the proposed choice will often lead the patient to agree to a certain technique. However, the patient's preference has to be considered.

C. The patient's emotional status is important, since psychological instability or apprehension may necessitate heavy premedication and avoidance of local or regional anesthesia.

D. A prolonged operative procedure under regional anesthesia, even with perfect pain relief, may be trying because of the discomfort of lying in one position for a long time.

E. Spinal and epidural anesthesia, in the majority of instances, is used for operations on the lower extremities, inguinal area, or lower abdomen. Recent ingestion of food, airway abnormalities, and hepatic, renal, or metabolic disease support a choice of spinal or epidural anesthesia. Contraindications are previous technical difficulties with spinal anesthesia, neurological deficits, backache, skin infections of the back, and the preoperative use of anticoagulants. Hypovolemia, severe anemia, and cardiovascular instability are lesser contraindications.

F. Postspinal (puncture) headache is due to decreased intracranial pressure following escape of cerebrospinal fluid through the dural opening after lumbar puncture. The headache is more severe in the head-up position and is more frequent in younger patients. Treatment consists of keeping the patient flat, administering analgesics, and carrying out IV hydration. The injection of 10 ml of fresh autologous blood into the peridural (extrathecal) space will seal the dural leak.

G. Epidural and caudal anesthesia are techniques that apply local anesthetics extrathecally. Indications and contraindications are essentially the same as those for spinal anesthesia.

H. Special considerations

   1. Respiratory insufficiency due to pulmonary abnormalities or neuromuscular or skeletal disorders, or central depression due to intracranial disease, drugs, or carbon dioxide retention, results in inadequate ventilation and impaired coughing and deep breathing. These patients are very susceptible to postoperative atelectasis. Narcotics are avoided in premedication because they depress alveolar minute volume, impair cough and sigh reflexes, and decrease sensitivity to carbon dioxide.

   2. Liver disease can influence the metabolism of anesthetic compounds. Acute hepatic disease is associated with a high mortality following anesthesia. Maximal improvement of liver function should be obtained prior to anesthesia. Values for serum albumin, prothrombin, sulfobromophthalein retention, and alkaline phosphatase should be minimally acceptable.

   3. Kidney failure affects excretion of anesthetic agents, acid-base balance, and water metabolism. Long-acting barbiturates, gallamine, and succinylcholine are avoided, since they all are excreted primarily by the kidney. Dialysis may restore relatively normal homeostasis preoperatively.

III. Anesthetic premedication

   A. The purpose of anesthetic premedication is to facilitate induction of, maintenance of, and recovery from anesthesia by administration of agents to:

   1. Decrease fear and anxiety.

   2. Reduce secretions in the air passages.

   3. Prevent undesirable reflexes (e.g., cardiac arrhythmias) due to:

   a. Afferent impulses from the trachea and the abdominal and thoracic cavities.

  b. Volatile agents.

  c. Succinylcholine.

4. Enhance analgesia during light anesthesia.

5. Decrease nausea and vomiting.

6. Aid in special techniques (e.g., chlorpromazine to facilitate hypothermia; diazepam for cardioversions).

B. General considerations

1. After premedication, patients should be awake but drowsy, free of anxiety, and cooperative.

2. Psychological rapport established during the preanesthetic visit will help to gain the patient's confidence and reduce the need for sedation. Frank discussion of the nature of the anesthetic, the operation, and immediate postoperative activities will help patient cooperation. Instruction, suggestion, and psychological support are important elements of preanesthetic preparation. The psychological preparation of a child and his or her parents is of utmost importance.

3. Age, sex, weight, and physical and psychological status dictate the dose of premedicants. The severely ill, aged, and debilitated patient requires fewer sedatives and analgesics.

4. In using a combination of drugs, keep each at a minimal dose to avoid depression of vital functions.

C. Effects of concomitant drug therapy

1. Potentiation (additive or synergistic effects) can be produced (e.g., barbiturates potentiate ethanol).

2. Enzyme inhibition produced by one drug can prevent metabolism of another (e.g., monoamine oxidase inhibitors prolong the action of meperidine).

3. Enzyme induction stimulation can lead to increased metabolism of another agent (e.g., phenobarbital stimulates metabolism of anticoagulants, requiring an increase in the dosage of the latter).

4. Plasma or tissue protein binding can be altered (e.g., chloral hydrate displaces coumarin from carrier protein, leading to increased anticoagulant effect).

5. Diuretics may cause a loss of potassium, producing abnormal responses to muscle relaxants or digitalis.

6. Monoamine oxidase inhibitors can cause a release of a mixture of catecholamines from nerve terminals.

7. Cessation of chronic drug therapy existing prior to anesthesia is frequently undesirable (e.g., antihypertensive agents should be maintained in order to avoid a state of hypertension). Safety lies in the knowledge that these drugs are being used.

8. Aminoglycoside antibiotics (neomycin, streptomycin, kanamycin, gentamicin) and others enhance the neuromuscular block created by nondepolarizing muscle relaxants.

9. Phenothiazine drugs potentiate opiates, cause peripheral vasodilation, and may produce severe hypotension during anesthesia.

10. Disulfiram (Antabuse) used in the treatment of alcoholism may have a synergistic depressant effect with thiopental.

D. Drugs used for premedication in adults are given in Table 8-1. Pediatric premedication is given in Table 8-2.

Table 8-1. Premedication

Trade Name	Generic Name	Dose	Administration Time (min before induction of anesthesia)	Action Desired	Side Effects and Potential Hazards
Short-acting barbiturates					
Nembutal	Pentobarbital	0.5–1.0 mg/kg IM	90–120	Sedation	Possible "excitement" if pain present; omit in patients with porphyria
Seconal	Secobarbital	0.5–1.0 mg/kg IM	90–120	Sedation	
Nonbarbiturate sedatives					
Doriden	Glutethimide	125–500 mg PO	90–120	Sedation	Tolerance and dependence
Noludar	Methyprylon	50–200 mg PO	90–120	Sedation	Habituation
Tranquilizers					
Phenergan	Promethazine	0.5 mg/kg IM	90–120	Tranquilization	Marked potentiation of narcotics and sedatives; use with caution in patients with Parkinson's disease
Valium	Diazepam	0.01–0.02 mg/kg IM	90–120	Tranquilization	
Vistaril, Atarax	Hydroxyzine	0.5–1.0 mg/kg IM	90–120	Tranquilization	
Inapsine	Droperidol	2.5–10.0 mg IM	30–60	Tranquilization	
Narcotics					
Morphine	None	0.01 mg/kg IM	45–60	Analgesia and sedation	Respiratory depression; omit in patients with respiratory disease
Demerol	Meperidine	0.5–1.0 mg/kg IM	45–60	Analgesia and sedation	
Fentanyl	Sublimaze	0.05–0.1 mg/70 kg IM	30–60	Analgesia	Muscular rigidity
Anticholinergics					
Atropine	None	0.4–0.6 mg/60 kg IM	45–60	Drying effect on airway secretions	Tachycardia; prevents reflex bradycardia
Scopolamine	None	0.4–0.6 mg/60 kg IM	45–60	Drying effect plus sedation and amnesia	
Glycopyrrolate	Robinul	0.1–0.2 mg IM	30–60	Drying effect	

Table 8-2. Pediatric Premedication

Body weight (kg)	Atropine (IM)	Meperidine (IM)	Morphine (IM)
0–10	0.1–0.2 mg	0	0
10–25	0.3–0.6 mg	20–50 mg	0
25–50	0.4–0.6 mg	0	6–10 mg

Suggested Reading

Eckenhoff, J. E., Bruce, D. L., Brunner, E. A., Holley, H. S., and Linde, H. W. Preoperative Judgments. In 1976 *Year Book of Anesthesia*. Chicago: Year Book, 1976. Pp. 117–131.

Acute Psychoses

I. General considerations

A. Preoperative psychological evaluation includes any history of previous emotional difficulties, drug ingestion, or alcoholism, as well as a mental status examination. Since many postoperative psychoses are depressive in nature and interfere with convalescence, elective operations should be postponed in cases of frank psychotic depression.

B. In psychoses the predominant behavior reflects lack of reality testing and one or more of the following:

1. Defects in consciousness, orientation, or judgment.

2. Inability to control behavior.

3. Disordered thinking.

4. Mood alteration.

C. The mental status examination includes investigation of:

1. Orientation (awareness of time, place, and person).

2. Level of consciousness (fluctuating, stable).

3. Judgment and intelligence (observed ability to manipulate numbers, words, arithmetic problems of addition and subtraction).

4. Memory (recent and early).

5. Communication (clear or distorted thinking).

6. Affect (mood is even and stable, depressive and withdrawn, or euphoric).

7. Motor changes (impulsive, aberrant discharges seemingly without provocation or withdrawn behavior).

II. Description of acute psychoses

A. There are **two categories** of psychoses: organic and functional. The functional psychoses are either affective (depressive or manic) or schizophrenic.

B. Depressive psychoses are the most frequent postoperative functional psychoses and involve the following:

1. Loss of esteem, self-depreciation, and suicidal thoughts.

2. Psychomotor changes, either retardation or agitation.

3. Affect changes, usually sadness or withdrawal.

C. **Schizophrenic disorders** include paranoid and catatonic reactions and other forms marked by:

1. **Thinking disorders:** delusions, loosened or incomprehensible associations, bizarre thoughts.

2. **Affect changes:** fear or panic, inappropriate affect.

3. **Sensory and motor changes:** visual or auditory hallucinations, bizarre and impulsive motor activity (including violence), states of autism and negativism.

D. **Organic brain syndromes** are recognized by marked or subtle deficits in cognition and awareness (delirium); deficits in orientation, memory, and intellectual functioning (acute and chronic brain syndromes); and conditions in which confusion, instability, and visual hallucinations are prominent (toxic psychosis).

III. Management of acute psychoses

A. The diagnosis and management of **organic brain syndromes** begins with the physician's awareness of mental status changes before or after operation. The diagnosis must take into account mental reactions to drugs, brain damage and aging processes, blood gas disorders, electrolyte disorders, nutritional and vitamin disorders, metabolic disease (e.g., sepsis, uremia, or hypothyroidism), acidosis, hepatotoxicity, alcoholism, ingestion of hallucinogens or amphetamines, and isolation (as in the intensive care unit syndrome).

1. Management should be aimed at eliminating the factors causing adverse mental reactions, e.g., hyponatremia, hypokalemia, uremia, hypoxia, hypercapnia, and drugs such as barbiturates and anticholinergics.

2. Postoperative psychoses are more common in the elderly than in the young. Elderly persons are more sensitive to drugs, relative malnutrition, shifts in electrolyte balance, and fluctuations in oxygenation of the cerebrum during and after an operation. Treatment should be directed to immediate search for and elimination of the offending drug, electrolyte imbalance, or cardiac imbalance that is reducing cerebral blood flow.

3. Psychological treatment of all organic syndromes should include continuous supervision in a well-lighted room, with adequate stimulation from staff and tranquilization with the lowest doses of diazepam (2–5 mg) or haloperidol (2–5 mg) that will control agitation.

4. Withdrawal reactions to opiates, alcohol, amphetamines, or hallucinogens may include delirium tremens (alcohol), convulsions (barbiturates, opiates), or paranoid states (amphetamines). If a patient manifests excitement or signs of cerebral irritability, sedate him or her with chlorpromazine, 75–100 mg IM, and continue to maintain adequate electrolyte, nutritional, and vitamin balance. Immediate psychiatric consultation is indicated.

5. The most common acute organic brain syndrome is **delirium,** characterized by obtunded consciousness and disorientation, coarse tremors, visual hallucinations, and fear. This is a medical emergency and requires an immediate search to uncover the interference with brain functioning (drug toxicity, impaired circulation, alcohol withdrawal, postsurgical state) that is causing the reaction. A diagnosis of delirium can be made early when patients complain of difficulty in concentration and thinking, soon to be followed by agitation, sleep disturbances, and frank confusion. Attendants and nurses are needed for constant supervision; use restraints only when necessary. Tranquilizers to be used for agitation include haloperidol, 2 mg tid for elderly patients, up to 5 mg tid for others. This drug is especially important for postoperative patients, since it causes the fewest hypotensive reactions.

B. The diagnosis and treatment of a **functional psychosis** begins with the finding that the mental status is clear. The patient's behavior demands immediate attention.

  1. Immediate therapy for the agitated or paranoid patient is isolation and restraint when necessary in a nonstimulating environment with continuous supervision and tranquilization with haloperidol, 2–5 mg IM q4h.

  2. Immediate therapy for a **psychotic depressive reaction** is to initiate protective care in a safe (windows screened) room, so that precautions against suicide can be enforced. Agitation can be controlled with diazepam, 5 mg q4h.

Suggested Reading

Altschule, M. D.   Postoperative psychosis. *Surg. Clin. North Am.* 49:677, 1969.

Small, S. M.   Psychological and Psychiatric Problems in Aged and High-Risk Surgical Patients. In J. Siegel and P. Chodoff (Eds.), *The Aged and High Risk Surgical Patient.* New York: Grune & Stratton, 1976.

Care of Drains and Tubes

I. Management of drains

  A. Drains are placed **prophylactically,** to prevent accumulation of fluids and to encourage the obliteration of dead space, or **therapeutically,** to promote escape of fluids that have already accumulated.

  B. Types of drains

   1. Gauze acts as a drain only as long as capillary action in the fabric can absorb fluid. As soon as gauze becomes saturated, it acts as a plug, rather than as a drain. Use gauze only under special circumstances: to pack a cavity to prevent its closure or to control diffuse oozing.

   2. Rubber is used as corrugated or flat strips or as hollow tubes (Penrose drain). A Penrose drain that has gauze within it forms a "cigarette drain." Remember that in a cigarette drain, material exits along and not through the gauze; the rubber acts as the conduit.

   3. Sump suction is used to accomplish drainage against the force of gravity. Sump drainage prevents skin damage from irritating secretions and permits accurate measurement of the volume of drainage removed. Sump drains are commercially available, but they also can be improvised with two rubber or plastic tubes tied side by side or one inside the other. The larger lumen drains the fluid to be aspirated, while the smaller lumen provides access for air, to prevent vacuum plugging of the drain. Properly placed sump drains can be used for irrigations: irrigating fluid flows through the air vent while intermittent suction continues. Sump drains are particularly advantageous in drainage of pancreatic, duodenal, jejunal, and ileal fistulas, as well as in drainage of the pancreas following trauma. One disadvantage of some sump drains is lack of pliability; pain and erosion of surrounding tissues may result. Sump drains should be fixed away from vital structures if long-term use is contemplated.

   4. Plastic tube drains made of inert Silastic are connected to closed gravity drainage (Foley bag) or to a suction apparatus (Jackson-Pratt); or they may be made of reactive plastic and attached to a suction apparatus (Hemovac, Reliavac).

C. General precautions

1. Drains act as two-way conduits. The benefits of prophylactic use of a drain must be weighed against possible ensuing infection. Careful dressing of the wound and removal of the drain as soon as possible reduce the likelihood of significant infection.

2. Because a drain permits bacterial ingress and prevents closure of a wound, it should never be brought through the operative incision.

3. A drain should always be fixed to the skin surface with sutures. If a drain has become detached from the skin surface, extreme care should be taken to refix it; otherwise, it may come out or become lost in the drained cavity.

4. A drain should not be placed through an area where fibrosis will cause impairment of function, such as across joint spaces or tendon sheaths.

5. Drains should not be placed in areas of bowel anastomosis to drain the anastomotic suture line, since this may increase anastomotic leakage.

6. A localized intraperitoneal abscess may be drained. Drainage of generalized peritonitis is usually of no benefit. However, continuous irrigation of the peritoneal cavity through multiple sump drainage may be useful in such patients. Keep in mind that drains placed into the peritoneal cavity may promote paralytic ileus or stimulate adhesions that secondarily result in mechanical bowel obstruction.

7. A drain that is too hard or stiff may cause pressure necrosis of surrounding tissues, especially one near a large blood vessel, tendon, nerve, or solid organ.

D. Removal of drains

1. A prophylactically placed drain should be removed as soon as drainage has subsided.

2. A therapeutically placed drain is kept in position until the drainage subsides. Then the drain is removed gradually—a few centimeters each day—to allow closure of the drain tract from its depth and thus prevent pocketing.

E. Use a drain whenever contaminated or infected material, blood, bile, lymph, or exudative or transudative accumulations are encountered or anticipated and are localized.

1. The drain used should be:

   a. Soft, so as not to erode the surrounding tissues.

   b. Smooth, so as not to permit fibrin to cling to it.

   c. Of a material, preferably radiopaque, that will not disintegrate and leave foreign bodies in the wound.

   d. Brought through a wound separate from the incision.

2. The stab wound that gives access to the drainage cavity should be large enough to permit free drainage.

3. The drain must be placed dependently if gravity alone is to accomplish drainage. A sump tube must be used to remove drainage "uphill," i.e., against the force of gravity.

4. The drain should be extracted straight through the abdominal wall to avoid kinking.

II. Nasogastric tubes.
Nasogastric tubes are used for aspiration of fluid or gas in the stomach and to prevent accumulation of swallowed air in the bowel. Suctioning through nasogastric tubes is one of the most important parts of the management of bowel obstruction or ileus from any cause. The tube is passed through the nose into

the nasopharynx and then down through the pharynx into the esophagus and stomach.

A. The placement of nasogastric tubes requires both skill on the physician's part and cooperation on the patient's. The patient should be advised beforehand about the purpose and the procedure. The tube is well lubricated and then advanced gently through the nostril into the nasopharynx. Then the patient is asked to swallow. With swallowing, the tube is advanced into the esophagus and then down into the stomach. Placement in the stomach is confirmed by aspiration of gastric contents or by auscultation of injected air.

B. A red rubber nasogastric tube should *not* be used. This is irritating and causes early esophagitis. At present, the Salem sump (Argyle) tube is the most widely used. This double-lumen tube has a central lumen for aspiration and a side vent for air entry. The tube may be connected to low continuous suction in cases of intestinal obstruction, but for routine use it may effectively be connected to gravity drainage (Foley bag). It should be noted that a single-lumen tube should be connected only to low intermittent suction.

C. The patency of nasogastric tubes should be checked every hour. Irrigate the tube with 30–50 ml of water, or reposition if necessary. To prevent injury, extreme care should be taken when irrigating or repositioning the tube after any kind of gastric or esophageal operation.

D. Complications

1. **Ulceration and necrosis of the nares** can be prevented by taping the tube properly to avoid any pressure over the skin, mucosa, or cartilage.

2. **Esophageal reflux, esophagitis, esophageal erosion, and stricture.** The placement of a tube through a gastroesophageal junction causes reflux of gastric contents (and bile) and may induce esophagitis, which ultimately results in stricture. The tube itself may also cause erosion of the esophageal mucosa. If erosion is superficial, it usually heals without any subsequent problem, but if the erosion is deep, it may result in stricture.

3. **Mouth breathing.** Because of the presence of tubes in a nostril, breathing through the nose is difficult, and thus the patient starts mouth breathing, which results in dry mouth and may lead to severe complications such as parotitis. Mouthwash should be given to the patient frequently.

4. The presence of nasogastric tubes **interferes with ventilation and coughing.**

5. **Loss of fluids.** Nasogastric suction may remove large amounts of fluids from the upper GI tract, resulting in depletion of chloride, potassium, and hydrogen ions. If the tube is inserted into the upper GI tract beyond the pylorus, or if there is transpyloric regurgitation of large amounts of biliary and pancreatic secretions, sodium depletion also may occur. If the patient is allowed to drink water or ingest ice chips, even in modest amounts, the resultant electrolyte loss may be increased significantly.

6. **Other complications.** The following are occasional complications of nasogastric intubation: otitis media, sinusitis, traumatic laryngitis and hoarseness; traumatic rupture of esophageal varices; knotting of the tube and inability to withdraw it; nasal bleeding from trauma to the mucous membranes during passage; pressure necrosis of the pharynx or the upper part of the esophagus opposite the cricoid cartilage; retropharyngeal or laryngeal abscesses.

III. Long intestinal tubes. Long intestinal tubes should be placed preoperatively or intraoperatively for decompression of dilated small bowel, to facilitate abdominal closure, or to splint the small bowel intraoperatively or postoperatively. Long tubes also can be used in patients with multiple recurrent episodes of obstruction or disseminated carcinomatosis.

A. There are **five types** of long intestinal tubes:

1. **Miller-Abbott.** 16 or 18 Fr double-lumen tubes with a distal balloon; one lumen is for suction, the other to fill and deflate the balloon at the distal end of the tube. The balloon is usually filled with mercury, less often with water or saline. The small suction lumen becomes plugged easily.

2. **Cantor.** 16 or 18 Fr single-lumen tube with a distal balloon; 1–2 ml of mercury is injected into the balloon. This is the best tube for long-term use. Multiple holes placed into the balloon with a 25- to 30-gauge needle will prevent overdistention with gas.

3. **Johnston.** Large, 26 Fr single-lumen tube with a steel weight at the distal end and no balloon. This is the best tube for initial decompression and short-term use.

4. **Baker.** 16 Fr double-lumen tube with a distal balloon (similar to Foley balloon concept) that can be inflated with fluid or air. The tube can be manipulated intraoperatively to decompress dilated small-bowel loops.

5. **A variety of tubes** incorporating wires or other means of manipulating the tube from outside the patient are available. They are usually single-lumen, with no balloon.

B. **Long intestinal tubes can only be passed if the bowel has peristalsis.** They cannot be passed into the small bowel in paralytic ileus or in late or complicated mechanical obstruction.

C. **Successful passage of a long intestinal tube** requires skill and effort.

1. Measure the distance from xiphoid to an earlobe; add 4 in. and note this distance from the tip of the tube.

2. A Miller-Abbott or Cantor tube (and balloon) should be well lubricated and then passed through the nose into the pharnyx. If a Cantor tube is being used, mercury can be placed in the balloon prior to placement through the nose. The tube is then passed into the stomach and advanced to the previously noted mark. If a Johnston tube is used, it is often too large to pass through the nose; if so, pass it through the mouth.

3. Progression of the tube from stomach to duodenum is helped by elevating the head of the patient's bed to 30 degrees and turning the patient to the right side. Fluoroscopy is not necessary in the routine case, but should the tube fail to advance, its position should be checked before abandoning long-tube treatment. Sometimes in this situation it is possible to place the tube in the region of the pylorus at fluoroscopy. When the tube is properly placed, the balloon of a Miller-Abbott tube is partially filled with air, mercury, or water. The remaining length of the tube is not advanced into the stomach but remains untethered outside the patient, so that peristalsis can advance it. The patient should be checked frequently to make certain that the tube is moving and that it is not plugged. Abdominal roentgenograms help to check the position of the distal tip of the tube. Once the tube passes the duodenum, it will advance rapidly to the point of obstruction. Once the tube has reached the mid–small bowel, a nasogastric tube should be inserted through the opposite nostril to aspirate gastric contents.

D. The tube is connected to **low intermittent suction** for proper decompression. Irrigation from time to time is necessary to maintain the patency of the tube.

E. **Withdrawal** of a long intestinal tube from the small bowel takes time. The tube simply cannot be pulled up all at once.

1. Withdraw about 6 in. of the tube, and fix the tube to the nose or cheek, so that this length cannot be reswallowed. After an hour or so, withdraw another 6 in. as before. When the end of the tube has been withdrawan into the stomach, it can be removed completely.

2. Once the tube has been withdrawn so that the bag is in the pharynx, it is desirable to grasp the bag with a hemostat and withdraw it through the mouth. The tube may be cut above the bag. When the bag contains a large amount of mercury or gas, considerable discomfort will result from pulling it forcefully out through the nose.

3. If the tip of the tube has passed the ileocecal valve, or if there is undue difficulty in removing the tube, cut the tube at the nose and allow it to pass per rectum. Operative removal of a long tube rarely is necessary.

F. Complications. Besides the complications associated with nasogastric tubes, long intestinal tubes have some unique complications.

1. Gaseous distention of the balloon is seen in long tubes with closed balloons, such as the Cantor tube. Diffusion of intestinal gas into the balloon causes the distention, making it difficult to remove. Rarely, bowel obstruction may occur, and laparotomy may be necessary. Multiple punctures with a small (21-gauge) needle in the proximal part of the balloon will prevent this complication.

2. Rupture of the balloon by irrigation through the lumen of the balloon rather than the suction lumen, or by the use of worn-out defective balloons, may cause spillage of mercury into the lumen of the intestine. Presence of metallic mercury in the lumen of the intestine is of no great consequence, but it may take a long time to pass.

3. Instillation of fluid in the balloon lumen may cause overdistention of the balloon, which may result in rupture of the intestine.

4. Reverse intussusception may occur during removal of the tube if the balloon cannot be deflated, or the tube is withdrawn rapidly, or both.

5. Perforation or strangulation of obstructed bowel must be listed as a complication of ill-advised or careless use of a long tube. Long intestinal tubes are extremely useful in situations in which they are indicated; however, they are no substitute for careful examination and application of good judgment in managing the patient with an intestinal obstruction (see Chap. 7).

IV. The Sengstaken-Blakemore tube. The Sengstaken-Blakemore tube is a multiple-lumen tube with esophageal and gastric balloons and is used to control bleeding esophageal varices.

A. Prior to insertion of the tube, blow up the esophageal balloon to 40 mm Hg, using an anaeroid manometer, and instill 300 cc of air into the gastric balloon. Test both balloons under water for leaks.

B. Place the tip of the gastric balloon at the xiphoid and note the marking at the side of the tube at the nose. Anesthetize the patient's nasopharynx, lubricate the tube, and pass it through a nostril into the stomach 15 cm beyond the mark noted at the nose.

C. Inflate the gastric balloon with 30–40 cc of air. Take an x-ray of the upper abdomen to be sure that the gastric balloon is in the stomach. After this, inflate the gastric balloon with 250–350 cc of air. *Do not inflate the gastric balloon in the esophageal lumen, or rupture of the esophagus may occur;* this is almost always fatal. Attach the main tube to 1¼-lb traction.

D. Lavage the stomach. Insert another nasogastric tube in the upper portion of the esophagus (if there is no esophageal suction incorporated in the tube). Connect this tube to intermittent suction.

E. If bleeding continues, inflate the esophageal balloon with air to a pressure of 30–40 mm Hg.

F. Recheck pressures in both balloons frequently.

G. If respiratory distress develops, the gastric balloon and esophageal balloon are to be deflated immediately.

H. If bleeding continues from the stomach, reevaluation is necessary. If bleeding is documented to be from varices and tamponade controls it, the esophageal balloon may be deflated at the end of 24 hr, but the gastric balloon should remain inflated on ¾-lb traction for another 24 hr. Following this, the gastric balloon is taken off traction and deflated, and the Levin tube is removed. The uninflated Sengstaken-Blakemore tube remains in place for another 24 hr.

I. If bleeding recurs, reinflate the balloons.

J. If no bleeding occurs, 24 hr after deflation of the gastric and esophageal balloons, the Sengstaken-Blakemore tube may be removed a half-hour after the patient has swallowed 2 oz of mineral oil to facilitate its removal.

V. Common bile duct T tubes

A. A T tube is placed for the following reasons:

1. For **decompression** and **drainage of bile** after exploration of the common bile duct, after choledocholithotomy, or in choangitis.

2. As a **splint** for repair of a common duct stricture.

3. In the event of a retained common duct stone, irrigation or infusion of saline through the T tube may facilitate passage of the stone. If that fails, the T-tube tract may be used for removal of the stone by inserting a Dormia basket under fluoroscopic observation.

4. Occasionally, **to form an external biliary fistula** in common duct obstructions not amenable to an internal bypass.

B. Long-arm T tubes have a limb that enters the duodenum through the ampulla of Vater. These tubes may obstruct the orifice of the pancreatic duct, producing pancreatitis. They permit reflux of duodenal content into the common duct, which may result in cholangitis. They are not generally recommended.

C. Any drainage tube within the common duct encroaches on the lumen. Any deposit inside these tubes increases the degree of obstruction, first in the tube and later in the duct itself; but the common bile duct has a remarkable capacity for dilation, and complete obstruction seldom occurs.

D. In the early postoperative period, deposits of biliary mud or blood clots may be flushed out easily by gentle irrigation of the tube with saline or water. Later, this becomes more and more difficult; ultimately, blocked T tubes have to be removed. Solvents such as ether or irrigating fluids other than saline should not be used. Recently, heparin solutions and chenodeoxycholic acid have been infused through T tubes and have been reported to dissolve retained stones.

E. T tubes occasionally may slip or be pulled out of the duct during removal of a dressing or movement of the patient. To avoid this, care should be taken during operation to leave some slack in the tube intra-abdominally, and the tube should be sutured to the skin.

F. When a tube becomes partially dislocated shortly after an operation, it is usually best not to remove it immediately, since it still may provide a track for escape of bile to the outside. In distal obstruction of the common duct, there usually is a large amount of bile drainage around the tube. If signs of bile peritonitis develop, the tube must be replaced operatively.

G. A cholangiogram through the T tube must be obtained prior to removal of the T tube. If the cholangiogram is normal and T-tube drainage is only 200–250 ml/day, the T-tube bag is elevated to shoulder level. If the patient experiences no pain in 48 hr, the T tube is clamped for 24 hr prior to its removal. Prophylactic antibiotic coverage is recommended for T-tube cholangiograms. Following the cholangiogram, the T tube should be connected to closed gravity drainage for several hours.

H. When larger T tubes are used, removal is facilitated if a V-shaped piece has been cut out of the tube opposite the external limb. Occasionally, difficulty is encountered in removing a T tube from the common duct. Gentle, persistent traction is needed. In particularly difficult situations, applying traction to the tube and then setting a clamp across it at skin level and having the patient walk about results in release of the tube. The T-tube tract may be used for manipulation and removal of retained common duct stones.

VI. Chest tubes

A. Intrapleural drainage tubes are placed in patients with chest trauma and after any intrathoracic operation, regardless of its magnitude. These tubes serve to remove (1) any accumulating fluid or blood, (2) any air leakage from lungs, and (3) any air entering the pleural space through the wound.

B. A **single tube** is used after nonpulmonary thoracic operations in which there is no injury to the lung and a major air leak is not expected. Usually, a polyethylene tube is placed through an interspace below the thoracotomy wound in the midaxillary line. The skin entrance wound is made one interspace below the interspace through which the tube is inserted into the chest. This permits the patient to lie either on the back or on the opposite side without kinking the tube. The intrapleural portion of the tube is placed posterior to the lung.

C. When air leakage, together with fluid, can be anticipated, **two chest tubes** may be required. One tube is placed as described in **B.** A second tube is introduced through a separate interspace below the thoracotomy wound and placed anteriorly in the pleural space.

D. **Chest tubes are not placed after pneumonectomy,** since transudative fluid is allowed to fill the empty space. Infrequently, a chest tube connected to a water seal is placed following a pneumonectomy if empyema is anticipated.

E. **In trauma patients,** or whenever a tube must be introduced into the chest by less experienced physicians, the safest method is the sixth intercostal space midaxillary line technique (see Fig. 25-19).

F. **Chest tubes must never be left open to atmospheric pressure,** since this produces complete pneumothorax.

G. Chest tubes should be connected either to water-seal drainage or to a chest suction apparatus. Water-seal drainage is useful when only minimal fluid or air drainage is expected. Suction drainage should be used whenever significant drainage of fluid or air is expected.

H. **Water-seal drainage** involves the placement of the external end of the drainage tube 1–2 cm below the surface of water in a container placed 15 cm below the patient's chest. During inspiration (increased negative intrapleural pressure), water is drawn up from the container into the chest and drainage tube, preventing entrance of air; during expiration or during coughing, as soon as intrapleural pressure exceeds the depth of the tube below the water surface (1–2 cm), air is blown out of the tube and bubbles away. The water seal thus acts as a one-way valve, permitting escape of air from the chest.

I. **Suction drainage,** either by the classic three-bottle technique or by one of the commercial devices incorporating this principle, is used whenever significant drainage of fluid or air is expected. Usually, 15–20 cm of effective negative suction is applied to the chest tube to produce gentle bubbling of air through the negative pressure-limiting tube.

The effective pressure relationship within the pleural space in this situation cannot be determined a priori, except within certain limits. If the pleural space and all tubing contain only air, the effective intrapleural suction pressure is that set externally, usually -15 to -20 cm H_2O. But if the pleural space and all tubing are filled with fluid, the effective intrapleural suction pressure is the sum of the negative pressure set externally plus the negative siphon pressure created in the tubes between the level of the chest and the level of the suction device; usually, this is of the order of -50 to -90 cm H_2O. These two situations (air-filled tubing and fluid-filled tubing) determine the limits of effective suction. Typically, the tubes are filled with slugs of fluid separated by air, and the effective intrapleural suction pressure falls somewhere between the limits outlined.

J. Chest tubes should be kept patent by frequent stripping, particularly when they are filled with fluid. If the tube must be irrigated, it should be done under strict aseptic conditions. Constant attention to maintenance of patency in chest tubes ensures prompt expansion of a collapsed lung and minimizes late pleural complications.

K. There is no rigid schedule for the removal of tubes. They are removed when it is apparent that the lung is well expanded, there is no air leak from the wound or the lung, and less than 150 ml of fluid is aspirated in a 24-hr period. In most nonpulmonary operations, the chest tube may be pulled the first postoperative day. In typical pulmonary resections without excessive air leakage, conditions permitting removal of the chest tube may be met between the second and fourth postoperative day. When the air leak initially is large, the tube may be needed for a longer period and should be clamped for 24 hr prior to actual withdrawal of the tube, to ensure that no further accumulation of air occurs.

L. Chest tubes are removed at the end of a deep expiration. At this point, the difference between atmospheric and intrapleural pressures is the least, minimizing the risk of significant pneumothorax. A previously prepared petrolatum gauze dressing is immediately applied to the wound as the tube is removed. A firm, dry gauze dressing is placed over the petrolatum gauze dressing for 12–24 hr and strapped to the chest wall with adhesive tape.

Suggested Reading

Cerise, E. J.   Drains in Abdominal Surgery: Their Use and Abuse. In W. Ballinger and T. Drapanis (eds.), *Practice of Surgery: Current Review*. St. Louis: Mosby, 1975.

Postoperative Fever

I. General comments

A. Any postoperative elevation of body temperature more than 1° above normal should be considered significant, and appropriate diagnostic studies should be undertaken to determine the cause. Blood cultures are indicated when the cause is in question or when there are signs of sepsis.

B. A diurnal variation in body temperature of approximately 0.5°C to 1.0°C is normal. The maximal temperature occurs in the late evening.

C. An increase in body temperature may be due to infection, pyrogens, acute endocrine stimulation, increased muscle activity, dehydration, loss of normal cooling mechanisms, or lesions in the anterior hypothalamus.

D. Heat is lost from the body in four ways:

1. **Radiation** accounts for 60% of the total loss and depends on the difference in temperature between skin and surroundings.

2. **Evaporation** of water from the skin and respiratory tract results in 25% of the total resting heat loss. This is the body's most useful means of dissipating heat.

3. Convection occurs when air currents pass over the body.

4. Conduction occurs when the body is in direct contact with a cooler object. Conduction and convection represent a small part of the total heat loss.

E. The functioning of the temperature-regulating "thermostat" in the hypothalamus can be altered by pyrogens, hormones, or trauma. During general anesthesia it is temporarily paralyzed.

F. The time at which an operative or postoperative fever begins may suggest its cause.

1. Fever beginning during an operation is usually caused by preoperative sepsis or hyperthermia (see **II**).

2. In the immediate postoperative period (first 6 hr) fever is usually produced by metabolic or endocrine abnormalities (thyroid crises, adrenocortical insufficiency), prolonged hypotension with inadequate peripheral tissue perfusion, atelectasis, or a transfusion reaction. Septicemia from operative manipulation of a bacterially contaminated area may result in fever and hypotension.

3. After the first 6 hr, pulmonary abnormalities provide the most common sources of fever until about the fourth to fifth postoperative day, at which time wound infections begin to appear.

4. Fever resulting from thrombophlebitis or urinary tract infection may appear at any time, but such fever is unusual before the second or third postoperative day.

G. The age of the patient may influence the magnitude of temperature changes. In children, trivial insults may result in high fevers or hypothermia. In the elderly, there may be a diminished response to infection or pyrogens.

II. Hyperthermia during anesthesia

A. Normally, the anesthetized patient loses heat at a greater rate than he or she produces it, resulting in a fall in body temperature.

B. Heat stroke, although rare during anesthesia, still occurs in overheated operating rooms. Predisposing factors are dehydration, preexisting fever, and the use of closed anesthesia systems.

C. Malignant hyperthermia is triggered in susceptible persons by certain inhalation anesthetics, such as halothane, or skeletal muscle relaxants, such as succinyccholine. It is characterized by **tachycardia, tachypnea, unstable blood pressure, acidosis, muscle rigidity,** and **high fever.** The incidence is approximately 1/15,000 in a normal hospital population undergoing anesthesia. **Treatment** consists of stopping inhalation anesthetic and muscle relaxants, hyperventilating with oxygen, administering procainamide and dantrolene sodium IV, and initiating cooling. Metabolic acidosis and hyperkalemia must be corrected. Diuresis should be established to prevent precipitation of myoglobin in the renal tubules.

III. Pulmonary problems

A. Patients who smoke or who have chronic bronchitis, emphysema, thoracic kyphoscoliosis, obesity, or asthma are predisposed to postoperative pulmonary complications.

B. Atelectasis and pneumonitis are the more common causes of postoperative fever. Atelectasis should be suspected in any patient with fever during the first 3 postoperative days.

C. Factors that tend to increase the incidence of postoperative atelectasis are narcotics (which depress the cough reflex), prolonged postoperative immobilization, splinting from pain or constricting bandages, pulmonary congestion and edema, aspiration of foreign material, and weakness of respiratory muscles.

D. **Postoperative atelectasis** is produced by inadequate ventilation or by obstruction of the tracheobronchial tree.

1. If atelectasis is allowed to persist, bacterial pneumonitis will supervene. The presence of leukocytosis usually indicates a complicating bacterial infection.

2. Postoperative atelectasis is diagnosed by the physical findings, which appear many hours before a characteristic picture is visible on a chest x-ray.

   a. The patient with postoperative atelectasis usually has tachypnea and tachycardia.

   b. Cyanosis and tracheal shift rarely are present unless massive atelectasis has occurred.

   c. Localized moist rales and diminished breath sounds with bronchial breathing are detected, especially posteriorly toward the lung bases.

3. **The treatment** of atelectasis is aimed at removing obstructing mucus and reexpanding the involved pulmonary parenchyma before bacterial infection supervenes. Preoperative instruction in deep breathing and coughing and postoperative use of incentive spirometry, which leads to airway expansion with deep inspiration, is essential.

   a. If atelectasis does not clear rapidly with conservative management, **tracheobronchial suctioning** or **transtracheal stimulation of coughing** should be instituted.

   b. **Bronchoscopy** performed with either the rigid or fiberoptic bronchoscope is ideal for removing plugs causing atelectasis. Sodium iodide (NaI) can be added to IV solutions to loosen secretions (500 mg NaI/liter, 500–1000 mg/day).

   c. **Antibiotics** are indicated only in patients with superimposed pneumonitis.

E. **Aspiration** during induction of anesthesia or at its termination may be obvious when it occurs but may go undiagnosed until fever and respiratory complications set in. Appropriate treatment as described under Pulmonary Aspiration should be begun immediately.

IV. Postoperative urinary tract infection

A. Factors that predispose to the development of infection are urinary stasis and the use of a urethral catheter.

B. **The organisms involved** usually are gram-negative enteric bacteria.

C. **The site of infection** usually is the urinary bladder (cystitis). Not infrequently, the infection then ascends directly to the upper urinary tract (pyelitis, pyelonephritis).

D. Any patient with a postoperative fever who has undergone a genitourinary operation or who has had a urethral catheter in place should be suspected of having a urinary tract infection.

E. **Symptoms** include dysuria, chills, increased frequency of urination, and pain localizing over the area of infection (flank, suprapubic).

F. A carefully obtained midstream urine specimen examined microscopically will show the presence of many leukocytes and bacteria. A specimen that contains only bacteria without white cells should be considered contaminated.

G. Following urological instrumentation, the patient may develop septicemia, heralded by a shaking chill and a sudden temperature elevation. Blood and urine cultures usually grow gram-negative bacilli. If hypotension or shock develops, elaboration of bacterial endotoxins should be assumed and treatment started immediately (see Chap. 14).

H. Unless infection is severe, **adequate hydration** should be the only treatment until culture and sensitivity studies of the urine are available.

I. If the patient is acutely ill or if septicemia is suspected, a **broad-spectrum antibiotic** should be started IV after adequate specimens of blood and urine have been taken for culture.

V. Wound infection

A. Postoperative wound infection usually is signaled by increasing local wound pain followed by daily temperature elevations (spike pattern) similar to those observed in patients with an abscess. The patient also may have tachycardia, chills, malaise, and leukocytosis.

B. Careful inspection of the wound discloses **marked tenderness and slight redness with enteric infections.** With staphylococcal infections, there is more obvious redness, swelling, elevated skin temperature, and, often, areas of fluctuation. Patients on immunosuppressive drugs may have few or no localizing signs.

C. **The location of the operative wound** is important because tissue resistance to infection and pathogenic organisms vary. Well-vascularized areas such as the scalp are generally resistant to infection, whereas poorly vascularized areas are prone to infection. Wounds about the head and neck are apt to become infected with streptococci, while wounds associated with colonic operations may be infected with anaerobic organisms.

D. **Clostridial myonecrosis** (gas gangrene) usually occurs dramatically during the first 24 hr after operation. One of the earliest symptoms is shock with tachycardia, fever, and hypotension. Skin discoloration (yellowish brown), crepitation, and a thin, brownish, malodorous discharge are characteristic of severe clostridial infections.

E. **Streptococcal wound infections** may result in fever as early as 48–72 hr after operation. Signs of spreading erythema are usually evident.

F. **Fever** appearing after the fourth postoperative day commonly is caused by wound infection by enteric aerobic (*Escherichia coli*) and anaerobic (*Bacteroides fragilis*) organisms or by staphylococci.

G. If the patient is undergoing antibiotic therapy for another reason or is receiving corticosteroids, infection may be present within the wound without many of the usual signs of inflammation.

H. Material found within the wound should be gram-stained and both aerobic and anaerobic cultures taken.

I. **Treatment** of a wound infection requires adequate drainage, which is best provided by widely opening the operative wound. A common mistake is to open only a small portion of the wound. With enteric infections, this leads to further spread of infection and necrosis of tissue.

K. After adequate drainage, any one of several solutions can be used to control bacterial growth and promote the formation of granulation tissue. Dakin's solution (one quarter to half strength), 0.5% silver nitrate solution, or Betadine solution can be used. If *Pseudomonas* organisms are present, acetic acid solution (0.25%) is the preferred agent.

L. Systemic antibiotics are used only when there is evidence of spreading cellulitis or systemic toxicity. Antibiotics should be started after cultures and Gram stains of the infected drainage have been done.

VI. Thrombophlebitis

A. **"Third day fever"** is a syndrome of sepsis caused by infection introduced through continuous IV lines with resulting acute thrombophlebitis. The **treatment** is removal of the offending line and administration of appropriate antibiotics for septicemia if present.

B. Thrombophlebitis of the lower extremities may be a source of fever in postoperative patients. The calves should be examined for deep tenderness and a positive Homan's sign. Adequate treatment, including anticoagulation, should be begun at the time of diagnosis to prevent pulmonary complications (see Chaps. 17 and 22).

C. When suppurative thrombophlebitis is present the entire length of the infected vein should be resected.

VII. Intra-abdominal abscess

A. Spiking fevers in the postoperative period may be the first sign of an intra-abdominal abscess.

B. A **physical examination,** during which the physician looks for changes in bowel sounds, deep tenderness, or a mass, is essential. Frequent rectal examinations may reveal tenderness and a pelvic mass. In postoperative gynecological patients, examination of the vaginal cuff is important.

C. Aerobic and anaerobic blood cultures should be obtained during fever spikes and, if possible, just before an anticipated spike.

D. Xray studies may aid in localizing the abscess.

   1. Fluoroscopy of the diaphragms may suggest a subphrenic abscess if one diaphragm is paralyzed or elevated.

   2. Sonography of the upper or lower abdomen may reveal a fluid-filled mass.

   3. A **CT scan** of the abdomen may localize an abnormal collection of fluid.

   4. An upper gastrointestinal contrast study may show compression or displacement of the stomach from a subphrenic abscess.

   5. Liver-lung scans may help in localizing subphrenic collections, or the liver scan alone may demonstrate intrahepatic abscesses.

   6. Gallium scans are subject to considerable error in the diagnosis of postoperative abscesses, since gallium may be picked up in areas of recent trauma or in an operative wound. In addition, postoperative ileus retards excretion of gallium that has been secreted into the colon lumen.

VIII. Miscellaneous causes of fever

A. Blood transfusions may result in fever. Minor febrile reactions, bacterial contamination, allergic reactions, or a transfusion reaction may be the cause. (See Chap. 15 for treatment.)

B. Dehydration may cause fever, especially in children. Treatment of the fluid imbalance will correct the fever.

C. Allergic reactions to antibiotics or other drugs may be manifested by fever alone or as part of a symptom complex. Use of the drug in question should be discontinued.

IX. General treatment of fever

A. Fever increases fluid losses and energy requirements. **Energy requirements** include the following:

   1. Sensible losses (sweat) increase by approximately 250 ml/day/degree of fever.

   2. Insensible losses (evaporation from the skin and lungs) increase by 50–75 ml/day/degree.

   3. Caloric requirements increase 5–8% for each degree rise in temperature.

B. Complications of fever occur in high-risk patients (children, the elderly, cardiovascular patients). The average patient, however, tolerates variations in body temperature.

C. The primary treatment of postoperative fever consists in treating its cause and not the fever itself. In high-risk patients, additional measures should be taken to control fever.

 1. Cooling mattresses and alcohol sponge baths will lower body temperature, but chilling must be prevented.

 2. Antipyretics such as salicylates lower body temperature by increasing heat loss primarily through sweating. Phenothiazines have a direct effect on the hypothalamus and cause peripheral vasodilation, which in turn lowers body temperature.

Pulmonary Aspiration

I. Types of aspiration

A. Particulate matter. Foreign bodies, as in "cafe coronary," commonly nuts, seeds, or coins.

B. Liquid material

 1. **Nongastric fluid.** Freshwater or saltwater drownings.

 2. **Gastric contents.** Mendelson's syndrome.

II. Frequency and magnitude

A. Foreign body aspirations occur most commonly in children younger than 15 yr of age (92%).

B. Drowning ranks second as a cause of accidental death in the age group younger than 15 yr.

C. Hospital stay is increased an average of 21 days in postoperative patients who aspirate.

D. The mortality of massive gastric content aspiration is reported to be 50–90%.

E. The incidence of aspiration is 10% in routine, elective anesthesia, but it is nearly 25% in emergency anesthesia.

III. Predisposing conditions

A. States of altered neurological status in which cough and gag reflexes are depressed predispose to aspiration. They include:

 1. General anesthesia.

 2. Trauma.

 3. Alcohol intoxication.

 4. Drug overdose.

 5. Seizure disorders.

 6. Cerebrovascular accidents.

 7. Cardiopulmonary resuscitation.

B. In **tracheostomies,** the incidence of aspiration is 70%. Glottic closure is somehow interfered with by tracheostomy.

C. **Esophageal motility disorders.** These include achalasia, diffuse esophageal spasm, and hiatal hernia with reflux.

D. Presence of nasogastric tube.

E. Tube feedings.

F. **Bowel obstructions,** including ileus, mechanical obstruction, and postoperative gastric dilation.

G. Esophageal balloon tamponade.

IV. Pathogenesis and pathophysiology

A. **Particulate matter** occludes an airway; hypoventilation of the distal segment occurs, followed by segment collapse, shunting, and hypoxia.

B. **Liquid nongastric aspirate.** The tonicity of the fluid and the amount aspirated are major factors.

1. With **hypotonic fluid** the following may occur: hypervolemia, hemodilution by rapid transalveolar absorption, electrolyte concentrations incompatible with life, massive hemolysis of red cells and tissue cells, hyperkalemia, death by ventricular fibrillation.

2. With **hypertonic fluid** there may be loss of water into alveolar spaces, hypovolemia, hemoconcentration, suffocation, hypotension, shock, death.

3. With **isotonic fluid** suffocation results from an increase in the alveolar-arterial gradient.

C. **Gastric content aspiration**

1. The toxic factor is hydrochloric acid.

2. The pH of fluid is important; above pH 2.5 there will be minimal reactions except as described previously for liquid aspirate.

3. Severe reactions can be caused by 50 ml of fluid with a pH of less than 2.5.

4. The toxic reaction is equivalent to that of a chemical burn.

   a. Fluid and blood from damaged capillary lining cells pour into the lungs.

   b. Surfactant from type II alveolar cell destruction decreases.

   c. Bronchospasm may occur as a result of irritation of larger airways.

   d. Pulmonary shunting and pulmonary artery pressure increase.

   e. The most common cause of death is respiratory failure.

V. Clinical presentation. The magnitude of the response depends on the nature, volume, frequency, and distribution of the aspirate.

A. **Symptoms and physical findings**

1. Dyspnea, cough, wheezing.

2. Fever, tachycardia, hypotension, shock, cyanosis, rhonchi, and rales in the lungs.

B. **Radiological picture**

1. Bilateral diffuse infiltrates (25%).

2. Unilateral infiltrate (42%).

3. Right upper lobe involvement if the patient is supine; right lower lobe involvement if the patient is semirecumbent or sitting.

4. Radiographic abnormalities rarely develop after 24–36 hr unless infection supervenes.

C. Laboratory findings

1. Leukocytosis, without infection, 12,000–15,000 WBC/ml^3.

2. **Hypoxia**

   a. Decreased PaO_2.

   b. Normal or decreased $PaCO_2$.

   c. Decreased $(a/A)PO_2$ ratio.

VI. Bacteriology of aspiration pneumonitis

A. Predominant organisms are those of oropharyngeal secretions.

B. Anaerobic organisms outnumber aerobic by 10 to 1.

C. Infecting floras are usually complex.

1. Anaerobic bacteria are the causative organisms in 87% of the patients; most commonly involved are *Peptostreptococcus, Bacteroides melaninogenicus* and *fragilis.*

2. The aerobic bacteria are usually gram-negative bacilli and *Staphylococcus aureus.*

D. Acid pneumonitis does not mean bacterial pneumonitis. Nearly 30% of patients have negative cultures.

VII. Management

A. Restoration of respiratory gaseous exchange.

1. Tilt the patient's head down.

2. Begin immediate pharyngeal and endotracheal suctioning.

3. Bronchoscopy is useful for particulate matter aspiration but rarely useful for liquid aspiration.

4. Do not lavage the lungs with saline, bicarbonate, or corticosteroids; this will only increase the extent of damage.

5. Mechanical ventilation is necessary if the state of consciousness, respiratory rate, or level of PaO_2 demands it.

6. Positive pressure is mandatory to maximize oxygenation.

7. Bronchodilators (e.g., aminophylline) are helpful if wheezing is present.

B. Restoration of effective circulating blood volume

1. A benefit from albumin in moderate doses has been demonstrated experimentally, but there is no clinical proof of its efficacy.

2. Close monitoring of central venous pressure, hematocrit, blood pressure, and urine output will determine the amount of fluid to infuse.

3. Diuretics and digitalis are **not** indicated unless pulmonary wedge pressure is elevated.

C. IV corticosteroids should be used in large doses **only** if they are administered within **5 min** of the event of aspiration; otherwise, they are useless. Intratracheal corticosteroids are not consistently helpful and are more bother than benefit.

D. Antibiotics

1. Broad-spectrum antibiotics are **not** indicated as a part of the initial treatment.

2. Use a specific antibiotic for an incriminating Gram stain or positive culture.

3. If another site of sepsis is present, of if the condition of the patient warrants, the antibiotics of choice are oxacillin (2 gm IV q4h) and gentamicin (3–5

mg/kg IV in three divided doses). Clindamycin is an alternative if the patient is penicillin sensitive.

E. The most effective form of treatment is **prevention.** All personnel caring for patients must be made increasingly aware of the possibility of aspiration in all patients.

Suggested Reading

Bartlett, J. G., and Gorbach, S. L.   The triple threat of aspiration pneumonia. *Chest* 68:560, 1975.

Bynum, L. J., and Pierce, A. K.   Pulmonary aspiration of gastric contents. *Am. Rev. Respir. Dis.* 114:1129, 1976.

Stewardson, R. H., and Nyhus, L. M.   Pulmonary aspiration: An update. *Arch. Surg.* 112:1192, 1977.

Tuong, T., and Cameron, J. L.   Cimetidine as a preoperative medication to reduce the complications of aspiration of gastric contents. *Surgery* 87:205, 1980.

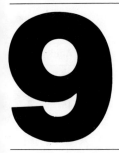

Fluid and Electrolyte Therapy

I. **Basic Physiology.** A rational and flexible approach to fluid and electrolyte therapy requires an understanding of body composition, electrolyte metabolism and acid-base balance.

A. **Body composition and compartments**

1. **Body water** varies from 45% to 80% of body weight, depending mainly on the amount of fat present (Table 9-1) and is divided into intracellular and extracellular compartments.

2. The **extracellular fluid (ECF)** is the fluid outside of cell membranes and contains most of the body sodium content. Extracellular water is divided into **interstitial** and **intravascular** compartments (Fig. 9-1). Body water and electrolytes interface with the environment through the intravascular space (blood and plasma). Maintenance of intravascular space is central to survival and should always be the first consideration in fluid and electrolyte therapy.

3. **Intracellular and extracellular ionic composition** is depicted in Figure 9-2. Of major importance are the following:

   a. **Sodium** is the major cation and osmotic component of the **extracellular** (interstitial and intravascular) compartment.

   b. **Potassium** is the major cation and osmotic component of the **intracellular** compartment.

   c. **Water** freely distributes through all body compartments (intracellular and extracellular) to bring the osmolality of all compartments into equilibrium. Therefore, measurement of osmolality in one compartment reflects osmolality in all compartments.

4. **Serum sodium concentration is the most convenient measurement of body osmolality.** An accurate approximation of plasma osmolality can be calculated from the following formula:

   $$POsm = 2 \times plasma\ (Na^+) + \frac{(glucose)}{18} + \frac{blood\ urea\ nitrogen}{2.8}$$

   a. **Elevation of serum sodium** concentration (body osmolality) means relative **lack of water.**

   b. **Depression of serum sodium** (body osmolality) means relative **excess of water.**

5. Body osmolality is usually maintained by intake and excretion of water mediated through thirst and the antidiuretic hormone (ADH) mechanism. Since hospitalized patients commonly lose direct control over their intake (nothing by mouth [NPO], nasogastric tubes, etc.), disorders of osmolality are common and frequently iatrogenic (and preventable).

B. **Electrolyte metabolism**

1. **Sodium,** as the major extracellular osmotic component, plays a central role in maintaining circulating vascular volume.

Table 9-1. Body Water Expressed as Percent of Body Weight

Build	Infant	Adult Male	Adult Female
Thin	80	65	55
Average	70	60	50
Obese	65	55	45

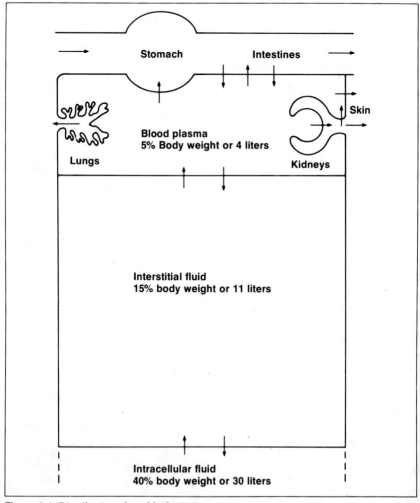

Figure 9-1. Distribution of total body water.

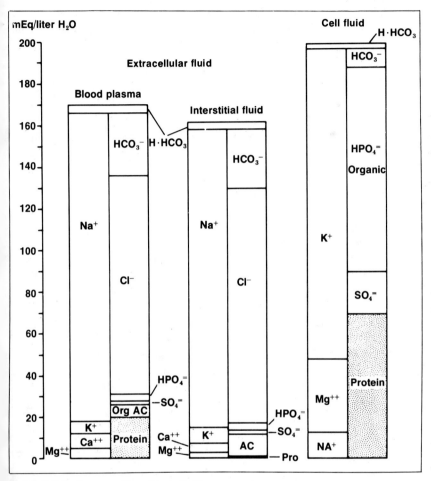

Figure 9-2. Ionic composition of body fluid components.

a. The extracellular volume usually is maintained by renal mechanisms of conservation of sodium.

b. The diagnosis of **sodium depletion** is the diagnosis of extracellular volume depletion and is based on clinical grounds and on measurements relating to central circulating vascular volume: central venous pressure and pulmonary artery wedge pressure. Sodium depletion is manifested by the clinical signs of hypovolemia, i.e., tachycardia, orthostatic hypotension, and shock. These signs are proportional to the degree of hypovolemia and can be used in planning corrections (Tables 9-2 and 9-3).

c. **The serum sodium concentration is not a measurement of sodium balance.**

d. **Sodium excess** is manifested by edema, hypertension, weight gain, and, eventually, by congestive heart failure. Avoiding sodium excess requires careful attention to the details of fluid and electrolyte therapy and knowledge of the patient's cardiac status.

Table 9-2. Response of Blood Pressure and Pulse to Hypovolemia

Blood Volume (ml)	Equivalent Percentage	Supine		Sitting	
		Blood Pressure	Pulse	Blood Pressure	Pulse
Normal	100	N	N	N	N
−500	−5	N	N	N	N or ↑
−1000	−10 to −15	N	N or ↑	N or ↓	↑
−1500	−20	N or ↓	↑	↓	↑ or ↓
−2000	−30	↓	↑ or ↓	↓↓	↑ or ↓

Table 9-3. Clinical Signs in Acute Saline Depletion

Magnitude of Deficit	Symptoms and Signs
Up to 450 mEq sodium (3 liters of ECF)	Furrowed tongue
	Neck veins collapse
	Increased hematocrit
	Urine sodium < 40 mEq/liter
	Tachycardia
	Anorexia
	Little or no thirst: craving for salt rare; serum sodium normal
More than 600 mEq sodium (more than 4 liters of ECF)	Marked increase in hematocrit
	Oliguria (prerenal)
	Hypotension (especially orthostatic)
	Apathy, nausea
	Some decrease in serum sodium
	If uncorrected and progressive: death in hypovolemic shock

  e. A **third space is a collection of ECF that is not functionally available** to normal mechanisms maintaining fluid and electrolyte balance. Examples of third spaces are intestinal content in paralytic ileus, tissue edema secondary to trauma or infection, and ascites. These spaces develop usually at the expense of the extracellular space; when they mobilize, the excess fluid is added to the extracellular space and may produce congestive heart failure. It is particularly important to realize that a third space cannot be altered by means of sodium and fluid restriction. Attempts to do so result in extracellular volume deficits that may be harmful to the patient.

 2. **Potassium** is the major intracellular cation. The major task in therapy is avoidance of potassium excess or depletion because of effects on cardiac and skeletal muscle contractility.

  a. **Hypokalemia** raises membrane excitation potentials, making nerve and muscle less excitable. Hypokalemia is life-threatening in patients on cardiac glycosides (digoxin, digitalis) (Fig. 9-3).

  b. **Hyperkalemia** decreases the excitation potential making them more excitable. Hyperkalemia may result in cardiac arrest and is a medical emergency.

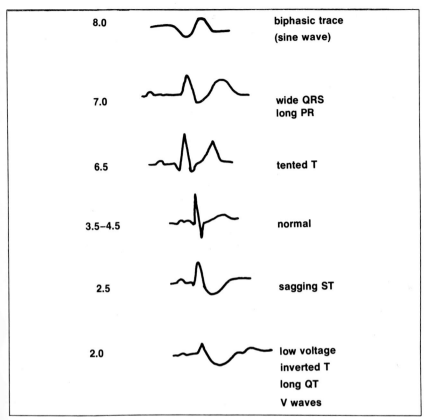

8.0	biphasic trace (sine wave)
7.0	wide QRS long PR
6.5	tented T
3.5–4.5	normal
2.5	sagging ST
2.0	low voltage inverted T long QT V waves

Figure 9-3. Changes in the ECG in hyperkalemia and hypokalemia. Serum potassium concentration is listed on the left, and typical ECG tracings are depicted in the middle of the figure. The abnormal features of the tracings are listed on the right.

    c. Only about 2% (60–80 mEq) of total body K^+ stores (3000–4000 mEq or 35–55 mEq/kg body weight) is present in the ECF of the normal adult. Total body stores depend on muscle mass and are less in women than men and less in patients who have undergone significant muscle wasting e.g., severely malnourished patients or patients who have been bedridden for long periods of time. Estimation of total body potassium becomes important when deficits must be replaced (Fig. 9-4).

    d. Hypokalemia impairs renal concentrating ability because of a decreased responsiveness to ADH. This accounts for the frequent observation of **polyuria** in patients with chronic K^+ depletion.

    e. Alterations in acid-base balance significantly affect K^+ distribution. **Acidosis results in a K^+ shift out of cells, causing an increase in serum K^+ concentration (Fig. 9-4). Alkalosis causes a K^+ shift into cells, resulting in a decrease in serum K^+** concentration. On the average, every 0.1-unit change in arterial pH results in a reciprocal change of 0.6 mEq/liter in plasma K^+ concentration. For example, a patient with a K^+ concentration of 4.4 mEq/liter and a pH of 7.00 would be expected to have a K^+ concentration of 2.0 mEq/liter if the pH were 7.40. Thus, a normal K^+ concentration in an

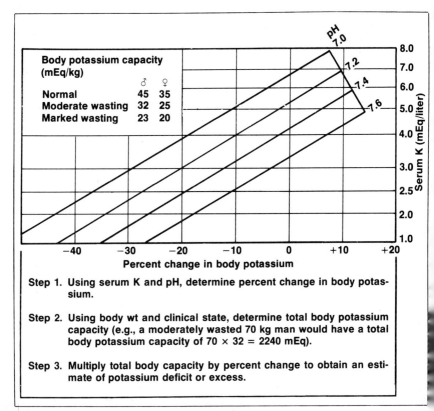

Step 1. Using serum K and pH, determine percent change in body potassium.

Step 2. Using body wt and clinical state, determine total body potassium capacity (e.g., a moderately wasted 70 kg man would have a total body potassium capacity of 70 × 32 = 2240 mEq).

Step 3. Multiply total body capacity by percent change to obtain an estimate of potassium deficit or excess.

Figure 9-4. Method of approximate calculation of depletion or excess of total body potassium.

acidotic patient would be indicative of K^+ depletion, and a normal K^+ concentration in an alkalotic patient would signify K^+ excess.

f. Insulin promotes entry of K^+ into muscle and hepatic cells. Elevation of plasma K^+ concentration stimulates insulin release. Conversely, insulin secretion is inhibited by hypokalemia.

g. The foregoing effects are important in three clinical settings:

  (1) Hypersecretion of insulin caused by a high carbohydrate diet (e.g., intravenous hyperalimentation) frequently results in hypokalemia.

  (2) The inducing of insulin secretion by means of IV glucose administration (or both insulin and glucose) is an effective therapy for hyperkalemia.

  (3) Patients with diabetes mellitus in whom there is reduced or absent insulin secretion are more prone to develop hyperkalemia than are normal persons.

h. Any condition of excessive cellular breakdown (e.g., trauma, acute vascular insufficiency, sepsis) results in release of intracellular K^+ and frequently in rapid elevation of plasma K^+ concentration.

3. Calcium is a major structural component of bone. There is usually no need to add calcium to short-term fluid and electrolyte therapy regimens.

a. Symptomatic **hypocalcemia** develops only in acute alkalosis (e.g., hyperventilation syndrome) or in hypoparathyroidism (see Chap. 13).

b. **Hypercalcemia** results from hyperparathyroidism, sarcoidosis, vitamin D intoxication, widespread osteolytic skeletal metastasis, or tumors producing a parathyroid hormone–like peptide product. Symptomatic hypercalcemia is treated by saline diuresis, calcitonin, mithramycin, and corticosteroids.

4. **Phosphate** imbalance rarely occurs except in the presence of **renal failure**. In patients with renal failure, hyperphosphatemia may present with psychological or neurological changes. These abnormalities almost always can be prevented by attention to serum phosphate concentration and administration of adequate phosphate-binding agents (e.g., Amphogel, Basogel). Chronic administration of these agents may cause severe constipation or bowel obstruction, so they should be combined with a regimen of stool softeners and cathartics.

5. **Trace elements: copper, manganese, magnesium, zinc.** Specific replacement of these elements should always be provided to patients on total parenteral hyperalimentation. The role of trace elements in homeostasis and in the metabolic response to stress is not completely understood, but deficiency states of each element have been described and may be fatal. These elements should be measured in patients on long-term hyperalimentation who develop unusual symptoms (e.g., rash, stupor).

C. Acid-base balance. Most enzymatic processes operate only within a narrow pH range (7.3–7.5). Normal metabolism produces approximately 15,000 mEq H^+/day. Mechanisms for the regulation of body pH must be operating for life to continue. They can be divided into three categories:

1. **Body buffer systems** constitute an important pool of absorbing capacity for H^+. They, in turn, can be divided into three subsystems: bicarbonate, hemoglobin, and tissue and bone. The addition of 100 mEq of H^+ to the body would be distributed as follows: 25% to the HCO_3^- system, 25% to the hemoglobin system, and 50% to tissue and bone. Body buffer systems rarely are impaired enough in acute situations to account for imbalances. Chronic states of anemia, renal failure, and osteoporosis theoretically may impair buffering capacity (e.g., by permitting severe states of acidosis or alkalosis associated with minor H^+ loads or deficits) but rarely appear important clinically.

2. **Renal mechanisms** function to maintain body pH by:

a. Reabsorbing filtered HCO_3^-, preventing loss of HCO_3^- in the urine.

b. Excreting 50–100 mEq H^+/day. Renal failure is associated with a state of chronic acidosis that is adaptive and allows for excretion of the maximum acid load of the particular degree of renal dysfunction. Attempts at total correction offer no advantage, since this state usually is adequately compensated by respiratory mechanisms.

3. **Respiratory regulation** occurs by elimination of CO_2 generated by the equilibrium $HCO_3^- + H^+ \rightleftarrows H_2O + CO_2$. Since CO_2 diffuses approximately 20 times more readily than O_2, severe respiratory impairment must occur before CO_2 retention occurs. Severely impaired respiration is associated with acute and chronic pulmonary parenchymal disease, with central nervous system depression of respiratory drive, and with severe impairment of respiratory motion (e.g., flail chest). Simple inspection of the patient usually suffices to determine if significant pulmonary impairment exists. If not, the acid-base state of the patient usually can be diagnosed by the serum HCO_3^- concentration. For accuracy, pH also should always be measured.

4. **Body pH** is expressed in the Henderson-Hasselbalch equation:

$$pH = 6.1 + \log \frac{HCO_3^-}{PCO_2} \quad \begin{array}{l} \text{(controlled by kidney)} \\ \text{(controlled by lung)} \end{array}$$

Table 9-4. Normal Acid-Base Values in Blood

Blood	pH	PCO$_2$	HCO$_3^-$
Arterial	7.37–7.43	36–44 mm Hg	22–26 mEq/liter
Venous	7.32–7.38	42–50 mm Hg	23–27 mEq/liter

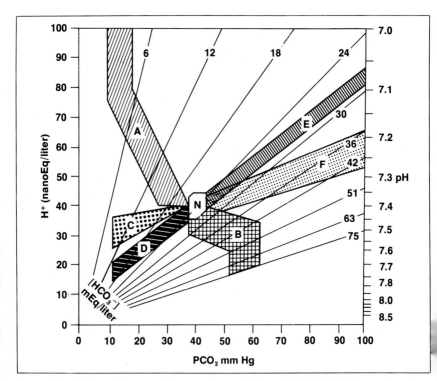

Figure 9-5. Acid-base diagram. The area of normal values is labeled N. The numbered lines represent HCO$_3^-$ concentration (mEq/liter). Progressive metabolic acidosis follows pathway A; metabolic alkalosis, pathway B. In acute respiratory alkalosis, values usually fall into area D; in respiratory acidosis, into area E. The effects of compensatory mechanisms bring values toward area C in chronic respiratory alkalosis and toward F in acidosis. (From Goldberg et al. *J.A.M.A.* 223:269, 1973. Copyright 1973, American Medical Association.)

Blood pH can be readily measured in most clinical laboratories, and when the pH is coupled with electrolyte and blood gas measurements, a diagnosis of acid-base abnormalities is usually simple. Table 9-4 shows the usual values for acid-base variables.

5. **Acid-base abnormalities** are classically divided into four categories of metabolic or respiratory acidosis or alkalosis (Fig. 9-5). These labels are useful in approaching acid-base imbalances, but, since the latter rarely occur in an uncompensated state, understanding the physiological mechanisms of compensation is important in diagnosis.

6. **Metabolic acidosis** results from a decrease in HCO$_3^-$ causing a decrease in pH and may occur:

a. From **overproduction of an organic acid** in:

(1) Diabetic ketoacidosis.

(2) Lactic acidosis of sepsis, shock, or poor perfusion due to vasopressor use.

(3) Salicylate, paraldehyde, methanol, or ethylene glycol intoxication; NH_4CL administration; or hyperalimentation, due to a relative excess of acidic amino acids.

b. From an **impaired renal excretory mechanism** in:

(1) Acute oliguric renal failure.

(2) Chronic renal failure.

(3) Renal tubular acidosis (distal, proximal).

c. From an **abnormal loss of bicarbonate** in:

(1) Diarrhea, intestinal intubation (past the pylorus), pancreatic or small bowel fistula.

(2) Cholestryamine.

(3) Ureterosigmoidostomy

(4) Acetazolamide (Daimox) therapy.

d. Metabolic acidosis almost always is at least partially compensated by stimulation of respiratory activity. This results in a decrease in PCO_2, bringing the $\dfrac{HCO_3^-}{PCO_2}$ ratio and the pH back to normal. If respiratory activity is not normal to begin with (e.g., central nervous system [CNS] injury, chronic obstructive pulmonary disease, flail chest), the patient cannot compensate and will become severely acidotic (hours to days). Eventually, renal compensation occurs by increased excretion of H^+. This effect is important in chronically acidotic patients with good renal function (a rare situation).

7. Metabolic alkalosis. A rise in pH due to accumulation of HCO_3^- is termed metabolic alkalosis. It can be produced either by retention of HCO_3^- or by loss of H^+ from the gastrointestinal (GI) tract or urine. The acid lost is produced from the intracellular dissociation of H_2CO_3.

$$CO_2 + H_2O \rightleftarrows H_2CO_3 \rightleftarrows H^+ + HCO_3$$

Therefore, for each H^+ lost, an equivalent amount of HCO_3^- is generated.

a. Causes of metabolic alkalosis are as follows:

(1) GI losses of H^+

(a) Vomiting or removal (suction) of GI secretions

(b) Congenital chloridiarrhea

(2) Renal losses of H^+

(a) Mineralocorticoid excess.

(b) Hypoparathyroidism.

(3) H^+ movement into cells in **hypokalemia.** As K^+ is lost from the extracellular space, K^+ moves out of the cells, and H^+ moves intracellularly to preserve electroneutrality. This results in extracellular alkalosis and a paradoxical intracellular acidosis. Replacement of K^+ reverses the process and corrects alkalosis.

(4) Bicarbonate retention

(a) $NaHCO_3$ administration.

(b) Massive blood transfusion.

(c) Milk-alkali syndrome.

(5) Plasma HCO_3^- increases also with profound volume contraction of the extracellular space. As NaCl and water are lost (e.g., through vomiting), the extracellular space contracts around a constant amount of HCO_3^- causing an increase in the relative HCO_3^- concentration. This is known as **contraction alkalosis.**

b. In patients with good kidney function, alkalosis would be rapidly corrected by the ability of the kidney to excrete HCO_3^-. Therefore, **metabolic alkalosis also requires an impairment of renal HCO_3^- excreting capacity** due either to decreased filtration of HCO_3^-, as in renal failure, or, more commonly, to increased reabsorption of filtered HCO_3^- because of volume or K^+ depletion.

c. In the presence of volume and K^+ depletion, H^+ secretion by the kidney is enhanced. The finding of an acid urine in the clinical setting of alkalosis is called **paradoxical aciduria** and is a useful observation because it is usually associated with about 20% decrease in total body potassium. This aids in planning replacement therapy of K^+.

d. Respiratory compensation for metabolic alkalosis acts by decreasing respiratory minute volume in order to increase PCO_2. Compensation is limited by the normal respiratory drive when PCO_2 reaches 60 mm Hg. In the normal person breathing air at sea level, the decreased respiratory minute volume results in a PCO_2 of about 65 mm Hg.

8. **Respiratory acidosis.** A fall in pH associated with a rise in PCO_2 is called respiratory acidosis.

a. Respiratory acidosis occurs from the following **causes:**

(1) Inhibition of respiratory drive

(a) Drugs: opiates, anesthetics.

(b) Oxygen administration in chronic hypercapnia.

(c) CNS lesions.

(d) Cardiac arrest.

(2) Disorders of respiratory muscles or the chest wall

(a) Muscle weakness: myasthenia, poliomyelitis, multiple sclerosis, aminoglycoside antibiotics (in conjunction with anesthesia).

(b) Morbid obesity.

(c) Thoracic trauma: flail chest.

(3) Disorders of gas exchange

(a) Chronic obstructive pulmonary disease.

(b) Pulmonary edema

(c) Hammon-Rich syndrome.

(4) Respiratory acidosis (and increased PCO_2), is **always associated with hypoxia.** This combination is **life-threatening,** since the rising PCO_2 will eventually result in respiratory depression, with attendant worsening of the hypoxia. Renal compensatory mechanisms are too slow to affect the outcome significantly. Except in cases of bronchospasm

(asthma), which can be readily reversed with pharmacological agents, mechanical respiratory support is usually needed. Delay in providing support is often fatal.

9. **Respiratory alkalosis.** A decrease in PCO_2 results in respiratory alkalosis.

   a. The **causes** of respiratory alkalosis are:

      (1) **Hypoxemia,** pulmonary diseases (e.g., pulmonary emboli), high altitude, congenital heart disease (right to left shunt), and congestive heart failure.

      (2) **CNS disorders,** i.e., subarachnoid hemorrhage.

      (3) **Psychogenic hyperventilation.**

      (4) **Salicylate intoxication.**

      (5) **Hypermetabolic states,** i.e., fever, thyrotoxicosis.

      (6) **Cirrhosis.**

      (7) **Assisted ventilation.**

      (8) **Sepsis.**

      (9) **Exercise.**

   b. The presence of **tachypnea** should suggest the diagnosis of respiratory alkalosis if the patient is found to be alkalotic. It is important to remember that tachypnea is the usual mechanism for compensation of metabolic acidosis. Once the presence of respiratory alkalosis is confirmed by measurement of blood gases and electrolytes, the cause must be determined. It is dangerous to assume that the condition is psychogenic in origin, since significantly morbid conditions (pulmonary embolus, sepsis) will be missed.

D. The **effects of trauma**

   1. Anesthesia and operations, as well as external violence, constitute forms of traumatic stress to which the body responds by **secreting additional aldosterone and antidiuretic hormone (ADH).** There is a reduction in renal capacity to excrete both water and sodium loads, and renal loss of potassium is increased.

   2. Trauma also results in **formation of edema** in and about injured tissues. The edema fluid is protein-rich and derived primarily from the plasma volume of the ECF compartment. Unlike normal ECF, traumatic edema is functionally sequestered as a third space and cannot readily be mobilized to meet body needs.

   3. In the past, there was a great deal of emphasis on the **general response** to stress: the demonstration in postoperative patients of a **decreased capacity to excrete sodium and water loads.** This led to recommendations that water and sodium intake be restricted in postoperative and post-traumatic patients.

   4. Conversely, until recently, there has been little or no emphasis placed on the body's **local response** to trauma, which is **functional loss of plasma volume.** This loss must be replaced in postoperative patients by providing sodium and protein-containing fluids.

   5. Much of the activation of ADH and aldosterone secretion in association with an operation is related not only to stress but also to preoperative restriction of fluid intake and inadequate replacement of fluid losses during and after operation.

   6. In general, daily maintenance fluid and electrolyte requirements are not altered by the fact of operation. The decreased capacity to handle sodium and water loads (the general response to stress) is balanced, in a sense, by the increased need for sodium and water to replace functionally lost traumatic

Table 9-5. Clinical Signs of Water Depletion

Magnitude of Deficit (adults)	Clinical Features
1.5 liters or less	Thirst
1.5–4.0 liters	Marked thirst
	Dry mouth
	Urine specific gravity increased
	Hematocrit, skin turgor, and blood pressure normal
4.0 liters or more	Intolerable thirst
	Marked hypernatremia
	Oliguria
	Body weight decreased
	Slightly increased hematocrit
	Apathy, stupor
	If not corrected: hyperosmolar coma, death

edema (the local response to stress). Fluid requirements of postoperative patients can be calculated just as for patients who have not been operated on, except in such special circumstances as administration of exogenous corticosteroids or a continuing state of inappropriate secretion of aldosterone (cirrhosis).

7. For most patients it is not necessary (and is possibly harmful) to restrict fluid and electrolyte intake markedly in the early postoperative period.

II. **Clinical states of fluid and electrolyte imbalance.** Imbalances rarely occur in pure form or in isolation: clinical problems are always mixtures. Nonetheless, it is conceptually convenient to compartmentalize clinical diagnosis and treatment on the basis of theoretical pure states. It is far easier to determine first if the patient has an excess, is normal, or has a deficit in total body water and then to make a separate determination, using other criteria, regarding the presence of an excess, normality, or deficit in total body sodium or potassium than to try to decide if the patient's problem is "hypotonic dehydration" or "acute desalting water loss." It must be reemphasized that the theoretical states discussed in this section rarely exist in pure form in patients. They are a conceptual and diagnostic convenience only.

A. **Water depletion**

1. Water depletion is caused either by unreplaced losses together with increased output (fever, osmotic diuresis, diarrhea) or by a lack of intake (NPO, coma).

2. A water deficit results in a decrease in volume of all body fluid compartments. Since solute content does not change, hyperosmolarity ensues. Osmoreceptors are stimulated, and secretion of ADH is increased. More water is resorbed from the distal renal tubule.

3. The chief symptoms and signs of water deficit are **thirst, oliguria, and hypernatremia.**

4. A rough initial working **estimate of the magnitude of water deficit** can be made from clinical data (Table 9-5) or by assuming that each 3 mEq of serum sodium concentration above the normal range represents a deficit of at least 1 liter of total body water.

5. In severe hyperglycemia, the serum sodium concentration will give a falsely low estimate of serum osmolarity. The estimate of water need based on the

serum sodium concentration should be mentally corrected by adding 500 ml of water for each 100 mg/100 ml blood glucose elevation above normal.

6. **Treatment of a water deficit requires provision of additional sodium-free water.** If water depletion is severe, at least one half of the estimated deficit should be replaced in the initial 12 hr of treatment.

7. **Water deficit (dehydration) frequently presents with concomitant ECF volume depletion.** In such cases, the patient is hypernatremic and also has clinical signs of hypovolemia (tachycardia, orthostatic hypertension, etc). As always, initial treatment should be aimed at correction of the ECF volume (sodium) deficit.

B. Water excess, water intoxication

1. Water excess frequently is **iatrogenic,** resulting from administration of electrolyte-free water to sodium-depleted patients or patients in whom ADH activity is increased, or from rapid administration of water in any situation in which oliguria exists. Water intoxication occasionally is caused by excessive intake (neurosis) or by injudicious administration of oxytocin (Pitocin) in an attempt to induce labor or stop bleeding from esophageal varices.

2. Water excess leads to an increase in the volume of all fluid compartments. Since body solute content is not altered, a state of hyposmolarity ensues. Hypothalamic osmoreceptors are inhibited, and pituitary secretion of ADH is decreased. The distal renal tubule resorbs less water, resulting in increased renal water excretion. These compensatory mechanisms are much less sensitive than those defending the body against a water deficit.

3. The symptoms and signs of water excess are related to both the degree of water overloading and the rate at which it develops. Moderate degrees of water excess often are well tolerated and clinically are asymptomatic. The only signs will be **a decreased serum sodium concentration, an increased urine volume, and an increase in body weight.** Pitting edema does not develop.

4. More marked water overloading causes swelling of brain cells and leads to nausea, vomiting, and ultimately to convulsions (water intoxication). These symptoms rarely appear unless the osmolar shift has been rapid and the serum sodium concentration is below 120 mEq/liter.

5. **Treatment** of water excess not complicated by convulsions requires only **restricting water intake;** it is not usually necessary to do anything more. IV ethyl alcohol will inhibit ADH secretion and may be useful in the treatment of some cases of water excess. In severe cases, induction of enforced solute diuresis with mannitol may be needed. If the patient is in renal failure and diuresis cannot be induced, dialysis is required. Convulsions should be treated by IV administration of small amounts (100–250 ml) of 5% sodium chloride solution. Convulsions or other CNS symptoms from water intoxication are the only good indication for use of IV hypertonic salt. Hypertonic salt is not the best treatment for a sodium deficit.

C. Sodium depletion

1. Severe sodium depletion may result from the following:

   a. Abnormal GI losses (suction, vomiting, diarrhea).

   b. Losses of ECF, either externally (burns, marked sweating) or internally as a third space (peritonitis, ascites, ileus).

   c. Excessive urine sodium wastage (diuretics, chronic nephritis, adrenal failure, vasopressin).

   d. Restricted dietary intake.

2. The symptoms and signs of sodium depletion are caused by decreased ECF volume (Table 9-3).

3. Changes in total body sodium content bear no reliable relation to serum sodium concentration.

4. Treatment of sodium deficit consists of restoration of ECF volume by **appropriate amounts of sodium-containing fluids.** Lost blood should be replaced with blood. Lost plasma should be replaced with single-donor, fresh-frozen plasma or plasma substitutes (e.g., albumin). Lost interstitial fluid (e.g., posttraumatic edema) should be replaced with electrolyte solutions. Exclusive replacement of plasma or blood loss with only electrolyte solutions requires about four times the volume of lost blood or plasma and results in overexpansion of the total ECF volume, since the distribution of sodium is not confined only to the plasma volume.

D. Sodium excess

1. Sodium excess usually is caused by abnormal renal retention of sodium—related to inability to excrete a sodium load (starvation, severe illness) or to increased sodium resorption (increased activity of aldosterone or other hormones with salt-retaining action [cortisone, estrogens, testosterone]). Acute hypernatremia occasionally follows absorption of intrauterine hypertonic saline administered to induce abortion.

2. The only reliable clinical sign of total body sodium excess is **edema.** Even this is relatively late evidence, since 400 mEq of excess sodium (i.e., about 3 liters of fluid) may accumulate before minimal dependent pitting edema is evident. **Weight gain** will parallel accumulation of ECF. While disability resulting from edema is minimal, it is undesirable because of the following: wound healing is impaired; plasma proteins are diluted, tending to bring about further sodium retention; and the patient is predisposed to develop heart failure and pulmonary edema.

3. Edema may, of course, be related primarily to other factors (increased hydrostatic pressure in CHF or in venous or lymphatic obstruction; increased capillary permeability in inflammation or allergic states; decreased plasma proteins in nephrosis and cirrhosis). These other abnormalities all bring about secondary renal sodium retention.

4. The hematocrit in sodium excess may be low but often is normal, since these conditions usually develop slowly. The serum sodium concentration usually is normal.

5. **Treatment** of sodium excess consists of **sodium restriction** and judicious use of **diuretics** and inotropic agents when indicated. In edema accompanied by marked hypoproteinemia, the protein deficit also must be corrected; otherwise sodium restriction alone will lead to a decrease in plasma volume. This is usually best accomplished by effective nutritional support.

6. Edema (sodium excess) accompanied by a low serum sodium concentration (water excess) is found in some severely debilitated patients. This situation is generally iatrogenic, resulting from efforts to treat a patient with "hyponatremia of severe illness" by administration of large amounts of salt or to treat an edematous patient with poor renal function by salt restriction. In such patients the kidneys have failed to respond to the osmotic stimulus to water excretion. This situation carries an extremely grave prognosis, since it means that the body has lost the ability to regulate its osmolarity. Treatment is aimed at maintaining a normal circulating plasma volume by judicious administration of plasma and sodium-containing fluids. The accumulating edema often will have to be ignored.

E. Potassium depletion

1. **Early signs of potassium depletion are vague:** malaise and weakness. Paralytic ileus and distention are seen in some hypokalemic patients. Muscular paresis appears only with extreme depletion. Postassium-depleted patient

are prone to develop ectopic atrial impulses or other signs of digitalis intoxication; hepatic coma may appear if the patient has liver disease; pseudodiabetic glucosuria may appear because of inability to transfer glucose across muscle cell membranes. ECG alterations are illustrated in Figure 9-3.

2. An approximation of the **magnitude of potassium deficit** can be obtained from an estimate of body potassium capacity and the measured blood pH and serum potassium concentration (Fig. 9-4).

3. **Potassium depletion is treated by parenteral administration of potassium salts.** Although large total amounts may be given in a single day when needed, the rate of infusion must be limited, so that transiently high venous blood concentrations do not affect the heart. In general, no more than 20 mEq of potassium should be administered per hour in very severe hypokalemia.

F. Potassium excess (hyperkalemia)

1. Life-threatening potassium excess usually is associated with **renal failure** and is potentiated by concomitant tissue destruction or by depletion of sodium or calcium. Less threatening increases in total body potassium are seen in adrenal insufficiency.

2. Elevation of serum potassium above 6 mEq/liter may stimulate secretion of aldosterone, which enhances excretion of potassium by the normal kidney. This corrective mechanism probably is not available in renal insufficiency.

3. If the serum potassium exceeds 7 mEq/liter, intercardiac impulse conduction is slowed: arrhythmia, bradycardia, and hypotension may be followed by diastolic cardiac arrest (see Fig. 9-3).

4. **Any patient showing a wide QRS complex, peaked T-waves or other evidence of hyperkalemic cardiac toxicity should be treated immediately** with IV calcium gluconate (antagonizes potassium), or bicarbonate (alkalization encourages potassium to shift into cells) and glucose plus insulin (potassium deposits with glycogen). These immediate treatment measures should be followed by administration of ion-exchange resins (Kayexalate) by enema. A fall in serum potassium usually may not occur for 30–60 min. If no fall occurs despite repeated Kayexalate enemas, dialysis will be necessary. To summarize: in case of **life-threatening hyperkalemia,** the following treatment should be given:

   a. Calcium gluconate, 1 amp. IV.

   b. $NaHCO_3$, 1 amp (44 mEq) IV.

   c. Glucose and insulin, 1 amp 5% D/W plus 10 units of regular insulin by IV push.

   d. Kayexalate, 50 gm in 70% sorbitol, as a retention enema. Repeat q1–2h. Total exchange is equivalent to 200 mEq K+.

   e. Hemodialysis or peritoneal dialysis.

G. Calcium and magnesium

1. Body reserves of calcium are mobilized readily from bone and are so great that **symptomatic hypocalcemia** develops only in acute alkalosis (e.g., hysterical hyperventilation) or in hypoparathyroidism (see Chap. 13).

2. **Chronic hypercalcemia** is seen in hyperparathyroidism, metastatic cancer, sarcoidosis, vitamin D intoxication, and similar states and results in formation of renal stones. Acute hypercalcemia producing coma is seen occasionally in hyperparathyroidism but more often is a result of widespread skeletal metastases (usually responds to corticosteroids).

3. **Magnesium** is the second most prevalent intracellular cation, but understanding of its metabolism in humans is incomplete. In experimental animals, mag-

nesium deficiency causes vasodilation and convulsions and is accompanied by myocardial necrosis. In humans, increased levels of serum magnesium are seen inconstantly in hypertension and chronic infections and more regularly in renal failure.

4. Other minor element deficiencies may occur in patients undergoing long-term parenteral nutritional support. In particular, copper and zinc deficiencies may present suddenly and be life-threatening. Blood levels of these elements should be measured if the patient's clinical status deteriorates inexplicably. Patients with zinc deficiency develop a total body rash and stupor.

H. Metabolic acidosis occurs whenever renal tubules fail to excrete sufficient hydrogen ion to maintain a normal serum pH. In acidosis caused by renal failure, GI losses, or ketosis, there is an increase in the so-called fixed acids (SO_4, PO_4, etc). In failure of oxidative metabolism, lactate is not converted to carbon dioxide and water for elimination via the lungs; "lactic acidosis" results. Respiratory attempts at partial compensation result in an increased rate and depth of breathing (Kussmaul's respirations); if respiratory compensation is impaired (emphysema, pneumonia, anesthesia), a combined metabolic and respiratory acidosis develops in which the serum HCO_3^- is nearly normal, but serum pH is very low.

1. Mild to moderate acidosis usually requires no specific therapy aimed at correcting pH. Therapy should be directed at the underlying cause of the acidosis. More severe acidosis (pH < 7.30, serum bicarbonate < 15 mEq/liter) requires treatment per se.

2. In **severe acute metabolic acidosis,** IV bicarbonate is preferred to lactate, since its effectiveness is not dependent on intermediary hepatic metabolism. The **amount of bicarbonate needed can be estimated from the formula:** body weight (kg) × 0.3 × (25 − measured serum bicarbonate) = mEq bicarbonate needed. One or two amps (44–88 mEq) of $NaHCO_3$ may be given immediately; the remainder of the calculated amount should be given over 24–36 hr. Ringer's lactate solution may be used in states of chronic acidosis but should not be given if hypoxia or shock is present (unless a volume deficit is the cause of shock) and should never be given to acidotic patients with liver failure. Care should be taken in administering bicarbonate in severe acidosis. Overly rapid administration (> 2 amp as an IV push) may result in seizures due to transient CNS acidosis occurring because CO_2 rapidly transverses the blood-brain barrier, while HCO_3^- does not (administration of bicarbonate lowers the respiratory drive, causing increased PCO_2; carbon dioxide then enters the CNS, causing decreased pH).

I. Metabolic alkalosis almost always is caused by **loss of acid gastric juice** and usually is accompanied by **hypokalemia.** Less frequently, metabolic alkalosis is caused by hypokalemia resulting from diuretic therapy, hyperaldosteronism, or a similar cause of renal potassium wastage. Partial pH compensation is rapidly achieved by a clinically inapparent decrease in ventilation, resulting in carbon dioxide retention, an increase in serum carbonic acid concentration, and partial restoration of the blood pH toward normal. Depression of respiratory minute volume can result in a PCO_2 of 60 mm Hg and a PO_2 of 65 mm Hg, even in patients with previously normal respiratory function. Beyond these partial pressures of CO_2 or O_2, respiratory hypoxic or hypercapnic drive overrides the pH compensating mechanism.

1. In all cases of metabolic alkalosis caused by loss of gastric juice, **replacement of chloride** is essential to successful therapy. Administration of saline solution is sufficient therapy in mild cases of metabolic alkalosis without hypokalemia, since the kidney will complete the job of correcting acid-base balance by retaining chloride and excreting sodium along with excess bicarbonate.

2. In moderately severe alkalosis, another problem arises. Besides potassium losses in gastric juice, there is an increase in renal potassium excretion to permit the tubules to retain hydrogen ion. In this situation, administration of potassium chloride IV is the preferred treatment, since it will correct both the potassium and the chloride deficits.

3. In severe metabolic alkalosis not responding to saline or potassium chloride alone, it may be necessary to use ammonium chloride. Ammonium chloride is given slowly IV in doses of up to 140 mEq (1 liter of the isotonic 0.75% solution). The blood pH should be checked frequently during ammonium chloride treatment. The use of ammonium chloride should be avoided in patients with compromised hepatic function, since it may precipitate hepatic coma. Severe metabolic alkalosis is the only definite indication for administration of ammonium chloride. Intravenous hydrogen chloride also may be used in this situation but should be administered via a central venous line. It usually is given as 0.05–0.15 N HCl solution (50–150 mEq H+/liter).

4. Severe or rapidly developing alkalosis may lead to **tetany** because of the pH-dependent decrease in available ionized calcium. If tetany occurs or appears imminent, 10 ml of calcium gluconate should be given slowly IV.

J. Respiratory acidosis is caused by pulmonary insufficiency, i.e., failure to excrete carbon dioxide via the lungs with normal efficiency (pneumonia, emphysema, fibrosis, central respiratory depression due to drugs, anesthesia, CNS trauma). It is usually accompanied by cyanosis. Retention of carbon dioxide leads to an increase in serum carbonic acid concentration and a fall in pH. In acute respiratory acidosis, the serum bicarbonate may not be elevated, since renal compensatory mechanisms have not had time to act. The diagnosis can best be made by measuring serum pH and PCO_2. In chronic respiratory acidosis, bicarbonate ion has been retained by the renal tubules, restoring the pH toward normal and, of course, resulting in an elevated serum bicarbonate concentration. **Treatment** in respiratory acidosis must be directed toward improving ventilation and aiding renal compensation. Respiratory acidosis in surgical patients normally requires ventilatory support.

K. Respiratory alkalosis results from hyperventilation and is seen in hysteria, early in salicylate poisoning, in some brainstem lesions, in patients hyperventilated by a respirator, and, occasionally, during general anesthesia. Patients undergoing neurosurgical procedures may be purposely hyperventilated because of the effect of hypocapnia in reducing cerebral blood flow (reduction of PCO_2 to 25–28 mm Hg will reduce cerebral blood flow approximately 20%). Below a PCO_2 of 23 mm Hg, oxyhemoglobin dissociation is significantly impaired.

1. Hyperventilation leads to a fall in alveolar carbon dioxide concentration and a decrease in serum carbonic acid concentration. Tetany is seen if alkalosis is severe.

2. Respiratory alkalosis in most clinical situations is short lived and well tolerated. When hyperventilation ceases, the carbonic acid concentration is rapidly restored, and pH returns to normal. Alkalosis of any degree may significantly impair cardiac output in patients with cardiac disease. Because of this, you may elect to treat such patients differently than patients with normal cardiac function.

3. If hysteria is the basis for hyperventilation, have the patient breathe into a paper bag. Other situations may call for the addition of small amounts of carbon dioxide to the inspired gas mixture. **The danger is in mistaking a compensating metabolic acidosis; (e.g., ketoacidosis) for respiratory acidosis.**

III. Diagnosis of imbalances. Diagnosis of the nature of imbalances present in the patient and an approximation of their magnitude are based on the history, clinical signs and symptoms, certain laboratory studies, and past clinical experience. Initial diagnoses always are more or less a guess. A more accurate diagnosis and an appreci-

Table 9-6. Approximate Electrolyte Composition of GI Secretions

Secretion	Usual Maximum Volume/Day	Sodium	Chloride	Potassium
		(mEq/liter in adults)		
Normal				
Saliva	1000	100	75	5
Gastric juice (pH < 4.0)	2500*	60	100	10
Gastric juice (ph > 4.0)	2000*	100	100	10
Bile	1500	140	100	10
Pancreatic juice	1000	140	75	10
Succus entericus (mixed small-bowel fluid	3500	100	100	20
Abnormal				
New ileostomy	500–2000	130	110	20
Adapted ileostomy	400	50	60	10
New cecostomy	400	80	50	20
Colostomy (transverse loop)	300	50	40	10
Diarrhea	1000–4000	60	45	30

*Nasogastric suction volume usually much less than this unless pyloric obstruction is present.

ation of the order of magnitude of any imbalance are obtained by assessment of the patient's response to the initial therapy.

A. Clues from the history

1. **Gastric outlet obstruction** (duodenal ulcer, pyloric stenosis) results in vomiting and produces alkalosis (loss of chloride and potassium) and hypokalemia (loss of potassium), as well as losses of water and sodium.

2. **Vomiting** secondary to a cause other than gastric outlet obstruction produces loss of water, sodium, and potassium. If there is any shift in acid-base balance it is toward metabolic acidosis. The electrolyte composition of various GI secretions is listed in Table 9-6.

3. **Diarrhea** (cholera, ulcerative colitis, ileostomy dysfunction) also results in loss of water, sodium, and potassium but tends to result in acidosis if the volume loss is severe.

4. **Burns** produce losses of plasma and ECF (water, protein, and sodium). The magnitude of fluid loss depends on the depth and extent of the burn.

5. **Sweating,** if excessive, causes appreciable loss of both sodium and water, results in shrinkage of the ECF volume, and eventually results in vascular collapse.

6. A **low-sodium diet** coupled with **diuretic therapy** commonly induces a moderate state of salt depletion and consequent hypovolemia that normally is of no consequence. However, when such patients are given a general anesthetic (which releases sympathetic vasoconstrictive tone), they may become hypotensive. **Potassium** also is lost as a result of diuretic treatment; unless potassium is replaced in the diet, hypokalemia ensues.

7. Loss of other sodium-containing fluids (e.g., ascites) rapidly can produce hypovolemia and acidosis.

B. Clinical signs and symptoms

1. Thirst is a very sensitive guide to the need for water

a. Thirst needs to be differentiated from dry oral mucous membranes. Dry mouth is relieved by gargling a small amount of water; thirst is not.

b. Thirst resulting from water depletion is such a compelling symptom that a patient who has access to water will promptly correct any deficit.

c. Clinical water depletion is found only in patients who are not able to drink water (feeble, comatose) or are prevented from drinking water (restrained, NPO). Patients also may have increased water losses caused by high fever, diarrhea, or osmotic diuresis (glucose in diabetic acidosis, mannitol, intravascular radiographic contrast agents).

2. Body weight

a. The importance of accurate, repetitive measurements cannot be overestimated.

b. Short-term (i.e., minute-to-minute or hour-to-hour) changes in body weight reflect changes in both ECF volume and total body water. Repetitive measurements of body weight are usually so clumsy to do that body weight is not a practically useful measure over the short-term except when using sensitive bed scales.

c. Longer-term trends in body weight over a period of days are a reasonably reliable guide to changes in total body water but should be interpreted in conjunction with other clinical and laboratory information; e.g., edema, electrolytes, serum proteins.

d. Measurements of body weight should be corrected for tissue losses in catabolic states (up to 500 gm/day) or for lean tissue gains in anabolic states (up to 150 gm/day). In most postoperative patients, a loss of at least 300 gm/day (about 0.5 lb) in body weight is expected.

e. Weight gain is interpreted as indicating water retention. Weight loss in excess of 300–500 gm/day indicates water loss. Therapy should not be based only on correcting changes in body weight; other signs are used to determine if shifts in water balance are of ECF origin or are of electrolyte-free water.

3. Jugular veins and central venous pressure (CVP) With the patient supine, the external jugular veins normally fill to the anterior border of the sternocleidomastoid muscle. These **veins provide a built-in manometer** for following changes in CVP.

a. A number of factors affect CVP. These include vascular volume, right ventricular function, intrathoracic pressure, and vascular tone.

b. Accurate interpretation of CVP can be made only by noting the response to fluid challenge or diuresis.

(1) A **high CVP** (> 14 cm H_2O) suggests volume overload or heart failure but can occur because of increased intrathoracic pressure or intense vasoconstriction due to hypovolemia or administration of vasoconstrictor drugs (levarterenol, epinephrine, vasopressin).

(2) A **low CVP** suggests hypovolemia but also may occur with acute left ventricular failure.

(3) In the absence of congestive heart failure (CHF), changes in neck-vein filling reflect changes in plasma volume. Since plasma volume is a part of the sodium-dependent ECF volume, alterations in filling of the neck veins are clues to changes in total body sodium content.

(4) The presence of CHF may be distinguished by the presence of **hepatojugular reflux.** The patient should be in a sitting-up or semi-reclining position for this test. Pressure on the abdomen over the liver causes a further increase in filling of the neck veins that persists as long as pressure is maintained. An expanded plasma volume in the absence of CHF will not produce a positive hepatojugular reflux test.

(5) In a supine patient, **flat neck veins reflect a contracted plasma volume and indicate a need for sodium-containing fluids.**

4. The **Swan-Ganz flow-directed catheter** and **measurement of pulmonary artery wedge pressure (PAWP)**

   a. **PAWP** accurately reflects left atrial pressure and left ventricular function except in the presence of severe mitral stenosis.

   b. A marked elevation in PAWP frequently occurs prior to overt CHF; alter therapy and thus avoid clinical CHF.

   c. A triple lumen catheter allows a variety of other measurements useful in the physiological management of acutely ill patients, e.g., CVP, cardiac output, mixed venous blood sampling, cardiac index.

   d. Because of the instrumentation required, Swan-Ganz catheters are best utilized in an intensive care unit. They can be inserted via a subclavian vein utilizing a Seldinger wire technique, or via a cutdown on an antecubital, external jugular, or shoulder cephalic vein.

5. **Tissue turgor**

   a. Decreased turgor should be interpreted as indicating a contraction of the interstitial fluid volume and a need for sodium-containing fluids. Unfortunately, tissue turgor varies with age, sex, race, complexion, and nutritional state. For observations to be meaningful, they must be done sequentially prior to the development of a fluid balance abnormality.

   b. The **tongue is the most reliable indicator of tissue turgor.** Normally, the tongue has a more or less single median furrow. Additional furrows that parallel the major median furrow appear with decreased interstitial volume. Mouth breathing, as occurs with nasogastric tubes, will cause tongue dryness, but not furrowing, in the absence of significant fluid deficits.

   c. Eyeball tension has been mentioned as an indicator of tissue turgor. Because physicians rarely have significant experience with this observation, it is unreliable.

6. **Blood pressure and pulse**

   a. Changes in these measures are influenced chiefly by changes in the circulating blood volume (see Table 9-2).

   b. Tachycardia is frequently the earliest sign of decreased vascular volume, followed by the appearance of postural hypotension and then hypotension when supine. In patients whose hemodynamic response is hampered by medications (propranolol, reserpine, etc.) or by a fixed cardiac rate (e.g., with cardiac pacemakers), severe hypotension is the first sign of hypovolemia.

   c. Bradycardia may accompany acute large losses in blood volume.

   d. Hypotension indicates a need for blood or sodium-containing fluids.

7. **Edema and rales**

   a. **Edema reflects an increase in interstitial fluid volume and implies that total body sodium is increased.** Edema is not produced by retention of water alone.

Table 9-7. Electrolyte Concentrations in Serum

Electrolyte	Normal Range (mEq/liter)
Sodium	135–145
Potassium	3.5–5.5
Chloride	85–115
"Bicarbonate"	22–29
Calcium	4.0–5.5 (9.0–10.6 mg/100 ml)
Magnesium	1.5–2.5
Phosphate	0.8–1.9 (2.4–4.8 mg/100 ml)

    b. Edema is not a very sensitive indicator of sodium balance. A 20% increase in total body exchangeable sodium may accumulate before edema becomes very obvious.

    c. Barely perceptible pitting edema indicates that total body sodium content has increased by at least 400 mEq (2.7 liters of saline).

    d. Rales in the absence of pulmonary disease indicate accumulation of alveolar fluid and imply heart failure, or an acutely expanded plasma volume, or both.

    e. When rales are caused by expansion of plasma volume, the acute increase in volume is at least 1500 ml.

C. Interpreting laboratory values (see Table 9-7).

  1. Serum sodium concentration

    a. Serum sodium concentration reflects solute concentration in all body compartments. It is a measure of the state of **total body osmolarity**. Unless there is a disparity between the proportions of salt and water gained or lost, body osmolarity will not change and the serum sodium concentration will be unaltered.

    b. Acute changes in body osmolarity most often are caused by changes in total body water content.

    c. In **water depletion**, all body fluid compartments contract proportionately in volume, increasing the concentration of all solutes. This is reflected in an **increase in serum sodium concentration**.

    d. In acute water depletion, the serum sodium concentration is a good guide to body need for water. Each 3 mEq of serum sodium concentration above normal indicates a deficit of at least 1 liter of water.

    e. A **decrease in serum sodium** concentration is due to **water excess**. Water excess due to stress-induced antidiuresis or to iatrogenic administration of only electrolyte-free IV solutions is seen frequently in surgical patients.

    f. Water excess is treated by restricting water intake. Administration of a hypertonic sodium solution is indicated only for convulsions (water intoxication). A concomitant sodium deficit may also be present but cannot be determined from the serum sodium. Diagnosis of a sodium deficit depends on signs of ECF depletion (see Table 9-3).

    g. Certain debilitated patients develop a low serum sodium concentration that is asymptomatic—the **"hyponatremia of severe illness"** or **"low salt syndrome."** The best treatment for this situation is no treatment at all. This syndrome is caused by a "resetting" of hypothalamic osmoreceptors; inappropriate secretion of ADH results in a chronic state of mild water excess. If one tries to raise the serum sodium concentration is such a situation by restricting water intake, signs of water depletion (thirst, oliguria) appear while hyponatremia persists. If one tries to raise the serum sodium concentration by administering salt, the salt is excreted via the kidneys; if not, the patient may become edematous, even while remaining hyponatremic.

h. The serum sodium concentration is not a reliable indicator of changes in total body sodium content or of sodium need in either acute or chronic imbalances.

i. **An increase in serum sodium concentration indicates a need for electrolyte-free water. A decrease in serum sodium concentration often indicates a need for restriction of electrolyte-free water intake;** sometimes there may be a need for administration of sodium-containing fluids to patients who are hypovolemic.

2. Hematocrit

a. Changes in hematocrit are interpretable in terms of fluid balance only when no changes are occurring in erythrocyte mass (i.e., no bleeding or hemolysis).

b. The whole-blood hematocrit provides a biopsy of both the intracellular compartment (erythrocytes) and the extracellular compartment (plasma).

c. The hematocrit changes little with disturbances of water balance, since, when only total body water changes, the erythrocytes (intracellular compartment) swell or shrink proportionately and in parallel with plasma volume (extracellular compartment). The percent volume of whole blood occupied by the erythrocytes (hematocrit) is not appreciably affected.

d. The plasma volume, as a part of the sodium-dependent ECF volume, changes in parallel with changes in total body sodium content. The erythrocytes (intracellular compartment) are little affected by changes in sodium balance. Therefore, **changes in total body sodium are associated with changes in hematocrit.**

e. In **sodium depletion,** the **plasma volume decreases and the hematocrit rises.** An initial rough estimate of the magnitude of sodium deficit may be obtained by equating each 3% increase in hematocrit value from normal with a deficit of 150 mEq of sodium. Considerable clinical judgment enters into the assumption of "normal hematocrit," i.e., what the hematocrit in a given patient would be if no imbalance were present. The magnitude of any imbalances estimated in this way should not be rigidly interpreted but used simply as a guide to initial treatment.

f. In **sodium excess,** the expected decrease in hematocrit is not regularly seen, usually because this disorder occurs over a long enough period of time to allow increased production of red cells by the bone marrow.

g. In situations of pure **water depletion** (dehydration), the hematocrit may be normal. Hemoglobin is a more reliable measure of the deficit, since the hemoglobin content of each red cell remains constant.

h. Over the short term and as long as hemorrhage is not occurring, **an increase in hematocrit is interpreted as indicating a need for sodium (saline).**

3. Serum potassium concentration

a. The serum potassium represents only a small fraction, about 1%, of the total body exchangeable potassium. Therefore, large changes in body potassium content can occur without producing a change in serum potassium concentration outside the normal range. Nonetheless, the serum potassium concentration, if properly interpreted, is a reliable but insensitive guide to potassium need.

b. Serum potassium is logarithmically related to total body potassium. Severe states of depletion may be reflected in only minor changes in serum potassium; in states of excess, small additions to the body potassium content can result in large (and dangerous) changes in serum potassium concentration.

c. Serum potassium concentration is increased in acidosis and decreased in alkalosis. This effect is caused by a shift in potassium out of (and hydrogen ion into) cells in acidosis, or a shift of potassium into cells in alkalosis without any change in total body potassium content. The approximate deficit or excess of potassium may be calculated from arterial pH and serum potassium using the nomogram in Figure 9-4.

d. Some hormones (vasopressin, thyroxine) raise the serum potassium concentration, while others (insulin, corticosteroids) lower it.

4. Blood pH

a. The diagnosis of acid-base abnormalities is markedly simplified by the use of an acid-base diagram (Fig. 9-5).

b. Blood pH is the most direct and accurate measurement of the state of acid-base balance. It should be used in preference to measurement of the serum bicarbonate.

c. Arterial samples should be used routinely. Venous samples have a lower normal value, and their range varies considerably, depending on the state of tissues peripheral to the site of venipuncture, making interpretation less reliable in acutely changing situations.

5. Serum bicarbonate concentration

a. Carbon dioxide combining power, usually reported as "CO_2," is the commonly available measure of bicarbonate concentration. Carbonic acid (H_2CO_3) concentration (dissolved CO_2 in blood) is measured as the PCO_2, or CO_2 tension, usually by means of a modified pH electrode. CO_2 content is the sum of bicarbonate (HCO_3^-) and H_2CO_3 and is measured manometrically.

b. For most clinical situations, measurement of the bicarbonate concentration in serum is adequate, although determination of arterial pH is simpler and more direct.

c. Clinical disturbances in acid-base balance were classically described in terms of the Henderson-Hasselbalch equation for the bicarbonate buffer system because bicarbonate was the only buffer anion that could be measured easily in serum. Such a description is adequate as long as one remembers how the pulmonary and renal mechanisms for hydrogen ion excretion influence the bicarbonate buffer system:

$$pH = pK + \log \frac{HCO_3^-}{H_2CO_3} \quad \begin{array}{l} \text{(controlled by kidney; measured as "bicarbonate")} \\ \text{(controlled by lung; equals } PCO_2 \times 0.03) \end{array}$$

d. Bicarbonate concentration is increased in respiratory acidosis and metabolic alkalosis; it is decreased in metabolic acidosis and respiratory alkalosis. As a general rule, the serum bicarbonate accurately reflects acid-base balance in the absence of pulmonary dysfunction.

6. Urine

a. Volume output

(1) Record urine output at least q8h in all patients on parenteral fluids. If there is a major imbalance, shock or any suspicion of renal insufficiency, record urine output hourly.

(2) Expected volume output is 1500 ± 500 ml/day (60 ± 20 ml/hr) in patients in a basal state.

Table 9-8. Urine Electrolyte Concentrations (Random Specimen)

Tubular Activity	Sodium (mEq/liter)	Potassium (mEq/liter)
Normal	> 40	> 40
Conserving (early)	10–30	20–30
Maximal retention	< 5	15–25

(3) Following trauma or stress, output may decrease transiently to 750–1200 ml/day (30–50 ml/hr).

(4) Excessive output (> 400–600 ml/hr) occurs with diabetes insipidus as a result of pituitary dysfunction due to trauma or CNS malignancy, or it can occur as a result of a primary renal abnormality (nephrogenic diabetes insipidus). Such conditions are dangerous because if insufficient salt and water replacement is given, shock will result.

(5) An output of 500 ml/day or less constitutes **oliguria.** In the absence of tubular failure or obstructive uropathy, oliguria is prerenal in origin and may be a result of either a deficit in ECF volume (total body sodium) or a deficit in total body water.

b. Urinalysis

(1) A random sample is sufficient. A 24-hr urine collection is not necessary to make any determination that is useful in managing fluid problems except in uncommon situations in which renal function may change rapidly, such as renal transplant rejection.

(2) **Specific gravity** reflects osmolar concentration of solutes in urine except when the urine contains significant amounts of abnormal solutes, such as protein, glucose, radiographic contrast media, or mannitol.

(3) As effective renal concentrating mechanism results in **high urine osmolality in states of water or sodium deficit.**

(4) **Iso-osmolar urine (specific gravity ≤ 1.010) and oliguria suggest a primary renal defect,** such as acute tubular necrosis or renal failure. Such situations should be elucidated with the aid of measurements of central hemodynamics (CVP, Swan-Ganz).

(5) **Urine pH** reflects the pH in serum and helps confirm a diagnosis of acidosis or alkalosis. There are several exceptions: paradoxical aciduria in hypokalemic alkalosis; alkaline urine secondary to infection with urea-splitting bacteria; and alkaline urine in renal tubular acidosis.

(6) **Urine electrolyte concentrations** are presented in Table 9-8. Sodium retention begins promptly on renal tubular stimulation by aldosterone, but maximal conservation requires 3–5 days of constant stimulation. When maximally stimulated, renal sodium excretion can be brought to zero. In the absence of marked diuresis, a **urine sodium concentration below 20 mEq/liter always indicates active conservation** that may be due to an actual or functional plasma or ECF volume deficit or to inappropriate secretion of aldosterone. Potassium retention is controlled by many factors (e.g., serum pH, tubular solute load, sodium balance) besides the state of total body potassium. Although some conservation of potassium occurs in hypokalemia, even with a large deficit in total body potassium there is still an **obligatory urinary loss of potassium of about 2 mEq/day.**

IV. Planning and execution of fluid and electrolyte therapy

A. Goals

1. Attain and maintain normal body composition and homeostasis.

2. Correct life-threatening imbalances (hypovolemia, hyperkalemia) as top priorities.

3. Avoid the complications of too-rapid correction or overcorrection (e.g., seizures due to overzealous treatment of acidosis, congestive heart failure due to over-administration of sodium [saline]).

4. Integrate fluid and electrolyte therapy with hyperalimentation therapy when indicated.

5. Construct easily understood and easily followed orders that can be quickly checked during therapy to assure correct composition and rate of infusion of the fluids being administered.

B. Guidelines for IV placement and maintenance

1. Placement of intravenous lines should be individualized to meet each patient's fluid and medication requirements.

   a. Avoid placement across joints.

   b. Use the nondominant arm when possible.

   c. Use central lines when administering hypertonic or sclerotic drugs (e.g., KCl in high concentration, antibiotics such as penicillin or cephalosporins).

   d. Avoid the use of the cephalic vein in the forearm when possible, especially in patients with renal disease in whom vascular access may become necessary, since this is the site of choice for future placement of an arteriovenous fistula.

   e. Inspect IV sites daily for signs of infection, and discontinue infusion if they are observed.

   f. Avoid leaving any peripheral IV cannula in place longer than 48 hours, to minimize septic phlebitis.

   g. Rotate IV sites, and use steel needles (butterfly) when possible.

2. **Suggested technique of placement**

   a. Apply venous tourniquets and select the vein to be used.

   b. Choose a steel needle or a plastic cannula for venipuncture, based on the considerations in the foregoing section.

   c. Tear tape as required for fixation prior to insertion of the IV line.

   d. Check that the IV solution is correct and the administration set is appropriate. Use a Volutrol if medications will be administered; use a set with Y-tubing if blood products are also to be needed. Prime the tubing, eliminating air bubbles.

   e. Prepare the site with an antibacterial solution (alcohol, chlorhexidine, povidone-iodine). Wear gloves or sterilize the fingers touching the prepared area on the patient. Avoid touching the actual site of puncture prior to or after placement of the IV needle.

   f. Insert and begin infusion.

   g. Fix the needle and tubing to the skin securely to minimize inconvenience to the patient and to avoid accidentally dislodging the needle.

h. Double-check to see that the infusion runs freely and that no evidence of infiltration has occurred.

i. Label the IV line with the date, so it can be changed at the appropriate time.

j. Inspect the IV line and proximal vein at least daily for signs of inflammation and infection.

C. Clinical approach to fluid therapy

1. Because it is not possible to decide in advance the exact requirements of any patient for fluids or electrolytes, and since it is clinically difficult to measure output of fluid volumes and electrolytes from some sources, practical fluid therapy, even in the most difficult situations, must involve a semiquantitative approach, not a series of exact balance studies.

2. Fluid and electrolyte **therapy is simplified if approached systematically.** To arrive at a plan of treatment in any situation, answers to these questions are needed:

   a. What **imbalances** are present now, and what is their probable magnitude?

   b. What **additional losses** can be expected during treatment?

   c. What are **daily maintenance requirements** for fluid and electrolytes?

   d. Most importantly, **what is the patient's most pressing problem?**

3. Within each of these categories—imbalances, expected losses, and maintenance—determine next the needs for the following:

   a. Electrolyte-free **water.**

   b. **Sodium** together with the water needed for its isosmotic solution (saline).

   c. **Potassium**

   d. Other electrolytes

   e. Acid-base adjustment.

   f. Blood and plasma products.

4. **Priorities** must be established in the treatment of fluid and electrolyte disorders. Therapy first must be directed toward correction of abnormalities that constitute the greatest threat to the patient's life. These are:

   a. **Restoration of circulating vascular volume (CVV).** Patients with normal cardiac reserve and hypotension (systolic blood pressure < 105 mm Hg) at rest (40% decrease in CVV) or patients who are normotensive but have an orthostatic drop of 20 mm Hg (20% decrease in CVV) need immediate vascular volume reconstitution.

   b. **Correction of hyperkalemia.** Because of its effect on cardiac condution, hyperkalemia carries a significant risk of fatal cardiac arrhythmias.

   c. **Correction of red cell mass (blood) deficits.**

   d. Overly rapid correction of some abnormalities, e.g., acidosis with IV $NaHCO_3$, carries a high risk of seizures because of rapid flux of PCO_2 into the cerebrospinal fluid (CSF) with resultant accentuation of CSF acidosis.

5. In the scheme to be outlined, three **assumptions** are made:

   a. **The patient is a "typical 70-kg man."** If the patient weighs more than 70 kg, no adjustments in fluid orders are necessary. If the patient weighs less than 70 kg, downward adjustments may be made using Figure 9-6 as a guide. In general, if renal function is adequate, i.e., creatinine clearance greater than 50 ml/min, no significant adjustments of maintenance fluids are required until body weight is less than 30 kg.

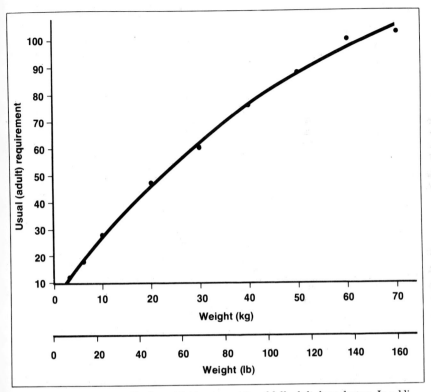

Figure 9-6. Relationship of body weight to percentage of full adult drug dosage. In addition to being useful in adapting fluid and electrolyte dosages for small adults and children, this curve also can be used to select a proper dose of any drug (sedatives and narcotics excepted). For patients weighing more than 70 kg, do not adjust the dosage upward.

b. **Renal function is adequate,** as indicated by a serum creatinine less than 2.0 mg/100 ml or creatinine clearance more than 50 ml/min. Children less than 2 yr of age have immature renal function, do not handle sodium well, and have higher proportional total body water than adults. The management of fluid and electrolyte therapy in these children should be done in consultation with a knowledgeable pediatric surgeon or pediatrician, as outlined in Chapter 19. Patients with acute or chronic renal failure should be managed as outlined in Chapter 11.

c. **Cardiac and hepatic function are normal.** Patients with cardiac or liver failure require downward adjustment in sodium and water allowances to minimize edema and ascites formation.

D. **Basic allowances (maintenance therapy)**

1. **Normal values** for basic allowances for adults are shown in Table 9-9.

2. The value for **daily urine volume** (1500 ml) is chosen as a convenient midpoint between the minimum volume (500 ml) with which the daily solute load (400–700 mOsm) can be eliminated and the maximum volume (20 liters) beyond which hypo-osmolality is induced in patients with normal renal function.

Table 9-9. Basic Daily Allowances

Loss	Water (ml)	Electrolytes (mEq)		
		Sodium	Chloride	Potassium
Urine	1500	150	90	40
Insensible	1000	0	0	0
Gastric	Previous volume	as measured	plus trend	10/liter

Table 9-10. Allowances for Losses Resulting from Fever, Environmental Temperature, and Hyperventilation*

Additional Allowance (per 24 hr)	Fever	Environmental Temperature (°F)	Respiratory Rate/Min
None	38.3°C (101°F) or less	85 or less	35 or less
500 ml water	38.4–39.4°C (101–103°F)	85–95	Over 35
1000 ml water	39.5°C (103°F) or more	95 or more	. . . . . .

*Corrections are additive; thus, a patient with fever of 38.8°C (102°F) (+500 ml) in an ambient environmental temperature of 86°F (30°C) (+500 ml) would have a total correction of +1000 ml water.

3. **Insensible losses** vary with ambient temperature and humidity, body temperature, and degree of integrity of the skin. However, 1000 ml/day of water covers most situations. Fecal losses rarely exceed 200 ml/day.

4. **Sodium requirements** may vary between as little as 500 mg (cirrhosis with ascites) and as much as 10–12 gm (usual daily intake in the United States; obligate loss in polyuric renal failure). The usual allowance of 150 mEq (6 gm) of sodium is a good midpoint for most surgical patients. The acute decrease from normal intake (250 mEq or 10–12 gm/day) to the lower level recommended by many texts (50 mEq or 2 gm) may result in clinical hypovolemia during the 24- to 48-hour period required for renal adjustment to the lower intake.

5. **Potassium losses** also may vary widely, but, in the absence of diuretic therapy or GI losses, 40–60 mEq/day is usually sufficient replacement. Serum potassium should be the only guide to potassium therapy. No allowances are made for acid-base corrections or for replacement of blood and plasma in the normal state.

E. **Additional losses during treatment.** Sources of additional losses during treatment may be:

1. GI secretion (see Table 9-6).

2. Increased insensible losses resulting from fever, high environmental temperatures, and hyperventilation (Table 9-10).

3. Increased water and salt loss from sweating (Table 9-11) or in cystic fibrosis.

4. Increased renal loss of water and salt from an enforced osmotic diuresis (mannitol, urea, low molecular weight dextran), or following arteriography or an intravenous pyelogram.

5. Formation of a third space of sequestered ECF in traumatized and postoperative patients.

Table 9-11. Allowances for Losses Resulting from Sweating

Degree of Sweating	Additional Allowance (per 24 hr)	
	Water (ml)	Sodium (mEq)
Moderate; intermittent	500	25
Moderate; continuous	1000	50
Profuse; continuous	2000 or more	75 or more

6. Plasma loss from burns, granulating wounds, chest tubes, and other drains.

7. **GI suction** is the most common and most important source of additional fluid losses during treatment of surgical patients. GI losses should be measured. Postoperative nasogastric suction usually produces 500–1000 ml/day. In most situations, the volume of GI fluid losses can be estimated in advance, the composition determined from Table 9-5, and the anticipated losses replaced as they occur.

8. Administration of each 12.5 gm of mannitol will enforce additional excretion of about 125 ml of water, 10 mEq of sodium, and 2 mEq of potassium. Prolonged use of mannitol leads to a predominant water deficit (hypernatremia), with an accompanying mild sodium deficit.

F. Guidelines for administration

1. Divide daily requirements equally and administer as readily available solutions (e.g., 5% D/W in 0.45 normal saline).

2. Number daily bottles sequentially (e.g., 1, 2, 3, etc).

3. Record daily weights, and keep a record of intake and output. Use body weight as check for intake and output balance.

4. Check serum electrolytes daily.

5. Serially assess clinical signs of hydration, i.e., thirst, skin turgor, edema, heart rate, and blood pressure changes with position.

6. Write orders at least daily, and adjust for patient needs. Avoid standing IV orders such as "5% D/W in 0.2 normal saline with 15 mEq KCl continuously at 125 ml/hr" which might continue indefinitely. Such orders breed oversights and lead to major iatrogenic imbalances. Review orders for critically ill patients more frequently than in other patients.

7. Carefully record unusual losses, such as ascitic fluid leaks, since they may quickly result in severe imbalances if not replaced.

8. Administer one half of estimated deficits in the first 24-hr period of replacement unless this restriction will not result in an adequate circulating volume or will permit persisting hypokalemia.

9. At the end of each treatment period, reevaluate the patient, and compare the actual with the expected results of treatment.

10. Limit potassium infusion to 20 mEq/hr to avoid cardiac arrest.

11. Except in cases of overt shock, when a physician will be in attendance, limit infusion rates to 500 ml/hr.

12. Add ascorbic acid and multiple vitamins to one bottle daily.

13. Take the cation content of antibiotics into consideration (e.g., sodium carbenicillin, potassium penicillin).

V. Examples of fluid management

A. Pyloric (gastric outlet) obstruction

1. **History.** A 55-yr old, 70-kg man with a long history of symptomatic duodenal ulcer enters the hospital with severe epigastric pain and vomiting present for 5 days. He has taken calcium carbonate to relieve pain. During the past 2 days, he has been thirsty and has drunk water copiously, most of which has been vomited. He now complains of severe thirst.

2. **Physical.** Temperature is 38.5°C (101.4°F), pulse 100, occasionally irregular, blood pressure 110/70, no postural hypotension. The oral mucous membranes, axillae, and groin are dry; the tongue is furrowed, skin turgor only fair; the patient is able to void only 30 ml of urine on admission. Urine specific gravity is 1.032, pH 6.0, Na 22, K 30, Hct 38%. Serum Na is 154, K 2.8. Arterial pH is 7.52. Gastric aspirate pH is 2.6.

3. **Diagnoses**

   a. **Severe water deficit.** 3000+ ml (history, hypernatremia, thirst, dry membranes, concentrated urine—the +9 mEq serum Na indicates at least a 3-liter total body water deficit).

   b. **Moderate sodium deficit.** 150–300 mEq (history, poor turgor, low urine Na, tachycardia).

   c. **Severe hypokalemia.** History, serum K, irregular pulse, paradoxical aciduria; using the nomogram in Figure 9-4, the change in body potassium is −11% [pH 7.52, serum K 2.8] and with a normal capacity of 3150 mEq [70 kg × 45] this indicates a total body potassium deficit of approximately 350 mEq.

   d. **Metabolic alkalosis.** History, alkali ingestion, hypokalemia, arterial pH.

4. **Fluid requirements for initial treatment period of 12 hr**

	Water (ml)	Sodium (mEq)	Potassium (mEq)
Half of deficits	1500	100	175
Maintenance	1250	25–50	20–40
Losses			
Temperature	250	....	....
GI suction	1000	60	10
	4000	185–210	205–225

5. **Fluid orders** (one of many possibilities; the large estimate for potassium needed in this treatment period cannot be met safely).

   a. **Bottle #1.** 1000 5% dextrose in 0.45% saline; run at 200 gtt/min; complete at 0130. If urine output more than 50 ml, continue with IVs as ordered; if urine output less than 50 ml, notify me.

   b. **Bottle #2.** 1000 5% dextrose in 0.45% saline; add 40 mEq KCl; run at 120 gtt/min; complete at 0400.

   c. **Bottle #3.** 1000 5% dextrose in 0.45% saline; add 60 mEq KCl; run at 60 gtt/min; complete at 0800.

   d. **Bottle #4.** 1000 5% D/W; add 60 mEq KCl plus 150 mg ascorbic acid; run at 60 gtt/min; complete at 1200.

   e. Measure and record CVP q15 min during bottle #1; if CVP rises over 12 cm saline, slow infusion to 50 gtt/min and notify me.

   f. Label all bottles: additives, time started, and time stopped.

   g. Save all bottles; place in box under patient's bed.

6. **Follow-up.** At the end of 12 hr of therapy the patient is much improved, although thirst persists. The temperature is 37.2°C (99°F), the tongue is no longer furrowed, and the axillae are questionably moist. Urine output has been 920 ml, specific gravity 1.028, pH 5.6, Na 40, K 36. Arterial pH is now 7.46. Nasogastric suction volume is 1000 ml with pH 3.0. Serum Na is 148, K 2.9.

7. **Reassessing** the situation, these diagnoses are made:

   a. **Moderate water deficit.** More than 1500 ml (persisting thirst).

   b. **Severe hypokalemia.** About 230 mEq deficit (history, paradoxical aciduria).

   c. **Mild metabolic alkalosis** (arterial pH). No change in the allowance for GI suction need be made, since the present rate of loss equals the estimate of 2000 ml/day; no allowance now need be made for fever. Requirements for the next 12 hr of therapy will be:

	Water (ml)	Sodium (mEq)	Potassium (mEq)
Half of deficits	750	....	115
Maintenance	1250	25–50	20–40
GI losses	1000	60	10
	3000	85–110	145–165

B. Peritonitis in a cardiac patient

1. **History.** A 72-yr old woman enters the hospital with a 3-day history of abdominal pain culminating in prostration a few hours before admission. She had severe congestive heart failure 2 yr previously and since then has been on digitalis, a low sodium diet, and a thiazide diuretic with potassium supplements.

2. **Physical.** She appears listless, has poor skin turgor, a furrowed tongue, and flat neck veins. Blood pressure is 99/50 mm Hg, pulse 116 and thready, temperature 38.9°C (102°F). Abdominal signs are those of peritonitis, and exploration is required urgently. She is unable to void; an indwelling catheter is placed and 50 ml of urine obtained. Urine specific gravity is 1.014, pH 5.5, Na 28, K 53, Hct 46%. Serum Na is 135, K 3.9, CO_2 20.

3. **Diagnoses**

   a. **Sodium depletion** 600 mEq (physical findings, hypotension, tachycardia, low urine Na).

   b. **Early metabolic acidosis** (low CO_2).

   c. **Mild water excess** (hyponatremia, history).

4. **Initial estimate of fluid requirements for 2 hr of therapy**

	Water (ml)	Sodium (mEq)	Potassium (mEq)
Half of deficits	2000	300	..
Maintenance	200	6	4
Losses			
Temperature	20	....	....
GI Suction	100	6	1
Third space	500	75	5
	2820	387	10

5. **Treatment.** A CVP catheter is inserted via the brachial vein; initial pressure is 5 cm saline. Since this patient requires very rapid correction, fluids (which also include appropriate antibiotics) are given by a physician in constant atten-

dance who monitors the CVP. Two liters of Ringer's lactate are given in the first 90 minutes, after which the patient's blood pressure is 130/80 mm Hg, pulse is 100, and CVP 9 cm. A third liter of Ringer's lactate is begun at a slower rate, and the patient is taken to the operating room. A perforated appendix with generalized peritonitis is found and appropriately treated.

6. **Follow-up.** Postoperatively, the patient is sweating, temperature is 38.9°C (102°F), blood pressure 110/70 mm Hg, pulse 110, Hct 42%. She has excreted 200 ml urine since admission. **Reassessing** the situation, make the following diagnoses:

   a. **Sodium depletion.** 450 mEq (history, tachycardia).

   b. **Mild metabolic acidosis** (probable).

   c. **Peritonitis.** Continuing development of a third space is to be anticipated.

7. **Estimated fluid requirements for the next 24 hr**

	Water (ml)	Sodium (mEq)	Potassium (mEq)
Half of deficits	1500	225	....
Maintenance	2000	50	50
Losses			
Temperature	500		
Sweat	500	25	....
GI Suction	600	60	6
Third space	1000	150	10
	6100	510	66

These requirements are too great to manage as a 24-hr treatment period in this patient. The next treatment period should be changed to 6–8 hr, using an appropriate fraction of the preceding estimates. At the end of this shorter first postoperative treatment period, a reassessment, including measurement of serum and urine electrolytes, is carried out, and new estimates of deficits are made to guide subsequent treatment.

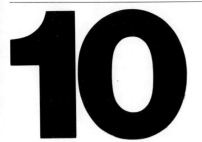

Surgical Nutrition

I. General principles governing nutritional requirements

A. The resting state for an adult male patient requires approximately 21 to 30 Cal/kg body weight/day. This will vary with the age of the patient. The younger patient will require a higher calorie per kilogram of energy supply than the elderly. An infant will need from 120 to 90 Cal/kg/day, while an elderly male will require approximately 18 Cal/kg/day. Caloric requirements are slightly less for females than for males.

B. Healthy young males who are fasting lose lean body mass more rapidly than do females, the elderly, and the debilitated.

C. **Sepsis** will increase these demands by 5–8% per each degree rise in temperature.

D. **Peritonitis,** even though associated with sepsis, imposes an additional caloric consumption of 20–40% over the resting state.

E. **Major fractures** of long bones will increase the caloric demand by 10–25%.

F. The greatest demands are those of **severe burn injuries** (second and third degree). The need for extra calories may be 40–100% of the normal intake.

G. In parenteral administration of nutrients, the major limiting factor is the utilization of **glucose** for calories, which maximally is 0.9 gm/kg/hr even with insulin administration.

H. **Protein requirements** for an average young adult will be 0.45 gm/kg/day. To minimize the catabolic effect of starvation, a ratio of 150–200 nonprotein calories/gm **nitrogen** must be reached before protein can be synthesized; more recent studies suggest that the calorie-to-nitrogen ratio should be higher. These nonprotein calories can be administered either as glucose or, when available, as fat emulsions.

I. To prevent essential **fatty acid** deficiency, it is necessary to have 2% of the total caloric intake as linoleic acid. Fatty acid deficiency is very common in children depleted of essential nutrition even for a short period of time. It is very uncommon in adults but still can be prevented by giving one to two bottles of fatty emulsion/ week. Patients who are on long term (>2 wk) total parenteral nutritional (TPN) therapy should have essential fatty acid replacement.

J. Young adults will require an infusion of 2.4 mEq of **sodium** and 2.0–2.3 mEq **potassium**/100 Cal/day. The cardiovascular and renal status of the patient often is a limiting factor in calculating the total requirements for hyperalimentation fluid. When using parenteral forms of nutrition, it is necessary also to replace calcium and phosphorus. Adults will require 200–400 mg calcium and 300–350 mg phosphorus/2500 Cal/day.

K. **Exact magnesium** requirements are not known with certainty. There appears to be no direct hormonal control of magnesium metabolism; serum levels depend on intake and renal output. Deprivation lasting more than 3–4 wk can lead to hypomagnesemia. The fall in serum magnesium is associated initially with neurological symptoms and later with gastrointestinal (GI) dysfunction (anorexia, nausea, and vomiting). For adults, the National Research Council recommends a daily dietary allowance of 25 mEq of magnesium; approximately one third of this is absorbed, so that 8 mEq enters the circulation. In infants, the recommended allowance range is 4–25 mEq/2500 Cal; thus, 1–8 mEq enters the circulation.

L. Iron supplements are given parenterally as an iron dextran once or twice a month. The estimated daily loss of iron in adults is 0.5–1.0 mg/day. For menstruating women, another 1 mg is added.

M. Trace elements. Trace elements can be replaced using a solution (Shils) that allows for replacement of zinc, copper, manganese, and iodine. Trace element solution, 1 ml in 1 liter of hyperalimentation fluid, is given once a day.

1. To compound trace element solution, measure the following:

  a. Zinc chloride, 651 mg.

  b. Cupric sulfate, 5 H_2O, 600 mg.

  c. Manganese chloride 4 H_2O, 234 mg.

  d. Sodium iodide, 10 mg.

  e. 1.0N hydrochloric acid, 0.55 ml.

  f. Sterile normal saline, 150 ml.

  g. Divide the total volume of 150 ml of sterile normal saline about equally into four sterile containers. Add approximately one half the measured amount of hydrochloric acid to each of two containers. Dissolve the zinc chloride in one of these containers and the cupric sulfate in the other. Dissolve the manganese chloride and the sodium iodide in each of the remaining two containers.

  h. Combine all previously dissolved ingredients. Mix well. Transfer to sterile vials through an 0.22-μ Millipore filter. Steam-sterilize for 30 min at 121°C (250°F).

2. The resultant **trace element solution** contains, in each milliliter:

  a. Zinc, 2.0 mg.

  b. Copper, 1.0 mg.

  c. Manganese, 0.4 mg.

  d. Iodide, 0.056 mg.

3. Trace element solutions are now commercially available in 10-ml sterile ampules. A typical solution contains:

  a. Zinc, 1 mg/ml.

  b. Manganese, 0.1 mg/ml.

  c. Copper, 0.4 mg/ml.

  d. Chromium, 4 μg/ml.

There is a scarcity of evidence that iodide is required in the average patient receiving total parenteral nutrition. However, if needed, sterile sodium iodide solution is available.

II. Indications for nutritional support

A. Patients who are **unable to maintain a normal state of nutrition** because of a variety of chronic disease conditions.

B. Patients in whom the **caloric demands of illness** are such that they cannot consume a meal in the usual fashion need nutritional support from either enteral (tube feeding) or parenteral (central or peripheral) hyperalimentation. The type of nutritional therapy depends on the ultimate outcome and goals that are planned for the patient. Patients who have an illness that requires nutritional support for a 1- to 3-wk period do well with peripheral administration of amino acids, glucose, and fat emulsion. Patients who should be considered for long-term nutritional therapy, either through a central venous line (parenteral alimentation) or by tube feeding using either gravity or a pump, include those who are losing large quantities of fluid or calories but who cannot eat for a variety of reasons:

1. Granulomatous disease of the bowel.

2. Short-bowel syndrome.

3. Large, upper GI tract fistulas.

4. Benign or malignant strictures of the upper GI tract.

5. Neurological disorders that prevent the patient from eating.

Patients with an anatomically and functionally intact intestinal tract who are unable to meet total needs by the usual oral means may require both parenteral and nasogastric tube feedings.

C. Patients whose **visceral protein is low,** as manifested by a decreased serum albumin or transferrin, or patients who are **anergic** after testing with standard skin test antigens.

1. The albumin range of 3.5–3.0 g/100 ml is considered evidence of minimal malnutrition, 3.0–2.5, of moderate malnutrition, and less than 2.5, of severe malnutrition. Albumin repletion will take a week or more of treatment before any response is seen.

2. A transferrin test is difficult to perform and is done by only a few laboratories. An estimate of serum transferrin concentration can be obtained by the following calculation: iron-binding capacity $\times$ 0.8 $-$ 43 = transferrin. Transferrin is a sensitive indicator of malnutrition and shows a rapid response to therapy. Patients with severe anemia due to chronic blood loss may have a low iron-binding capacity.

3. Lack of a reaction to skin test antigens is associated with increased postoperative morbidity and mortality. Patients in a nonimmunosuppressed state tested with streptokinase-streptodornase, mumps, intermediate strength tuberculin, and *Trichophyton* antigens who fail to show at least a 1-cm wheal in 48 hr to one of these compounds are considered to be anergic and to have a moderate to severe state of malnutrition.

D. Many patients with an **anatomically altered but functionally intact intestinal tract (short-bowel syndrome,** internal and external fistulas) can be given tube feeding regimens with the use of low-bulk "elemental" diets. Such diets also are helpful in patients with an **anatomically intact but functionally altered intestinal tract** (ulcerative colitis, regional enteritis, pancreatitis, biliary fistula).

E. Patients whose illness is considered to be terminal, in whom prolonging life is the only aim of therapy, should not be considered candidates for prolonged nutritional support, especially if a central or peripheral form of parenteral administration is anticipated. However, this form of therapy is a distinctive adjuvant to care of patients who show evidence of recovery or have tumors that respond to chemotherapy or further surgical treatment.

III. Tube feeding

A. **Routes of administration** include nasogastric intubation, gastrostomy, and jejunostomy.

B. **Tube feeding formulas.** There are three categories from which to select a specific tube feeding formula:

Table 10-1. Tube Feeding Prepared from Food

Type of Food and Content	1 Cal/ml
Baby food (meat)	210 ml
Egg	50 ml (frozen)
Applesauce	120 ml
Orange juice	240 ml (reconstituted)
Instant potato granules	50 gm
Refined cereal	100 ml
Oil	45 ml
Milk	960 ml
Strained carrots	100 ml
Dextrose	60 gm
	2000 ml
Percentage of calories	
Protein	16
Fat	40
Carbohydrate	44
Osmolarity (mOsm/liter)	567

1. **Commercially prepared** nutrient solutions. These are supplied in premixed form. These formulas contain 1 Cal/ml; the protein is derived from either casein or soy. Their major appeal is ease of preparation. Sufficient minerals and vitamins are supplied in the formula for maintenance requirements, but supplements may have to be added when excess losses so dictate. Their major **disadvantages** are the cost and the occurrence of diarrhea when concentrations of more than 1 Cal/ml are required.

2. **Blenderized feedings** can be concocted from baby foods or any table food soft enough to be liquified, or a commercial preparation may be chosen; blenderized tube feedings supply calories in a balanced manner and are better tolerated. A whole food diet that can be prepared easily and inexpensively is presented in Table 10-1.

3. **Low-bulk diets**

   a. The protein is supplied as one of the following:

      (1) Crystalline amino acids (Vivonex).

      (2) Casein hydrolysate (Flexical).

      (3) Egg albumin (Precision LR).

   b. All contain the eight essential amino acids plus a number of nonessential amino acids and are similar to solutions used for IV hyperalimentation. The **advantages** of these diets are:

      (1) The composition is known precisely.

      (2) There is almost complete absorption.

      (3) Minimal digestion is required (important in short-bowel syndrome).

      (4) Pancreatic, biliary, and gut secretions are diminished (important in inflammatory bowel diseases, fistulas, pancreatitis).

(5) Stool bulk is lessened (important in ulcerative and granulomatous colitis).

(6) Losses through fistulas are minimized.

c. While these diets may be given PO, poor patient acceptance during long-term maintenance, in spite of a choice of flavors, eventually prompts introduction via a feeding tube. In full-strength dilution there is 1 Cal/ml, and osmolarity varies from 500 to 1200 mOsm/liter, depending on the flavor.

C. Method of tube feeding

1. Start with a dilute (one quarter strength) solution and maintenance volumes and gradually increase the concentration every 2–3 days. Excess water must be provided to prevent hypernatremia and azotemia, which can lead to severe osmotic dehydration; for every milliliter of tube feeding one should calculate at least 0.5 ml of water in excess to prevent this problem. Thirst is an early indicator of serum hyperosmolarity and a need for additional water but is lacking in the obtunded or comatose patient.

2. A constant infusion of diet over a 24-hr period is preferred and can be accomplished by either gravity drip or mechanical pump (such as the Barron); bolus feedings of 200–400 ml q4h are less desirable. Tube feedings must not be allowed to stand at or above room temperature for more than 2–3 hr in order to prevent bacterial overgrowth. If a continuous infusion is contemplated, a means of cooling must be provided. For the same reason, no more than a 24-hr requirement should be prepared at any given time.

3. Gastrostomy and nasogastric tubes should be aspirated twice a day to check for gastric retention and then lavaged with saline to clean the tube of inspissated food material mechanically. Gastrostomy and jejunostomy tubes need time to seal and generally are not safe for infusion until 3 days after insertion. Every 3 days the skin around the tube should be washed and the tube sterilely dressed and securely taped to the skin to prevent accidental dislodgment.

IV. Parenteral nutrition

A. General comments. Parenteral nutrition can be administered by two routes:

1. So-called hyperalimentation, or total parenteral nutrition, through a **central venous catheter,** necessitating the insertion of a catheter into the superior vena cava under strict aseptic conditions (see Fig. 25-9). Insertion of a long-term catheter tunnel underneath the anterior chest wall and placed into the superior vena cava through the cephalic vein is an alternative. This is the patient's lifeline, and attention to details in its placement and care will prevent most serious and possibly life-threatening complications.

2. An isotonic, iso-osmolar amino acid solution, with or without electrolytes, for **administration via peripheral veins** is now available, usually in a 3.0 or 3.5% solution providing approximately 5.6 gm of nitrogen/liter. Nonprotein calorie requirements are made up with 10% glucose and IV fat emulsions, usually in the proportions 40% carbohydrate and 60% fat. Total support by this form of therapy requires administration of considerable volumes of fluid and is probably limited to very short-term therapy.

B. Preparation of nutrient fluid

1. All the preparation of the nutrient materials should be carried on in the pharmacy under strictly aseptic conditions, whether it be for central or for peripheral administration. (The preparation of the peripheral fluid is simpler than for the central, since the isotonic amino acids come with electrolytes premixed.)

2. The actual formulation of the fluid for central administration is the diluting of an amino acid solution (8% or 7%) with a 50% solution of glucose so as to arrive at a final amino acid mixture of between 3.5 and 4.25%, with approximately

23–25% glucose. This will give a calorie-to-nitrogen ratio of better than 150 Cal/gm nitrogen.

3. Additives

a. Sodium, 30–40 mEq, as a phosphate or bicarbonate.

b. Potassium, 40–50 mEq, as a phosphate or chloride.

c. Magnesium sulphate, 8 mEq.

d. Calcium gluconate, 9 mEq (must be added last and slowly to avoid insoluble calcium phosphate precipitation, which forms because of the acidic pH of the solution).

e. Vitamins

(1) To utilize the carbohydrates and amino acids in hyperalimentation fluid efficiently, adequate amounts of water-soluble (B and C) vitamins are necessary. Water-soluble vitamins have no serious toxic effects, even in renal insufficiency. To one bottle/day of hyperalimentation fluid, addition of 5 ml of the commercial parenteral vitamin preparation MVI plus 1–2 mg of folic acid will more than meet requirements for water-soluble vitamins.

(2) Care should be exercised in administration of the fat-soluble vitamins (A, D, E, K), since they produce toxicity with overdosage. Only one bottle of hyperalimentation fluid each day should contain the fat-soluble vitamins. Vitamin K, 10 mg, should be administered twice weekly; additional vitamin K can be given if indicated by serum prothrombin studies. Administration of fat-soluble vitamins to patients on parenteral nutrition for more than 4–6 wk should be limited to once or twice a week.

(3) For patients on long-term parenteral nutrition, 1000 μg of vitamin B_{12} is given monthly.

4. The final formulation of the nutrient fluid is as follows:

Volume	1100 ml
Calories (non-nitrogen)	1000
Protein equivalent	30–35 gm
Nitrogen equivalent	5.5–6.25 gm
Potassium	40 mEq/liter
Sodium	40 mEq/liter
Magnesium	8 mEq/liter
Calcium	10 mEq/liter
Chloride	50 mEq/liter
Phosphate	20 mMol/liter

C. Administration

1. The administration of hypertonic nutrient fluid **through a central line** has to be done carefully to avoid a hyperosmotic state. The osmolarity of a bottle of hyperalimentation fluid is over 1000 mOsm. The starting infusion rate should be 50–100 ml/hr, depending on the patient's cardiovascular-renal status; this will give anywhere from 1200–2400 Cal/day. The increases should be in steps of 25–50 ml/hr every 2–3 days to permit the cardiovascular system and pancreas to adjust to the increased osmolarity and glucose load. The infusion volume should be increased continually until the desired caloric intake is reached.

2. When using **peripheral hyperalimentation** to decrease the fluid volume, one must increase the caloric portion contributed by fat. The usual recommended dosage of fat is approximately 1–2 gm/kg body weight/day. The recommended ratio of fat to carbohydrate is 40–60%. This more closely approximates the normal oral diet in this country. The glucose can be supplied as either 5 or 10% dextrose. The care of the catheter-skin junction is the same as for the central line. The intravenous fat can be pulsed through this line, since there are several different Y-type injection lines on the market with one-way valves, which will prevent fluid backing up into one of the two lines. Glucose cannot be given with fat because it will cause the emulsion to break down.

3. Each bottle should hang at room temperature no longer than 8 hr. All others are kept in a refrigerator, and none should be kept longer than 24 hr. In fact, if the desired infusion rate has not been met for one reason or another at the end of a 24-hr period, it should be noted how much the patient has taken in, and the remainder should be discarded.

4. A final filter should be placed on each infusion unit. These are now available in line filters of 0.22-μ pore size that do not require a pump to allow for adequate flow rates.

5. If the nursing personnel are diligent in watching the flow rate, gravity drip is satisfactory. However, in many institutions, especially in pediatric units, it will be necessary to use a volume-type infusion pump to maintain the proper infusion rate.

6. Diabetic patients. If the patient has latent or frank diabetes, or if the pancreas does not produce enough insulin to handle a glucose load, as in patients with chronic fibrocalcific pancreatitis, exogenous insulin is necessary. We recommend only the use of the subcutaneous route and of regular insulin, 5–10 units for 3+ and 4+ urine sugars. Especially in septic patients, ability to handle glucose is impaired, and higher doses of insulin will have to be used. In these patients, giving small doses of NPH insulin may reduce overall insulin needs. We avoid the addition of insulin to bottles of hyperalimentation fluid because of adsorption of insulin on the surface of the bottle, tubing, or plastic bag, reducing its effectiveness.

7. Discontinuation. When stopping hyperalimentation fluid, especially when given centrally, it is necessary to decrease the flow rate in a stepwise fashion, thus allowing the body to readjust to smaller fluid volumes and particularly to a lesser glucose load.

D. Complications

1. Catheter. Numerous complications related to the catheter and its placement have been reported, including pneumothorax, hydrothorax, hemothorax, brachial plexus injury, subclavian and carotid artery injury, catheter embolus, tracheal perforation, subclavian internal jugular vein thrombosis, arteriovenous fistula, air embolus, thoracic duct injury, and cardiac perforation and tamponade. All these complications can be prevented by meticulous attention to the details of placing the catheter and its care.

2. Sepsis

a. Contamination of the catheter puncture site due to improper technique during insertion, e.g., not using a sterile scrub of the area or failure to use a mask and gloves while placing the catheter. Catheters indwelling more than 3 wk should be changed. For long-term hyperalimentation, a Broviac catheter should be inserted into the superior vena cava (see Fig. 25-9).

b. Long-term placement may be associated with superficial infection around the catheter site that could migrate internally. Pericatheter problems can be minimized by cleaning the puncture site and changing the dressing q48h.

c. Catheter seeding from distant foci during bacteremia, especially in chronically ill patients who have been receiving antibiotics for some time.

d. Solution contamination due to a break in aseptic technique, either on the ward or in the pharmacy.

3. Metabolic disorders

a. Hyperosmolar nonketotic hyperglycemia and acidosis are associated with improper administration, e.g., too rapid an infusion rate or not allowing time for the pancreas to adjust to the glucose load before increasing it further. These same problems occur with tube feedings and can be avoided by increasing the extra water intake, e.g., 0.5 ml for every 1.0 ml of tube feeding.

b. Hypoglycemia may be due to a combination of exogenous insulin overdose along with endogenous insulin overproduction. We therefore recommend the administration of insulin subcutaneously as regular insulin on a rainbow system (see **C.6**).

c. Latent unrecognized diabetes appears particularly in the geriatric patient and in patients with chronic pancreatic insufficiency.

d. Hyperammonemia may appear in patients with chronic liver disease and in pediatric patients because of inadequate liver function.

e. Renal failure may be potentiated in patients with chronic renal disease. This complication can be lessened by decreasing the amino acid load and using a small volume of fluid while still giving the calories needed to prevent catabolism.

f. Calcium, phosphate, and magnesium overload or deficiency appears especially in chronic renal disease and can be minimized by monitoring the serum values.

g. Anemia during long-term therapy can be avoided by administering parenteral iron, vitamin B_{12}, and folic acid.

h. Cardiac arrhythmias are rare. When present, they are usually associated with electrolyte abnormalities, especially hypokalemia.

i. Acidosis can be associated with decreased peripheral perfusion, renal failure, or diabetic ketoacidosis. It also can be a complication of the use of crystal amino acid solutions, which usually are highly acidic.

j. Coma can result from rapid administration, either parenteral or enteral, of hyperosmolar fluid, which produces dehydration and hypernatremia.

k. Hypervitaminosis is most likely to occur when fat-soluble vitamins are given with every bottle of fluid over long periods.

l. Zinc deficiency may appear after several weeks of total parenteral nutrition in the already depleted patient. It is manifested by erythema, vesicles, pustules, and erosions. Clustering of these lesions occurs around body orifices and perineum, over the genital region, and on the hands and feet. Zinc deficiency can be treated by adding trace elements to the solution, as discussed earlier.

m. Essential fatty acid deficiency is seen in patients who are chronically debilitated and have been on long-term parenteral nutrition. The clinical manifestation of this problem is a scaling exematoid dermatitis that may be confused with psoriasis. The treatment and prevention is administration of fat emulsion IV two to three times/wk.

n. Aspiration of gastric contents may occur in patients with weak gag and cough reflexes who are being fed intragastrically. Place the patient in the sitting position and avoid nighttime infusions.

o. Cramps, nausea, and vomiting often are related to jejunostomy feedings that are too great in volume and concentration.

p. Diarrhea, dehydration, and azotemia are caused by hypertonicity of the nutrient solutions, especially when low-bulk diets are infused into the jejunum. Start with a dilute solution (0.25 Cal/ml) with additional supplies of water. The presence of small amounts of fat (less than 8%) may lessen diarrhea by increasing gastric emptying time.

q. Increased quantities of electrolytes will be needed to replace abnormal losses and for anabolism of new protein.

r. Bleeding most often is caused by hypoprothrombinemia resulting from inadequate vitamin K intake.

s. Fluid retention is seen when the source of body energy is converted from oxidation of fat (starvation) to carbohydrates (feeding). The intermittent use of diuretics will control water retention; water retention is more refractory if there is concomitant hypoalbuminemia.

t. Other complications are tube dislodgment, intraperitoneal leakage, skin infection and erosion, intestinal obstruction (jejunostomy), mucosal erosions with bleeding, and faulty tube placement into the ileum.

V. Investigations indicated for all forms of therapy

A. Laboratory

1. Electrolytes (sodium, potassium, magnesium, carbon dioxide), glucose, and blood urea nitrogen daily for the first 7 days, then every third day.

2. Serum total protein, albumin, uric acid, calcium, phosphorus, alkaline phosphatase, and serum glutamic-oxaloacetic transaminase every 3 days for the first week and then twice weekly thereafter.

3. A complete blood count weekly, including hematocrit and white count with differential.

4. Serum osmolarity every day for the first week and then at least twice weekly.

5. Ammonia twice the first week and then once weekly.

6. Urine sugar and acetone qid the first week and bid thereafter. Urine osmolarity qid the first week and once a day thereafter.

B. General measurements

1. Weight, every morning.

2. Strict intake and output.

3. Body length and head circumference in infants, every day.

Suggested Reading

Ballinger, W. F. *Manual of Surgical Nutrition.* Philadelphia: Saunders, 1975.

Elwyn, D. H. Nutritional requirements of adult surgical patients. *Crit. Care Med.* 8:9, 1980.

Fischer, J. E. *Total Parenteral Nutrition.* Boston: Little, Brown, 1976.

Shils, M. E. Guidelines for total parenteral nutrition. *J.A.M.A.* 220:1721, 1972.

Stephens, R. V., and Randall, H. T. Use of a concentrated balanced, liquid elemental diet for nutritional management of catabolic states. *Ann. Surg.* 170:642, 1969.

Winters, R. W., and Hasselmeyer, E. G. *Intravenous Nutrition in the High Risk Infant.* New York: Wiley, 1975.

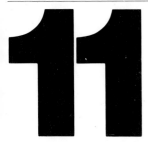

Acute Renal Failure

I. Types of renal failure. Acute renal insufficiency is the rapid deterioration of glomerular filtration, which causes nitrogenous wastes to accumulate in the body. Often, but not always, there is a decreased urinary flow rate. The causes of acute renal failure may be prerenal, postrenal, or renal parenchymal in origin. In patients experiencing a sudden decrease in renal function, several questions must be answered (Table 11-1).

   A. Prerenal azotemia results from **underperfusion** of the renal arterioles.

   1. The kidney responds appropriately to underperfusion by retaining sodium to reexpand effective circulating blood volume. Since the kidney retains salt in an effort to reexpand blood volume, the urinary concentration of sodium and chloride will be low (0–20 mEq/liter).

   2. Extracellular fluid volume may be expanded (congestive heart failure) or contracted (dehydration). There is always, however, decreased effective renal artery perfusion.

   3. The underperfused kidney produces renin, which causes arterial vasoconstriction and raises renal artery blood pressure. Secondary aldosteronism accompanies the contraction of effective arterial blood volume, causing urinary potassium concentration to be high.

   4. Urine osmolality is greater than serum osmolality in prerenal azotemia.

   5. Reabsorption is stimulated in patients with prerenal azotemia. Since the kidney can reabsorb urea, blood urea nitrogen (BUN) rises more than serum creatinine; the BUN-creatinine ratio is usually more than 10 in prerenal azotemia.

   6. Patients with protracted vomiting or diuretic therapy have a metabolic alkalosis superimposed on prerenal azotemia. These patients will have sodium loss in the urine (as $NaHCO_3$), and urine chloride concentration will remain low. In such patients, the combination of high sodium and low chloride in the urine has the same clinical connotation as the combination of low sodium and low chloride in patients with volume contraction not suffering from metabolic alkalosis.

   7. **Treatment.** Prerenal azotemia is always secondary to some other problem. Treatment is aimed at the primary cause of renal underperfusion. Fluid losses from the gastrointestinal tract, genitourinary tract (excessive diuresis), or skin or secondary to hemorrhage must be replaced. Prompt administration of fluids will restore renal function to the level existing prior to the insult if ischemic renal injury has not occurred. However, if underperfusion is due to a decrease in effective rather than absolute blood volume (as in congestive heart failure), administration of fluids is contraindicated; renal function will be restored only when cardiac function improves.

   8. Patients with nephrotic syndrome may have a mild prerenal azotemia. Volume contraction occurs as a consequence of decreased plasma oncotic pressure.

Table 11-1. Investigation of Acute Renal Failure

Question	Indicated Tests
Is vascular volume adequate?	Ultrasound, central venous pressure, pulmonary artery wedge pressure
Is cardiac function adequate?	Ultrasound, central venous pressure, pulmonary artery wedge pressure, cardiac output, thallium heart scan
Is the urethra patent?	Insert or check Foley catheter; cystogram
Do kidneys have blood flow?	Isotope renogram, arteriogram
Are the kidneys obstructed?	Ultrasound, retrograde pyelogram

9. Patients with severe liver disease may develop hepatorenal syndrome, a severe example of prerenal azotemia. Successful treatment of the renal failure depends on successful treatment of the liver failure.

10. Diuretics are appropriate in the treatment of congestive heart failure. Otherwise, the use of diuretics in prerenal azotemia is to be condemned. The use of powerful loop diuretics (furosemide, ethacrynic acid) to enforce urine output only contracts the effective blood volume and makes prerenal azotemia worse.

B. Acute parenchymal renal failure

1. The **causes** of acute parenchymal renal failure include acute tubular necrosis (ATN), toxin-induced renal failure, glomerulonephritis, hypertension, renal artery occlusion, and a multitude of disorders affecting the intrarenal vasculature, glomeruli, tubules, and interstitium.

2. **ATN** is often seen in the absence of an identifiable histological abnormality and might better be thought of as reversible acute tubular dysfunction. Pathophysiologically, ATN is associated with volume contraction secondary to hypotension, cardiovascular collapse, hemorrhage, or toxins, often combined with hemolysis or rhabdomyolysis.

3. **Prevention of ATN** can best be accomplished by prevention of volume contraction. Once the insult has occurred, the patient must be carefully supported until recovery occurs. Attempts at lessening the severity of ATN with diuretics or fluid challenges usually fail. If obstruction of the renal tubules by hemoglobin breakdown products is considered a possibility, early osmotic diuresis with mannitol should be effective in lessening the severity of ATN.

4. Since the tubules are diseased, there is impaired urinary concentrating ability and decreased reabsorption of sodium. Urine osmolality tends to equal that of plasma; the urine sodium concentration is above 40 mEq/liter. The urine may contain casts or renal tubular epithelial cells.

5. Usually, ATN can be divided into an **oliguric phase** and a **diuretic phase.** Some patients, however, develop acute renal failure without the initial oliguric phase. Such **high-output renal failure** is seen with methoxyflurane nephropathy and often with aminoglycoside renal toxicity. Combined aminoglycoside and cephalosporin therapy may cause renal toxicity significantly in excess of that of aminoglycosides alone.

6. The **oliguric phase** lasts from days to weeks, during which time 24-hr volume varies between 50 and 400 ml/day. Oliguria rarely lasts longer than 1 mo. The presence of anuria is atypical and suggests another disorder (cortical necrosis, urinary tract obstruction, renal artery occlusion).

7. The **diuretic phase** begins with a gradual increase in urine volume that results from diuresis of accumulated edema fluid rather than from inability to conserve fluids and electrolytes. Accumulated urea also may act as an osmotic

diuretic. Occasionally, diuresis may be massive and require large amounts of replacement fluid.

8. Recovery of glomerular function may lag behind in the diuretic phase. The initial urine volume increase may not be accompanied by a fall in BUN or creatinine. After several days, however, BUN and creatinine will fall; BUN rises first and falls last, making it a more sensitive indicator of renal failure.

C. Postrenal (obstructive) uropathy must be considered in any patient who develops acute renal failure or even diminished urinary output. Permanent impairment of renal function develops if total upper urinary tract obstruction persists more than 7 days. Early diagnosis is desirable; delay in diagnosis may lead to permanent decompensation of the lower urinary tract.

1. An intravenous pyelogram should be obtained in the **hydrated** patient. Renal visualization may be obtained even with a serum creatinine as high as 5–7 mg/100 ml. There is no place for deliberate dehydration of patients receiving contrast material.

2. Rectal and abdominal examinations must be performed as part of the initial physical examination of all patients. If there is a question of bladder distention or prostatic enlargement, a urethral (Foley) catheter should be sterilely inserted; if urinary retention is present, the catheter may be connected to a closed drainage system.

3. If the renal pelves and ureters have not been visualized by intravenous pyelography, prompt bilateral retrograde pyelography should be performed.

4. Postobstructive diuresis may follow relief of urinary tract obstruction. The basis of the diuresis is multifactorial. An osmotic diuresis will occur because of accumulated BUN. A saline load diuresis will also occur to clear accumulated edema fluid. Replacement of large amounts of fluid and electrolytes will only perpetuate the diuresis; fluid requirements should be calculated to provide for normal urine output (see Chap. 9). Occasionally, impaired tubular reabsorption of salt and water due to long-standing obstruction will be present. Excretion of high volumes of urine in this situation will lead to circulatory collapse if fluid and electrolytes are not replaced. Replacement of fluids initially can be given hourly as 80–90% of the previous hour's urine output using 0.5 normal saline.

II. Management of acute renal failure

A. Hemodialysis

1. From the moment potential renal failure is diagnosed one must prepare for potential **vascular access.** All lines must be removed from one arm and the arm marked "do not touch." No blood drawing or infusion lines of any sort should be permitted in this arm. Adherence to a policy of sparing one arm for vascular access will avoid a major problem for the patient, dialysis unit, and vascular surgeon.

2. Dialysis should be performed **early** in acute renal failure. Management will be more difficult if the patient is allowed to become uremic before dialysis is instituted. There is little to be gained by heroic attempts to manage renal failure without dialysis. **Patients with acute renal failure, especially postoperatively or following trauma, need frequent dialysis.** Hemodialysis is preferred to peritoneal dialysis in patients who are severely catabolic or who have suffered extensive tissue destruction (trauma, postoperative) resulting in release of large amounts of K^+ into the extracellular fluid.

3. Hemodialysis is generally conducted under systemic anticoagulation. Hemodialysis can be performed with only regional heparinization if systemic anticoagulation must be avoided (e.g., postoperatively). However, the surgeon should be aware that patients often become systemically anticoagulated during and after regional heparinization.

B. Peritoneal dialysis

1. Peritoneal dialysis uses the peritoneal membrane to separate the dialysate from the bloodstream. Since a foreign body (the dialysis catheter) is being implanted transcutaneously, maintenance of sterility is extremely important. Acute dialysis catheters (Tenkoff or Travenol) may or may not have a Dacron felt cuff; chronic catheters have two Dacron felt cuffs to help prevent infection. Implantation of the Silastic dialysis catheter may be performed surgically under anesthesia or at the bedside using a trocar. The bladder must be empty It is best not to treat patients with skin infections or any gastrointestinal disorder (ileus, intra-abdominal adhesions) with peritoneal dialysis.

2. After catheter placement, antibiotics are added to standard dialysate solution which is warmed to 38°C (100.4F) and run in and out of the peritoneal cavity using sterile technique in 500–1000 ml exchange volumes, accomplishing two exchanges/hr. Later, in chronic peritoneal dialysis, the exchange volume may be increased to 2000 ml and three exchanges done each hour. In children, the exchange volumes are necessarily smaller (100–500 ml).

3. Each liter of standard peritoneal dialysate solution contains 130 mEq Na^+ 96.5mEq Cl^-, 0 mEq K^+, 3.5 mEq Ca^{++}, 1 mEq Mg^{++}, 38 mEq acetate, and 15 gm dextrose. This fluid will remove Na^+, Cl^-, K^+, phosphate, Mg^{++}, and water Dextrose and calcium are absorbed, and serum pH rises. If more fluid removal is required, then a dialysate with 45 gm/liter of dextrose can be used Peritoneal dialysis is usually performed for 36–48 hr two or three times/wk as needed.

4. Peritoneal dialysis is useful in patients with severe acute pancreatitis Potassium, 4mEq/liter, heparin, 5000 units/liter, and antibiotics are added to standard dialysate (15 gm/liter dextrose) solution. Dialysis is run frequently during the first 1–4 days following diagnosis.

C. Diet.
It is traditional to institute protein restriction in renal failure. With hemodialysis, protein restriction is not required. Catabolic patients should receive protein supplements. Hyperalimentation and hemodialysis are compatible (see Chap. 10). Potassium restriction is important in the management of renal failure before institution of hemodialysis but may be liberalized after hemodialysis begins.

D. Fluid management

1. Patients with acute renal failure generally receive too much fluid. Overhydration leads to both hypertension and edema formation.

2. In addition to the replacement of gastrointestinal and urinary losses, maintenance fluid intake should be restricted to 10 ml/kg/day. Additional fluid can be provided for excessive insensible losses. Monitoring of weight daily permits evaluation of hydration; the same scale should be used each day for accuracy

3. Overhydration will cause an elevated central venous pressure, pulmonary edema, and increase in heart size. Cardiac output, tissue oxygenation, and circulation time, however, are normal. Administration of digitalis will not correct the abnormalities of overhydration; digitalis should be given only if true congestive heart failure is present—and then in reduced doses. Frequent monitoring of serum digoxin concentration is necessary to prevent toxicity.

4. Hypertension in acute renal failure is a consequence of overhydration. Dialysis will remove salt and water. Markedly elevated blood pressure must be controlled quickly; IV hydralazine (10–40 mg q6h) or methyldopa (Aldomet (250–1000 mg q6h) can be used initially; for life-threatening hypertension, IV diazoxide (300mg) should be given. If the blood pressure does not promptly fall a constant infusion of sodium nitroprusside (100 mg/liter 5% D/W) should be started and run at a rate sufficient to lower the blood pressure; *do not exceed 8 μg/kg/min.*

E. Electrolytes

1. Urinary sodium losses should be measured and replaced. Many patients develop hyponatremia secondary to overhydration. Fluid restriction coupled with hemodialysis can correct hyponatremia.

2. Hyperkalemia is a major problem in acute renal failure and represents a potential emergency. In acute renal failure, particularly in postoperative or trauma patients, serum potassium can climb rapidly. Potassium should not be replaced in acute renal failure unless hypokalemia is present, and, even then, replacement should be limited to identifiable losses. Potassium-containing drugs (particularly penicillin) should be avoided.

3. The electrocardiographic (ECG) findings of hyperkalemia may lag behind the rise in serum K^+ but are predictive of toxicity. Peaked elevation of the T wave, a prolonged Q–T interval, QRS widening, and a prolonged P–R interval precede the development of a sine wave and cardiac arrest in acute renal failure (see Chap. 9).

4. Sodium polystyrene sulfonate (Kayexalate) is an exchange resin that will bind K^+ in the gastrointestinal tract. It may be given orally or as an enema; 15–60 gm in 50–250 ml of fluid can be given qid. Sorbitol 20% administered concomitantly will prevent the constipation caused by oral Kayexalate.

5. A **serum K^+ more than 6.5mEq/liter is an emergency.** In addition to administration of Kayexalate, the patient should be given glucose and insulin. A rapid IV push of 25 mg of glucose and 8–10 units of regular insulin usually will lower the serum K^+. The effect is caused by a shift of potassium from the extracellular to the intracellular space. Administration of IV $NaHCO_3$ (45 mEq) also will lower serum K^+ and should be combined with the glucose-insulin therapy. Hemodialysis should be started as soon as possible. If the serum K^+ reaches 7.5mEq/liter, or if significant ECG changes are present, IV calcium (5–10 ml 10% $CaCl_2$) should be given slowly. Calcium will antagonize the effect of K^+ on the myocardium. The treatment may need to be repeated q30–120 min.

6. With loss of renal function, retention of dietary phosphorus occurs because of diminished excretion. Control of dietary phosphorus intake and administration of phosphate-binding gels are generally instituted when serum phosphate concentration becomes elevated. Antacids containing aluminum hydroxide are used to bind phosphorus; the dosage is adjusted to produce a lowering of serum phosphorus. Magnesium intake must be restricted in patients with renal failure. Many common antacid preparations contain large amounts of magnesium and are therefore contraindicated. **Antacids useful in renal failure** include Amphogel, Basaljel, and ALternaGEL. Antacids contraindicated in renal failure (they contain Mg^{++}) include Maalox, Riopan, Mylanta, Aludrox, Gaviscon, and Gelusil.

   An increase in the serum Mg^{++} level may result in neuromuscular weakness, loss of deep tendon reflexes, complete heart block, hypertension, and respiratory depression. Calcium administered IV antagonizes the action of Mg^{++} on the myocardium in the same way that it antagonizes the action of K^+.

7. Most patients with acute renal failure develop asymptomatic hypocalcemia. Serum albumin also falls in catabolic patients, so that the ionized calcium fraction may only be modestly depressed.

8. Metabolic acidosis occurs in all patients with renal failure due to the reduced renal excretion of acid metabolites. Hemodialysis usually controls bicarbonate concentration, but $NaHCO_3$ should be administered IV for serum HCO_3^- levels less than 15 mEq/liter.

F. Anemia. Patients with chronic renal failure develop secondary anemia but usually require only rare or intermittent transfusion. In acute renal failure, however, especially in the postoperative patient, it is best to keep the hematocrit above

Table 11-2. Drug Therapy in Renal Failure

Drug	Dosage in Renal Failure (Ccr <30 ml/min)	Dosage in Uremia (Ccr <10 ml/min)	Effect of Hemodialysis
Acetaminophen	NC	NC, nephrotoxic	WD
Acetazolamide	Not effective	Not effective	?
Adriamycin	NC	NC	?
Aldomet	250–500 mg q8–12h	250–500 mg q12–18h	60% removed
Allopurinol	200–300 mg/day	200 mg/day	WD
Amikacin	7.5 mg/kg q(9 × Ccr)h	7.5 mg/kg q(9 × Ccr)h	WD
Aminophylline	NC	NC	WD
Amitriptyline	NC	NC	None
Amoxicillin	0.5 gm q8h	0.5 gm q16–24h	WD
Amphotericin B	NC	Modest reduction	None
Ampicillin	5–20 mg/kg/day in 2–4 doses	5–20 mg/kg/day in 2–4 doses	40–80% removed
Aspirin	Short course only	Short course only	WD
Azathioprine	NC	NC	Moderately dialyzed
Barbiturates, short acting	NC	NC	Poorly dialyzed
Barbiturates, long acting	NC	Reduce dose markedly	WD
Bleomycin	Reduce dose	Avoid	?
Carbenicillin	4–16 gm/day in 2–4 doses	4–16 gm/day in 2–4 doses	2 gm/day while on D; 20–40% removed
Cefamandole	NC	1 gm qd	WD; 0.5 gm after D
Cefazolin	NC	0.5 gm LD, then 250 mg qod	WD; 250 mg after D
Cefoxitin	NC	1 gm q12–24h	WD; 1 gm after D
Cephalexin	NC	0.5 gm LD, then 0.5 gm qd	WD; 0.5 gm after D
Cephaloridine	Do not use—nephrotoxic	Do not use	WD
Cephalothin	NC	2 gm LD, then 1 gm q12–24h	2 gm qd on D, 20–40% removed

Cephapirin	NC	30 mg/kg in 2 doses	WD, 15 mg/kg after D and then bid
Chloral hydrate	NC	NC	?
Chloramphenicol	NC	Decrease dose 10%	WD
Chlordiazepoxide	NC	NC	Poorly dialyzed
Chlorpropamide	NC	Do not use	Poorly dialyzed
Cimetidine	NC	300 mg q12h	?
Cis-platinum	Do not use	Do not use	WD
Clindamycin	NC	NC	None
Cloxacillin	NC	NC	None
Codeine	NC	NC	?
Colchicine	Short course only	Short course only	Poorly dialyzed
Coumadin	NC	NC	?
Cyclophosphamide	Reduce dose	Avoid	Dialyzed
Diazepam	NC	NC	Poorly dialyzed
Diazoxide	?	?	WD
Dicloxacillin	NC	?	None
Digoxin	LD 0.5–1.5 mg, then 0.125 mg/day maintenance	LD 0.5–1.5 mg, then 0.125 mg qod maintenance	None
Doxycycline	NC	NC	Minimally dialyzed
Erythromycin	NC	NC	None
Ethacrynic acid	NC	NC	?
Ethambutol	7–15 mg/kg/day	5 mg/kg/day	WD
5-Fluorocytosine	25–50 mg/kg q12h	25–50 mg/kg q24–36h	WD
5-Fluorouracil	NC	Reduce dose	WD
Furosemide	NC	NC	None
Gentamicin	1 mg/kg q(8 × Ccr)h	1 mg/kg q(8 × Ccr)h	30–50% removed
Gold	Do not use	Do not use	None
Griseofulvin	NC	?	?
Guanethidine	NC	NC	None
Haloperidol	NC	?	?

Table 11-2 (Continued)

Drug	Dosage in Renal Failure (Ccr <30 mg/min)	Dosage in Uremia (Ccr <10 ml/min)	Effect of Hemodialysis
Heparin	NC	NC	None
Hydralazine	NC	Decrease dose 25%	?
Hydrochlorthiazide	Ineffective	Ineffective	?
Indomethacin	NC	NC	?
INH	NC	200–300 mg/day	Moderately dialyzed
Insulin	NC	Decrease dose	None
Kanamycin	7.5 mg/kg q(9 × Ccr)h	7.5 mg/kg q(9 × Ccr)h	WD; 7 mg/kg qod after D
Levodopa	NC	NC	?
Lidocaine	NC	NC	None
Lincomycin	NC	0.5 gm q24–36 h	Poorly dialyzed
Lithium	4–5 mEq q12h; monitor levels	4–5 mEq qd; monitor levels	WD
Meperidine	NC	NC	?
Meprobamate	NC	NC	Poorly dialyzed
Methenamine mandelate	NC	Do not use	?
Methicillin	NC	1–2 gm q8h	None
Methotrexate	Reduce dose	Avoid	?
Metronidazole	NC	Decrease dose	?
Minoxidil	NC	NC	?
Morphine	NC	NC	?
Nafcillin	NC	NC	None
Nalidixic acid	NC	Do not use	?
Nitrofurantoin	Do not use	Do not use	WD
Oxacillin	NC	NC	None
PAS	NC	Do not use	?

		≥10 million units/day in 2–3 doses	5–20% removed
Pentazocine		NC	?
Phenothiazines	NC	NC	None
Phenylbutazone	NC	Do not use	Poorly dialyzed
Phenytoin Sodium	NC	NC (or increase)	None
Probenecid	Do not use	Do not use	?
Procainamide	NC	Dose q8–12h	WD; dose after D
Propoxyphene	NC	NC; nephrotoxic	WD
Propranolol	NC	NC	None
Quinidine	NC	NC	None
Reserpine	NC	Decrease dose	None
Rifampin	NC	300 mg qd	None
Sisomicin	1 mg/kg q(8 × Ccr)h	1 mg/kg q(8 × Ccr)h	1 mg/kg after D
Spectinomycin	Do not use	Do not use	?
Spironolactone	Do not use	Do not use	?
Streptomycin	1g LD, then 0.5 gm every 2–3 days	1g LD, then 0.5 gm every 2–3 days	WD
Tetracycline	Do not use	Do not use	Slightly dialyzed
Thiazide	Ineffective	Ineffective	?
Ticarcillin	2 gm q4h	2 gm q12h	WD; 2 gm after D
Tobramycin	100 mg q(6 × Ccr)h	100 mg q(6 × Ccr)h	WD; 1 mg/kg after D
Tolbutamide	NC	NC	None
Triamterene	Do not use	Do not use	?
Trimethoprim	40 mg q12h	40 mg qd	WD
Sulfonamides	Usual dose as LD, then ½LD bid	Same as in renal failure	WD; LD after D
Vancomycin	1 gm/day	1 gm q7d	Poorly dialyzed
Vinblastine	NC	NC	?
Vincristine	NC	NC	?

NC = no change; WD = well dialyzed; LD = loading dose; D = dialysis.

30%. A rapid decrease in hematocrit is not consistent only with acute renal fail ure, and a source for blood loss should be sought.

G. Neurological manifestations

1. Uremia causes dysarthria, asterixis, tremors, myoclonus, and generalized sen sorial clouding. Delirium with hallucinations, tetany, and frontal lobe depres sion appears later. Convulsions occur late in uremia and are either focal or generalized motor seizures. Elevated serum concentration of penicillin can exacerbate any of the neurological disorders in uremia.

2. Uremic convulsions are treated acutely with 10–20 mg of diazepam (Valium IV over 3–5 min. Acute respiratory arrest can occur with such treatment, so one should be prepared to ventilate the patient. Phenytoin sodium (Dilantin can be given IV acutely but is not immediately effective; it should be given PO 100 mg, 2–4 times each day to help prevent future seizures. Phenobarbitol 90–180 mg/day, is useful in preventing both acute and chronic seizures. If these drugs fail to control acute uremic convulsions, an IV bolus injection of 100 mg of lidocaine, followed by an infusion of 30 μg/kg/min, may control the seizures.

3. After either hemodialysis or peritoneal dialysis, a **dysequilibrium syndrome** commonly occurs. Patients complain of headache, nausea, and muscle cramp and display agitation, irritability, and even delirium, obtundation, or convul sions. The signs and symptoms are directly related to the rapidity and com pleteness of the dialysis and are most common during the first few dialyses. A shift of water into the brain causes the dysequilibrium syndrome. More gentle less efficient early dialyses allows the patient to become better adapted to the fluid changes occurring during dialysis.

H. Drugs.
Excretion of many drugs depends on renal clearance; the dosage must be reduced in renal failure to avoid toxicity (Table 11-2). Only some drugs are re moved by hemodialysis; others are rendered ineffective by renal failure and should not be used. Drugs with potential renal toxicity should be avoided in acut renal failure so as not to compound the renal disease.

Suggested Reading

Appel, G. B., and Neu, H. C.   The nephrotoxicity of antimicrobial agents. *N. Engl. J. Med.* 296:663, 722, 784, 1977.

Dornfeld, L., and Narins, R. G.   Pre- and postoperative renal failure. *Urolog. Clin North Am.* 3:363, 1977.

Merrill, J. P.   Acute Renal Failure. In M. B. Strauss and L. G. Welt (eds.), *Diseases o the Kidney.* Boston: Little, Brown, 1971.

Ranson, J. H. C., and Spencer, F. C.   The role of peritoneal lavage in severe acut pancreatitis. *Ann. Surg.* 187:565, 1978.

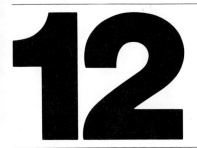

Respiratory Insufficiency

I. General comments. The process of **respiration** involves not only the exchange of oxygen and carbon dioxide through the lungs but also exchange and appropriate utilization in the tissues. This requires adequate function to meet demands in the lungs, the circulation, and the cellular enzyme systems. **Pulmonary failure** indicates the inability of the lungs to exchange oxygen and carbon dioxide with ambient air to maintain the PO_2 above 60 mm Hg or the PCO_2 below 49 mm Hg.

II. Pathophysiology of respiration

  A. Definitions: ventilation

    1. Tidal volume (V_T) is the volume of gas (ml) inspired or expired during each average ventilatory cycle.

    2. Minute volume (V_M) equals the tidal volume × cycles/min.

    3. Dead space (V_D) is the volume of inspired gas (ml) that does not cause arterialization of venous blood. It includes the mouth, nose, trachea, upper bronchi (anatomical); endotracheal tubes and connecting tubes (mechanical); and gas in poorly perfused alveoli (physiological).

    4. Alveolar ventilation ($\dot{V}_A$) equals the volume of gas actively exchanging with pulmonary venous blood:

$$\dot{V}_A = (V_T - V_D) \times rate$$

    5. Total vital capacity (VC) is the maximal volume of gas that can be voluntarily expelled from the lungs after a maximal inspiration.

    6. Functional residual capacity (FRC) is the volume of gas remaining in the lungs after a passive expiration.

    7. Compliance (V/P) is the volume change of lungs and thorax/unit change in either pleural or airway pressure. Decreased compliance means stiffer lungs.

    8. Resistance is the pressure differential produced by a unit change in flow (cm H_2O/liters/sec). Resistance is primarily a function of small airways and is markedly increased by secretions or bronchospasm.

  B. Definitions: perfusion

    1. Cardiac output (CO or $\dot{Q}t$) is the volume of blood ejected from the heart per minute (liters/min). CO is measured by thermodilution using a Swan-Ganz catheter or by dilution of indocyanine green dye injected IV.

    2. Cardiac index (CI) equals the cardiac output divided by body surface area (liters/min/m²).

    3. Oxygen content (C) is the quantity of oxygen carried in blood (ml O_2/100 ml blood) where:

$$O_2\ content = (Hgb \times 1.306 \times \frac{Sat\ (\%)}{100}) + (PO_2 \times 0.0031)$$

4. **Ventilation-perfusion ratio ($\dot{V}A/\dot{Q}$).** The volume of blood perfusing a given lung area should be appropriate to the volume of ventilation to this area in order to produce well-oxygenated pulmonary venous blood without excessive and wasteful ventilation. Regions with a high $\dot{V}A/\dot{Q}$ (e.g., after pulmonary embolus decreases perfusion) are excessively ventilated, and, as noted, the volume of gas that does not participate in gas exchange is called **physiological dead space.** Conversely, regions with poor ventilation but adequate perfusion (e.g., atelectasis) receive more blood than can be adequately oxygenated, thereby allowing desaturated blood to enter the pulmonary veins. This is physiologically identical to blood that is **shunted** past the pulmonary capillaries via the anatomical pathways, such as, the thebesian veins or intrapulmonary arteriovenous shunts. The physiological and anatomical shunts cause arterial hypoxemia.

5. **Alveolar-arterial oxygen difference P(A-a)O_2.** If all pulmonary arterial blood exchanges uniformly with alveolar (A) gas, then systemic arterial blood (a) should have the same oxygen concentration as alveolar gas (A). It does not, because of the normal presence of low$\dot{V}A/\dot{Q}$ areas in the lung and of small anatomical shunts. The difference, P(A-a)O_2, is an expression of this discrepancy. Usually, arterial blood gases are measured directly, and the **alveolar gas composition** is calculated using the equation:

$$PAO_2 = (PB - PH_2O)\, FIO_2 - \frac{PaC}{RQ}$$

where PB = barometric pressure; PH_2O = partial pressure of water (47 mm Hg at 37° C); FIO_2 = fractional inspired O_2 (0.21 on room air); and RQ = respiratory exchange ratio $\frac{CO_2}{O_2}$ = 0.8 (average).

6. **Shunt fraction ($\dot{Q}s/\dot{Q}t$).** This value usually is calculated while breathing 100% oxygen, which theoretically converts all low $\dot{V}A/\dot{Q}$ regions to 100% oxygen (FIO_2 = 1.0), eliminating these regions as a cause of hypoxemia and leaving only anatomical shunts to be measured. This practice has fallen into disuse because low $\dot{V}A/\dot{Q}$ areas may collapse while inspiring pure oxygen, and the calculated shunt values become spuriously high. The shunt equation can be calculated using lesser inspired oxygen concentrations, provided alveolar PO_2 is expected to produce 100% hemoglobin saturation (i.e., above FIO_2 = 0.3). However, the value obtained then will include low $\dot{V}A/\dot{Q}$ areas as part of the shunt value.

$$\dot{Q}s/\dot{Q}t = \frac{CcO_2 - CaO_2}{CcO_2 - C\overline{v}O_2}$$

where CcO_2 = O_2 content of blood in pulmonary capillary, CaO_2 = O_2 content of blood in arterial blood, and $C\overline{v}O_2$ = O_2 content of mixed venous blood.

C. The **diagnosis** of respiratory insufficiency is based on both clinical and laboratory findings. Proper therapy must be instituted without delay, occasionally, when the need is urgent, without completing the usual complement of diagnostic procedures.

1. The **history** should seek possible known pulmonary problems, such as obstructive or restrictive disease, bronchitis, asthma, pneumonia, aspiration, or recent trauma, in addition to intake of drugs that may depress respiration.

2. **Physical examination.** Anxiety, confusion, agitation, diaphoresis, tachycardia, and hypertension may be present in the early stages of respiratory insufficiency. Such findings in an ill patient are highly suggestive of impending disaster and should be investigated immediately. When tachypnea, nasal flaring, wheezing, use of accessory muscles, or stridor is present, the diagnosis of respiratory insufficiency is established, and active treatment is indicated. The presence of cyanosis, bradycardia, or hypotension is a late sign indicating imminent cardiac arrest.

Table 12-1. Indications for Respiratory Therapy

Measurement	Normal Values	Active Therapy Indicated*	Mechanical Ventilator Support Indicated
Respiratory rate	12–20/min	20–35	>35
Vital capacity	65–75 ml/kg	15–60	<15
V_D/V_T	0.25–0.40	0.40–0.60	>0.60
PaO_2	75–100 mm Hg (room air)		<70 (on mask O_2)
$PaCO_2$	35–45 mm Hg	45–50	>50

*Active therapy means close observation, suctioning of secretions, supplemental O_2 by mask, bronchodilators as needed, and supplemental humidity.

   3. Indications for mechanical ventilator support include:

   a. Loss of mechanical function of the chest or diaphragm (flail chest, lacerated diaphragm).

   b. Neurological syndromes (head trauma, Guillain-Barré, myasthenia gravis).

   c. Acute decompensation of chronic lung disease.

   d. Aspiration of gastric contents.

   4. Functional measurements aid the diagnosis and therapy of respiratory insufficiency. The indices in Table 12-1 exclude patients with chronic obstructive pulmonary disease (COPD) and chronic hypercapnea.

D. Causes of respiratory insufficiency are multiple. Knowledge of possible causes may allow one to predict which patients will need close observation or earlier ventilator support.

   1. Depressed ventilation occurs with the following:

   a. Upper airway obstruction by stenosis, edema, or foreign body.

   b. Decreased lung expansion due to flail chest, pneumothorax, or hemothorax.

   c. Drugs and anesthetics that depress respiratory muscle activity by local or central actions (e.g., morphine, pancuronium, heroin, barbiturates).

   d. Head or spinal cord injury with loss of respiratory control and muscular effort.

   2. Lung parenchymal abnormalities include:

   a. Atelectasis

   b. Sepsis associated with endotoxins or other vasoactive substances and leading to loss of capillary integrity.

   c. Aspiration causing inflammation and infection of the lungs.

   d. Iatrogenic fluid overload, drowning, left heart failure, non-cardiac pulmonary edema.

   e. Pulmonary embolus.

   f. Shock and multiple blood transfusions.

III. Prevention. Prevention of respiratory insufficiency, especially in patients facing elective surgery, is worth the effort. Pulmonary complications are most common after operations in the abdomen or thorax.

A. History. Preexisting **respiratory disease** and **smoking** are the most significant factors contributing to postoperative complications, followed by **obesity, advanced age,** and **site of operative incision** (upper abdominal > lower abdominal > extremities). Careful inquiries regarding previous respiratory problems, dyspnea, orthopnea, cough, sputum production, exercise tolerance, and allergies are needed, as is a detailed smoking history.

B. The **physical examination** should evaluate the following:

1. The level of consciousness.

2. The ability to cooperate with respiratory maneuvers, such as chest clapping, incentive spirometry, or intermittent positive-pressure breathing.

3. The presence of cyanosis or clubbing, muscle wasting or weakness.

4. The patient's **ability to cough** (needs to be tested specifically); many people do not know how to cough voluntarily.

5. In addition to the character of breath sounds, the chest examination should evaluate diaphragm excursion by percussion (normal > 5 cm), the need to use accessory respiratory muscles, and the expiratory time after maximal inspiration (normal < 4 sec).

C. Laboratory examinations

1. A **chest x-ray** is mandatory when respiratory symptoms are present, or a general anesthetic is planned.

2. If the patient has a productive cough, **sputum** for **Gram stain** and **culture** should be obtained.

3. **Pulmonary function** may be measured if abnormalities are detected in the history or physical examination. Measurements should include the forced expiratory volume in 1 sec (FEV_1) and the response to bronchodilators.

D. Therapy is directed toward increasing the patient's ability to improve existing abnormalities and clear secretions and thus prevent atelectasis. The emphasis is on educating the patient to cough and deep-breathe effectively and to use respiratory devices appropriately.

1. The **incentive spirometer** is the most successful device for attaining optimal lung inflation at the least cost.

2. **Chest physiotherapy** will assist in clearing secretions, especially when combined with **bronchodilators.**

3. **Antibiotics** may be necessary in chronic bronchitis to treat infected sputum.

4. **Hydration** should be adequate to prevent inspissation of secretions; clearance of secretions may be augmented by the use of a heated nebulizer.

IV. Treatment of respiratory insufficiency and failure. The cause (e.g., pneumothorax, airway obstruction, or fluid overload) should be identified and specifically treated. If it is not immediately evident, or if initial treatment is not effective in reversing respiratory insufficiency and respiratory failure is likely, secure control of the airway and mechanical support is indicated. Delay may be dangerous.

A. Airway management. In an emergency, placement of an oropharyngeal airway and ventilation by bag and mask often will be adequate and is preferable to attempts at endotracheal intubation by inexperienced personnel.

1. Orotracheal intubation is the fastest route for airway control but requires oral instrumentation and is difficult in awake patients. It is most useful for intubation of short duration. This technique has almost eliminated the necessity for an emergency tracheostomy.

2. **Nasotracheal intubation** is traumatic to nasal tissues but more comfortable during use and more secure than orotracheal intubation. It is most useful for nonemergent circumstances in patients who may require prolonged intubation.

3. **Choice of tube.** Select a low-pressure, soft-cuff design. The cuff should be inflated just enough to prevent air leak. A small controlled air leak is preferable to overinflation of the cuff, which risks tracheal injury.

4. **Complications of endotracheal intubation**

   a. **Inhibition of mucociliary action** to clear secretions. The patient is dependent on suctioning by attendants.

   b. **Tracheal stenosis** caused by necrosis at site of balloon inflation.

   c. **Airway obstruction** by inspissated secretions or an overinflated cuff balloon.

5. **Tracheostomy** provides long-term airway control, effective removal of secretions, and increased patient comfort, and it prevents laryngeal damage and stenosis. It should be considered **after 1 wk of endotracheal intubation** if the patient will require more than a few more days of airway control, and it should be used in **massive facial trauma** and in respiratory failure due to **upper airway tumors.**

6. **Complications of tracheostomy**

   a. **Occlusion.** The tracheostomy tube may have to be removed and replaced if the soft balloon overrides the end of the tracheostomy tube, or if secretions occlude or narrow the tube or produce a ball-valve type of occlusion.

   b. **Aspiration.** Swallowing mechanisms are discoordinated after tracheostomy, leading to aspiration of saliva and a consequent need for frequent suctioning.

   c. **Tracheoesophogeal fistula** is rare but can be caused by overinflation of the cuff.

   d. **Hemoptysis** may occur from tracheitis (relatively common) or erosion of the tube into the innominate artery (uncommon but potentially lethal). Major bleeding around or through a tracheostomy tube several days after placement indicates a need for exploration of the neck and upper mediastinum.

B. **Mechanical ventilation** with a respirator is useful for increasing alveolar ventilation, decreasing or eliminating the work of breathing, restoring functional residual capacity, and maintaining open airways.

1. **Respirator terminology**

   a. **Volume controlled.** A preset volume of a gas is delivered over a wide range of pressure (Bennett MA-1, MA-2; Engstrom; Servo). This type of respirator is most useful for long-term support.

   b. **Pressure controlled.** Gas is delivered until a preset pressure is achieved (Bird Mark VII, Bennett PR-1).

   c. **Continuous mandatory ventilation** ventilates the patient at a set tidal volume and regular rate.

   d. **Assisted ventilation.** A preset tidal volume is delivered when the patient actively initiates a respiratory effort.

   e. **Intermittent mandatory ventilation** allows the patient to breathe at his or her own rate and V_T, but, in addition, the respirator delivers a preset volume, usually at a rate less than the patient's existing respiratory rate.

   f. **Intermittent demand ventilation** is the same as intermittent mandatory ventilation, except that the augmented volume is delivered synchronously with inspiratory effort.

2. Initial ventilator settings

a. Tidal volume (VT) should be 12–15 ml/kg. This is substantially greater than normal, but it helps to prevent atelectasis and decreased compliance.

b. The **rate** should be 10–12/min. In agitated patients with respiratory distress, the rate may need to be much higher for the initial few minutes, decreasing as acceptance of the ventilator occurs.

c. Inspired oxygen concentration (FIO_2) should start at 0.50 unless the patient is known to need more oxygen.

d. Sensitivity is the setting that allows the patient to initiate an assisted breath. It should not require excessive effort; 2 cm H_2O below zero airway pressure is a usual setting. The proper sensitivity setting during positive end expiratory pressure (PEEP) ventilation is controversial but should probably remain near zero.

e. Sigh at a high VT is not necessary, but at a low VT (< 8 ml/kg) a sigh cycle with a volume 50–100% greater than the VT should be set at a rate of 4–8 times/hr.

f. Alarms usually are present for excessively high or low pressures and must not be turned off.

3. Subsequent ventilator adjustments. Arterial blood gas values, along with the patient's acceptance of the ventilator, help to determine appropriate settings. Tidal volume, flow rate, respiratory rate, FIO_2, dead space, and sedation of the patient should be altered to make the patient comfortable and to achieve the following blood gas values:

a. A **PO_2** of 65–90 mm Hg. Only minimal additional oxygen-carrying capacity is added by achieving a PO_2 of 100 mm Hg or greater, while the risk of oxygen toxicity to the lung parenchyma is increased.

b. A **PCO_2** of 35–45 mm Hg and a **pH** of 7.35–7.45. Respiratory alkalosis, the most frequent abnormality during mechanical ventilation, is deleterious and should be avoided.

4. Positive end expiratory pressure (PEEP)

a. Indications. A PO_2 less than 60 mm Hg with FIO_2 more than 0.40 prophylactically in patients at high risk of developing atelectasis or hypoxemia.

b. Beneficial effects of PEEP include increased FRC, prevention of small airway closure, improved $\dot{V}A$, less $\dot{V}A/\dot{Q}$ imbalance, and less shunt ($\dot{Q}s/\dot{Q}t$).

c. Deleterious effects of PEEP less than 5 cm H_2O probably are nonexistent. Above 5 cm H_2O, PEEP may cause decreased cardiac output due to increased intrathoracic pressure and depressed myocardial function, increased interstitial pulmonary edema, a shift of perfusion away from well ventilated areas, and an increased likelihood of pneumothorax. Measurement of cardiac output, oxygen delivery, and shunt fraction are required to balance benefits and risks optimally.

5. Monitoring of patients receiving mechanical ventilation is aimed at avoiding complications and measuring changes in the disease state.

a. A **daily chest x-ray** is required to check endotracheal tube position and to look for evidence of pneumothorax, fluid overload, pneumonia, or atelectasis.

b. Arterial blood gases should be determined every time a change in respirator settings is made, whenever the patient's condition changes, and at least twice a day to detect early changes in the patient's condition and possible ventilator malfunction.

c. **Fluid balance** is followed by recording accurate daily intake and output and patient weight and measuring serum sodium and hematocrit.

d. **Pulmonary artery and wedge pressure** should be measured in patients with PEEP more than 5 cm H_2O, cardiovascular instability, or increased pulmonary interstitial fluid.

e. **Spontaneous VT and VC** measurements are needed to determine when weaning is possible.

f. **Peak inspiratory pressure** will allow calculation of effective compliance.

6. **Weaning** is the process of removing mechanical support as the patient regains the ability to provide adequate, spontaneous ventilation.

   a. **General considerations**

      (1) The pathological process that caused respiratory failure must be improving or resolved.

      (2) Factors that decrease ventilatory ability, such as pain, flail chest, respiratory alkalosis, and nutritional depletion, must be controlled.

      (3) Factors that increase requirements for oxygen, such as fever and sepsis, should be controlled.

      (4) Oxygen delivery should be optimal after hypotension, shock, anemia, and metabolic alkalosis are corrected.

   b. **Criteria** suggesting that an attempt at weaning may succeed include:

      (1) VC is more than 10 ml/kg.

      (2) FEV_1 is greater than 10 ml/kg.

      (3) VD/VT is less than 0.5.

      (4) Shunt fraction is less than 15–20%.

      (5) For COPD patients, arterial blood gases should approximate the usual values in that patient while still on the respirator.
      Failure to meet any of these criteria suggests that weaning efforts should be delayed.

   c. **Technique #1** is most useful in patients who have been intubated for a short period or whose ventilatory ability is recovering rapidly.

      (1) Inform the patient of the procedure and the expected results.

      (2) Place T piece on the endotracheal tube and insufflate with gas of high humidity and an FIO_2 of 20% above the concentration used during ventilator assistance.

      (3) Initially leave the patient off the respirator for 10–20 min at the first trial. Progressively lengthen the time as tolerated. Do not force to exhaustion.

      (4) Measure VT and arterial blood gases at the end of the trial period.

      (5) Continuous positive airway pressure (CPAP) of 3–5 cm H_2O may assist in maintaining lung inflation and avoiding airway closure.

   d. **Technique #2** is useful in patients who are less able to cooperate, have been on a ventilator for a prolonged time, are debilitated, or have chronic lung disease.

      (1) Switch the ventilator to the intermittent mandatory ventilation or intermittent demand ventilation mode.

      (2) Set the rate below the patient's spontaneous rate (usually 4–8/min) and set VT at 12–15 ml/kg.

      (3) Decrease the rate as tolerated. Some patients with COPD may require very slow weaning.

  e. Weaning should be terminated and the ventilator reconnected if:

   (1) Blood pressure increases or decreases more than 20 mm Hg.

   (2) Pulse increases more than 20/min or is more than 120/min;

   (3) Respiratory rate is over 35/min.

   (4) V_D/V_T is more than 0.6.

   (5) PO_2 is less than 60 mm Hg.

   (6) PCO_2 is more than 50 mm Hg (except COPD patients).

   (7) The patient's breathing becomes labored, or excessive anxiety occurs.

C. Circulatory management is important because the transport and delivery of respiratory gases is as crucial to cellular function as is ventilation to gas exchange in the lung.

 1. Cardiac output should be monitored in every unstable patient because significant depression may occur with both mechanical ventilation and PEEP. Cardiac output is directly related to O_2 delivery and, when increased, can compensate for hypoxemia. Also, as cardiac output decreases, mixed venous O_2 falls (assuming an unchanged metabolic rate), and hypoxemia may therefore occur even if lung parenchymal disease and shunt remain unchanged.

 2. Hemoglobin transports oxygen and carbon dioxide, and an adequate amount (> 10 gm/100 ml) is important to prevent a needless increase in cardiac output. Oxyhemoglobin dissociation should be kept normal by avoiding metabolic alkalosis and hypocarbia.

 3. Fluid balance should be adequate to support cardiac output (a wedge pressure of 10–14 mm Hg). However, if pulmonary capillary damage exists (aspiration, sepsis, noncardiac pulmonary edema), the lowest wedge pressure should be maintained that allows adequate blood pressure and perfusion. Fluid overload causes pulmonary edema, hypoxia, and decreased compliance and may prevent successful weaning.

D. Adjunctive treatment includes such features of patient care as:

 1. Frequent **position change** and **skin care** to prevent pressure necrosis (decubitus ulcer or bedsore). The supine position should be used sparingly because it decreases FRC and allows secretions to collect in the dependent bronchi.

 2. Nutrition should be provided by either the enteral or parenteral route early in the patient's course (see Chap. 10).

 3. Sedation and **pain relief** are important to make the patient comfortable mentally and physically. Excessive sedation should be avoided. Pharmacological paralysis (pancuronium, curare) rarely is indicated and can be dangerous by producing **total** dependence on mechanical ventilation and medical attendants. Occasionally, patients who fight the respirator or are physically violent may benefit from total control induced by pancuronium.

V. Adult respiratory distress syndrome is respiratory insufficiency or failure associated with increased capillary permeability to fluids and protein, resulting in pulmonary edema, cellular infiltration of lung parenchyma, increased shunt fraction, and ventilation-perfusion imbalance. Predisposing factors are diverse but include sepsis, aspiration, shock, trauma, pancreatitis, drug overdose, viral infection, increased intracranial pressure, cardiopulmonary bypass, exogenous toxic agents, and disseminated intravascular coagulation. Adult respiratory distress syndrome is not a sufficient diagnosis in itself and does not mandate a specific form of therapy. The various components of the syndrome must be identified and acted on appropriately, i.e., fluid overload, infection, pulmonary artery hypertension, or hypoxia.

Suggested Reading

Bartlett, R. H., Gazzaniga, A. B., Wilson, A. F., Medley, T., and Wetmore, N. Mortality prediction in adult respiratory insufficiency. *Chest* 67:680, 1975.

Surgical Endocrinology

The Diabetic Patient

I. General information

A. The stress of anesthesia and operation exacerbates the patient's glucose intolerance, and the frequent necessary modifications in food and fluid intake during this period further complicate management.

B. To maintain nutrition and prevent ketoacidosis and hypoglycemia, it is imperative that the patient receive a **minimum of 100 gm of carbohydrate daily** and that **adequate insulin be continuously available** to promote utilization of these carbohydrate calories. It should never be forgotten that caloric intake and insulin availability must always be considered together. A liter of 5% D/W contains 50 gm of carbohydrate.

C. It is important that the diabetic patient be in the best possible nutritional balance at the time of operation. Therefore, if the operative procedure is not urgent, it should be delayed until the following are evaluated and controlled: diabetic state, nutritional status, hydration, and electrolyte status. This often requires 2–6 days of hospitalization before operation.

D. Even when the need for operation is urgent, a few hours should be taken to correct **ketoacidosis,** if possible. Operative mortality is high for patients in ketoacidosis; even a short period of intensive therapy with fluids and insulin will improve the prognosis. Ketoacidosis may mimic acute surgical conditions, particularly appendicitis. This is another reason for delaying any procedure until ketoacidosis is treated.

E. Because of individual variations in the renal threshold for glucose, the frequent difficulty in complete bladder emptying in the perioperative period, and the hazards of catheterization of the diabetic patient, one should depend predominantly on **plasma glucose and ketone** determinations. These should be obtained at least q6h for 1–3 days after operation for better evaluation of the patient's diabetic control.

F. Hypoglycemia is a more hazardous condition than hyperglycemia. When there is no hyperketonemia, moderate hyperglycemia (200–250 mg/100 ml) is not hazardous and should be expected during the early postoperative period. However, marked hyperglycemia can lead to an osmotic diuresis, dehydration, and hyperosmolarity and should be avoided. Some diabetic patients who have had neurosurgical procedures, and those receiving corticosteroids or hyperalimentation, are especially prone to develop marked hyperglycemia and hyperosmolality. These conditions should be anticipated and treated with increased doses of insulin and IV fluids.

G. While moderate hyperglycemia is acceptable in the operative and immediate postoperative period, there is evidence that elevated plasma glucose levels may alter leukocyte and fibroblast function, predisposing to infection and poor wound

231

healing. Insulin deficiency can also aggravate the postoperative catabolic state. Therefore, the plasma glucose level optimally should be maintained between 100 and 200 mg/100 ml, as long as this does not lead to severely hypoglycemic periods.

H. Diabetic patients are particularly liable to staphylococcal and mixed gram-negative infections. In a diabetic patient, the usual body antibacterial defense mechanisms may be insufficient to prevent a gross wound infection that, with the same degree of contamination, would not be clinically apparent in a nondiabetic person. Any apparent infection should be defined by culture and vigorously treated with appropriate antibiotics.

I. Insulin requirements may fall abruptly after an infection is drained or at the termination of a pregnancy (by delivery or abortion). The physician should anticipate this by decreasing the insulin dose to one third the previous dose. Supplemental insulin can be given later if this reduction is too great.

II. Minor operation under local anesthesia. Generally, no alteration in diabetic management is necessary here. If the patient must omit a meal for the procedure, however, the carbohydrate content of that meal (approximately 50 gm, or 1000 ml 5% dextrose in water or saline solution) should be given IV over a 4- to 6-hr period.

III. Major operation

A. Diabetes adequately controlled with diet and NPH or lente insulin

1. Prior to the operation. No change in insulin or diet regimen is necessary.

2. On day of operation. Management is most convenient if the procedure can be done in the early morning, although adjustments in the following regimen can be made if this is not possible.

a. In the early morning

(1) Omit breakfast.

(2) Start an IV infusion of 1000 ml 5% glucose in water or saline solution to be infused over a 6- to 8-hr period.

(3) Give approximately one third to one half the patient's usual daily dose of NPH or lente insulin subcutaneously.

b. On completion of operation

(1) Continue IV infusion with 5% glucose in water or saline solution, so that the patient receives a total of approximately 100 gm of glucose in 2000 ml of fluids in the first 24-hr period. Modifications, of course, may have to be made, depending on the fluid and electrolyte needs of the patient, but be certain to include at least 100 gm of glucose daily.

(2) Give regular insulin q4–6h based on blood (or urine) glucose levels. The first determination should be done as soon as the patient arrives in the recovery room. The dose should be based on the patient's response to previous doses of insulin. As a start, 10 units of regular insulin can be given for plasma glucose over 250 mg/100 ml, and 15 units for glucose over 350 mg/100 ml. Some authorities recommend giving the remainder of the patient's usual NPH or lente insulin after surgery, but the presence of long-acting insulin injected at different times can complicate further management.

(3) Give oral fluids and food as soon as the patient's condition permits.

3. On days following operation

a. If the patient cannot be fed orally, or oral intake is inadequate, give an IV infusion of 5 or 10% glucose in water or saline to a total of 200 gm of carbohydrate daily, and divide the usual dose of NPH or lente insulin into two equal doses given 12 hr apart. Obtain a serum glucose determination q6h during this period, and give supplemental insulin as needed to maintain an acceptable plasma glucose level (100–250 mg/100 ml). Lower the dose of lente or NPH by about 20% if hypoglycemia occurs.

b. Resume the usual preoperative diet (or a diet comparable in calories) and the preoperative daily dose of insulin as soon as the postoperative condition permits.

B. Poorly controlled diabetes without ketosis. The operative procedure can be delayed 2–6 days.

1. Preparation for operation

a. Diet. Provide 200–300 gm of carbohydrate and at least 30 Cal/kg of ideal body weight daily, with the diet divided into three meals and a bedtime snack.

b. Insulin

(1) If the patient is already on lente or NPH insulin, continue or increase the usual dose. Patients not on insulin can be started on 10–15 units of lente or NPH.

(2) Check urine specimens for glucose and ketones a half hour before each meal, or obtain a **stat** plasma glucose about 1 hr before each meal and at bedtime.

(3) Give supplemental regular insulin before each meal, based on blood or urine sugar. About 10 units of insulin initially can be given for glucosuria of 1% (3+) or more or a plasma glucose over 250 mg/100 ml, but subsequent doses should be modified based on the patient's previous responses. If the patient remains hyperglycemic throughout the day on this regimen, the next day's NPH or lente insulin can be increased by 5–10 units.

(4) For patients in whom the use of insulin may be temporary, the newer, highly purified pork insulin may be advantageous because it minimizes development of insulin antibodies.

c. When the patient's diabetes has been stabilized (serum glucose 150–250 mg/100 ml) on this regimen, proceed with the elective operation.

2. On day of operation

a. Omit breakfast.

b. Give fluids and insulin as described in **1.a.**

3. On days following operation. As surgical stress diminishes, the insulin dose can gradually be decreased, unless the patient becomes hyperglycemic. If continued insulin is necessary, an internist should be consulted prior to discharge to provide continuing follow-up, and the nurse and dietician should be asked to give appropriate patient education.

C. Poorly controlled diabetes with minimal or no ketosis. Operation within a day is urgent.

1. Preparation and during operation

a. Give IV infusions of saline or 5% glucose in saline or water (depending on serum glucose), so that the patient receives about 100 gm of glucose in 24 hr. Additional fluid and electrolyte replacement prior to the operation may be necessary to correct deficits.

b. Give crystalline insulin subcutaneously q6h, starting with 10 units. Check the serum or urine for sugar and ketones. Increase the insulin dose by 5–10 units for serum glucose in excess of 200 mg/100 ml or for a 3+ or 4+ urine sugar reaction, and reevaluate the dose requirement 4–6 hr later. A negative urine reaction for glucose may indicate a need for reduction in the dose, but insulin should not be omitted completely as long as IV glucose is being given.

2. On days following operation. Continue the postoperative regimen outlined in **B.3.**

D. Severe ketoacidosis

1. The patient in severe ketoacidosis is a very poor risk for any operation except incision and drainage of an abscess or a similar urgent procedure.

2. A delay of 4–6 hr is imperative (much longer if possible) to initiate correction of ketoacidosis and fluid electrolyte imbalance. Frequent doses of crystalline insulin, or continuous intravenous infusion of insulin, will be required. Further details on the management of severe ketoacidosis are beyond the scope of this discussion. Immediate consultation with an internist or endocrinologist should be obtained.

3. As soon as severe ketoacidosis has improved, the patient should be managed as outlined in **C.**

E. Diabetes well controlled with an oral hypoglycemic agent

1. This condition generally requires insulin during the stress of the surgical period unless the diabetes is very mild.

2. Discontinue chlorpropamide the morning before operation, and discontinue other shorter-acting agents the evening before operation.

3. On the day of the operation, measure plasma glucose prior to surgery and urine or plasma glucose q4–6 h subsequently. Give 10 units of regular insulin for plasma glucose over 200 mg/100 ml or urine glucose over 1% (3+). Modify further doses by the initial response. As previously noted, the use of highly purified pork insulin may be preferable if insulin use is likely to be temporary.

4. When the stress of the surgical period is over, the patient may be returned to the previous oral regimen.

F. Diabetes that cannot be controlled by the usual measures.
Although most diabetes is managed readily by the foregoing procedures, some persons with unusual insulin resistance may not respond. On surgical services, this is most common in recipients of renal transplants who are given large doses of corticosteroids. In such patients, continuous intravenous infusion of regular insulin may be useful. An infusion pump is highly desirable. Dividing the plasma glucose by 100 (150 for patients not on glucocorticoids) gives the initial hourly infusion rate in units; plasma glucose is measured q2–3h and the infusion rate adjusted if needed. Consultation with an endocrinologist or internist is recommended.

Suggested Reading

Meyer, E. J., Lorenzi, M., Bohannon, N. V., Amend, W., Feduska, N. J., Salvatierra, O., and Forsham, P. Diabetic management by insulin infusion during major surgery. *Am. J. Surg.* 137:323, 1979.

Rossini, A. A., and Hare, J. W. How to control the blood glucose level in the surgical diabetic patient. *Arch. Surg.* 111:945, 1976.

Steinke, J. Management of diabetes mellitus and surgery. *N. Engl. J. Med.* 282:1472, 1970.

The Patient on Corticosteroids

I. General information

A. Normal adrenal cortices secrete about 20 mg of hydrocortisone daily.

B. A patient's ability to withstand stress, surgical or otherwise, depends on the ability of the adrenals to respond by markedly increasing the output of hydrocortisone (up to 10 times the basal amount).

C. A patient who is receiving corticosteroids currently, or who has received them for more than 1–2 wk within the 6- to 12-mo period prior to the operation, has an unpredictable degree of functional adrenocortical suppression. These patients should be considered to have iatrogenic adrenocortical insufficiency at the time of operation and should be managed accordingly.

D. The same type of management should be employed for patients who have previously undergone adrenalectomy, patients with spontaneous adrenal insufficiency and patients who are to undergo adrenalectomy.

E. It is important to recognize (1) that these patients will need large amounts of hydrocortisone or cortisone readily available to all tissues at all times during the stress of the surgical period, and (2) that **short-term excess of glucocorticoids is relatively harmless, but short-term deficiency during stress can be fatal.**

F. Cortisone acetate is poorly absorbed when given IM, whereas IM hydrocortisone sodium succinate and phosphate are well absorbed. However, both cortisone acetate and hydrocortisone are effective when given orally.

II. Patients with adrenal insufficiency undergoing operation or patients undergoing adrenalectomy. The following outline includes a planned excess of corticosteroids given by more than one route to assure continuous availability during the period of maximal stress.

A. Day of operation

1. 2 hr preoperatively: hydrocortisone succinate or phosphate, 100 mg IM.

2. One half hour preoperatively: hydrocortisone succinate or phosphate, 100 mg IM.

3. One half hour preoperatively: Start hydrocortisone succinate by continuous IV drip, 100 mg q8h for 24 hr.

4. Immediately after operation: hydrocortisone succinate or phosphate, 50 mg IM q4h.

B. Days following operation

1. Days 1 and 2: hydrocortisone succinate or phosphate, 35 mg IM q4h (see **C.1**).

2. Days 3 and 4: hydrocortisone succinate or phosphate, 25 mg IM q4h (see **C.1**).

3. Days 5 and 6: hydrocortisone succinate or phosphate, 20 mg IM q4h (see **C.2**).

4. Days 7 and 8: hydrocortisone succinate or phosphate, 15 mg IM q4h (see **C.2**).

5. Days 9 and 10: hydrocortisone succinate or phosphate, 10 mg IM q4h (see **C.2.**).

6. Day 11 and thereafter: maintenance dosage for patients with known adrenal insufficiency; discontinuance of cortisone in patients minimally suspected of corticosteroid-induced adrenocortical suppression and therefore treated only during surgical stress.

C. Modifications

1. If patient is receiving IV fluids during the early postoperative period, the daily dose of hydrocortisone may be given by **continuous** IV drip.

2. When the patient can tolerate and retain oral feedings without difficulty, corticosteroid medication can be given PO as **cortisone acetate** in the same dosage as listed in **B.,** above.

3. The preceding regimen of dose reduction in **B.,** above, is a general guide, to be modified to each patient's needs, as judged by clinical status (especially the presence or absence of fever, pain, or other stress), blood pressure, and serum electrolytes.

4. Amounts of cortisone or hydrocortisone greater than 100 mg daily exert adequate mineralocorticoid effects. When the daily dose is reduced below 100 mg, 9α-fluorohydrocortisone, 0.1 mg PO daily, should be added to the regimen.

5. The cortisone dose reduction regimen for patients who have undergone adrenalectomy for Cushing's syndrome generally must proceed more slowly than average, and the dose often cannot be reduced below 50 mg daily for several weeks.

6. Conversely, in patients with questionable adrenocortical suppression because of past corticosteroid therapy, the postoperative corticosteroid dosage may be reduced more rapidly and often may be discontinued within 4–7 days.

7. The addition of potassium (40–80 mEq daily) to the IV fluids and later to the oral intake is helpful in preventing potassium depletion.

III. Minor procedures. Patients undergoing procedures such as tooth extraction or biopsy should receive 50–100 mg of cortisone acetate PO, or 50–100 mg of hydrocortisone succinate or phosphate IM, about 2 hr before the procedure and 50–100 mg about 4 and 8 hr after the procedure. Generally, the patient's maintenance regimen can be resumed the following day.

Suggested Reading

Fariss, B. L., Hane, S., Shinseko, J., and Forsham, P. H.   Comparison of absorption of cortisone acetate and hydrocortisone hemisuccinate. *J. Clin. Endocrinol. Metab.* 47:1137, 1978.

Thorn, G. W., and Lauler, D. P.   Clinical therapeutics of adrenal disorders. *Am. J. Med.* 53:673, 1972.

Acute Hypercalcemia (Hypercalcemic Crisis)

I. **Recognition.** Serum calcium levels normally are 8.5–10.5 mg/100 ml. Increases of serum calcium to 11–13 mg may be associated with only vague symptoms: tiredness, easy fatigability, constipation, polyuria, nocturia, and polydipsia. As serum calcium progressively increases, more toxic symptoms appear, and a life-threatening situation exists: anorexia, nausea and vomiting, dehydration, prerenal azotemia, calcium nephropathy with renal failure, and somnolence progressing to stupor and coma. Remember that 40–50% of serum calcium is bound to protein, primarily albumin, and it is the ionized calcium (usually not measured) that is important in regulating biological processes. This means that patients with hypoalbuminemia may have a relatively low total serum calcium but an elevated ionized fraction of calcium. Therefore, it is essential that serum albumin concentration be known when interpreting total serum calcium concentration.

II. Diagnosis. Acute hypercalcemic crisis is a syndrome seen primarily in patients with (1) hyperparathyroidism and (2) neoplasms associated with bone metastases. Parathyroid hormone (PTH) levels usually are not elevated with bone metastases, although some neoplasms produce excess PTH or a PTH-like hormone, resulting in hypercalcemia without bone involvement. Rarely do the other causes of hypercalcemia listed in **C** produce crises except when certain drugs are superimposed or when hypercalcemia is exacerbated by dehydration.

III. Major causes of hypercalcemia

A. Primary hyperparathyroidism (adenoma or hyperplasia).

B. Neoplasms associated with osteolytic lesions: breast, lung, kidney, ovary (PTH not elevated).

C. Neoplasms secreting PTH or a PTH-like hormone, or an osteoclast-activating factor: The tumor source may be the kidney, lung, ovary, pancreas, or a sarcoma.

D. Multiple myeloma.

E. Sarcoidosis.

F. Drugs. Vitamin D intoxication, thiazide diuretics, estrogens (particularly when used in the therapy of breast cancer), excess Ca^{++} intake in combination with antacids (milk-alkali syndrome).

G. Immobilization (especially in Paget's disease of bone).

H. Acute osteoporosis.

I. Idiopathic hypercalcemia of infancy.

J. Hyperthyroidism.

IV. Treatment. Acute hypercalcemic crises can be fatal and must be treated promptly. Serum calcium can be decreased by (1) increasing calcium excretion, (2) decreasing bone resorption, and (3) decreasing calcium intake. The most judicious and practical methods currently in use are listed in Table 13-1.

A. Rehydration with saline infusion and diuresis with furosemide, accompanied by careful monitoring of central venous pressure, body weight, urine output, and serum electrolytes (particularly K^+ and Mg^{++}), is the initial treatment of hypercalcemic crisis. Oral phosphate may be used if a response is not immediate, but only when serum phosphorus is not already elevated and renal function is adequate. Phosphate in a retention enema may be helpful when the oral route cannot be used. *Intravenous phosphate is hazardous and should be used only when other agents have failed to moderate the acute hypercalcemic crises.*

B. Other agents used to lower serum calcium

1. Mithramycin (25/kg/day IV), previously reserved for patients with neoplastic disease, has proved effective and safe for moderating severe hypercalcemia. Any calcium-lowering effect usually is seen in 12 hr, with a peak effect at 36 hr, sometimes lasting for many days. The toxic effects of this drug usually have been in patients on long-term antitumor therapy. Since repeated daily administration is rarely needed, this drug is relatively safe when calcium concentrations remain dangerously elevated (above 13–15 mg/100 ml) after fluids, diuretics, and oral phosphates. Mithramycin is not suitable for long-term use in primary hyperparathyroidism.

2. Corticosteroids may lower serum Ca^{++} in some diseases, but the response is inconsistent and the onset slow. Patients with vitamin D intoxication, lymphomas, sarcoidosis, myeloma, or breast carcinoma as a cause of hypercalcemia may be benefited by corticosteroids.

3. Calcitonin, a peptide hormone used in the treatment of Paget's disease, lowers serum calcium primarily by inhibition of bone reabsorption. The dosage of

Table 13-1. Preferred Methods of Treatment of Hypercalcemic Crisis

Agent	Dosage and Route	Mechanism of Action	Complications and Remarks
0.9% Saline	100–200 ml/hr IV	Rehydration; increased urinary Ca excretion.	Na and H_2O overload, congestive heart failure. Monitor central venous pressure, body weight.
Furosemide (Lasix)	20–100 mg/hr IV (must be given with 0.9% saline infusion)	Induced diuresis; increased urinary Ca excretion.	Volume, K^+, and Mg^{++} depletion; renal failure if oliguria not responsive. Monitor weight, central venous pressure, urine, electrolytes; replace appropriately.
Inorganic phosphate (Neutra-Phos)	1–3 gm/day PO or through nasogastric tube	Binds Ca in gut, increases Ca movement into bone.	Monitor serum phosphorus, creatinine, magnesium, and urine.
Phosphate-phosphorus in glucose* (Inphos)	50 mmol in 500–1000 ml 5% dextrose q6–12h IV	? Deposition of $CaPO_4$ salts.	*Hazardous:* Avoid hyperphosphatemia > 5 mg/100 ml because of possible soft tissue calcification. Do not use in renal insufficiency.
Corticosteroids (prednisone)*	40–80 mg/day starting dose	Decreased bone reabsorption; ? anti–vitamin D	Delayed effect; reserved for vitamin D intoxication, lymphomas, sarcoidosis, myeloma, and breast carcinoma.
Mithramycin*	25 μg/kg/day IV (observe effect of single or ½ dose)	? Antitumor or PTH antagonist (no increase in urinary calcium)	Effect in 12–24 hr; may be given for 5 days. Hepatotoxic, nephrotoxic, thrombocytopenia.

*Adjunctive therapy. Use after rehydration, furosemide, and possibly oral phosphate.

calcitonin-salmon (Calcimar) varies. The therapeutic effects are variable and usually transient. Allergic reactions are possible.

4. Edetate (EDTA), given IV, lowers serum Ca^{++}, but the effect is transient, requiring administration of additional EDTA, and each dose increases the risk of renal tubular damage.

5. Sodium sulfate infusion offers no advantage over phosphates and may be less effective.

Parathyroid Insufficiency

I. General comments

A. Parathyroid insufficiency following thyroidectomy occurs *transiently* in 8% of surgically treated patients; symptoms may persist for 3–6 mo but eventually clear completely. Symptomatic hypoparathyroidism occurs transiently in 70% of patients having excision of abnormal parathyroid glands. This state is probably a result of compromise of the blood supply of the remaining normal parathyroid glands.

B. If the operative procedure was a parathyroidectomy for hyperparathyroidism associated with an elevated alkaline phosphatase or with overt bone disease, postoperative hypocalcemic tetany may be particularly severe because of the rapid uptake of calcium by osteoblasts. Continual adjustment of postoperative calcium and vitamin D therapy in these patients is required until the alkaline phosphatase has returned to normal.

C. Permanent hypoparathyroidism or tetany as a complication of thyroid or parathyroid surgery is uncommon. The incidence following operations for benign thyroid disease is less than 1%; following operations for thyroid cancer, it is 5%.

D. Symptoms are related to neuromuscular irritability secondary to hypocalcemia. Initially, the patient may exhibit only nervousness, irritability, and personality changes. Later, tingling of the extremities may appear, followed by paresthesias, muscle cramps, and numbness.

E. Chvostek's sign often is positive, and tendon reflexes are hyperactive. Carpopedal spasms and a positive Trousseau's sign appear only later.

F. Laryngeal stridor or **convulsions** may supervene at any time, without marked warning symptoms.

G. There may be **ECG evidence of hypocalcemia** manifested by a prolonged Q–T interval.

H. The **diagnosis** is confirmed by determination of the serum calcium. Levels below 7 mg/100 ml (3.5 mEq/liter) in the absence of alkalosis are usually symptomatic and require treatment. Occasionally, a patient may be seen with a low-normal serum calcium who still exhibits a positive Chvostek's sign.

II. Treatment

A. Blood for a serum calcium determination should be drawn before any therapy is given.

B. If symptoms are severe, 1 gm (10 ml) of 10% calcium gluconate should be given **slowly** IV with electrocardiographic control. Slow administration of calcium is emphasized, especially if the patient is receiving digitalis, so that acute hypercalcemic cardiac arrest will not ensue.

C. Oral calcium salts (calcium gluconate or lactate powder or wafers), 12 gm/day in divided doses, is the mainstay of therapy and all that will be required in the majority of patients.

D. Should signs of hypocalcemia persist after oral calcium therapy, vitamin D is indicated. The usual starting dose of calciferol (vitamin D_2) is 50,000 units daily. Occasionally, doses of vitamin D up to 500,000 units/day may be required.

E. Oral antacids such as magaldrate (Riopan) and magnesium-aluminum hydroxide (Maalox) that bind phosphates will permit enhanced absorption of dietary calcium and should be given with meals.

Thyroid Storm

I. Definition. Thyroid storm can be described as a marked augmentation of the symptoms of thyrotoxicosis. It is now thought to be due to markedly increased serum levels of triiodothyronine (T_3) and thyroxine (T_4) (singly or in combination), combined with hypersensitivity of beta-adrenergic receptors.

II. Symptoms. The symptoms may occur following any operation in the hyperthyroid patient and occasionally following operations in a euthyroid patient who has been pretreated with iodine. They include:

A. Hyperpyrexia, which may be severe (41.6–42.2°C [107–108°F]).

B. Tachycardia, 160–200 beats/min.

C. Nervousness, irritability, frank psychosis.

D. Vomiting and diarrhea.

E. High-output cardiac failure, the most common cause of death.

III. Treatment

A. Prevention is the cornerstone of therapy. Propylthiouracil is administered preoperatively to convert the toxic patient to euthyroidism. Beta-adrenergic blockage with propranolol, 20–40 mg tid, is more rapid-acting but does not treat the primary disease, only its effects.

B. When the syndrome has developed, **immediate treatment** consists of:

1. Symptomatic therapy for hyperpyrexia: cooling mattresses and oxygen.

2. Beta-adrenergic blockade with 1–2 mg of propranolol slowly IV as a test dose under cardiac monitor control after adequate volume restoration, followed by titration of the patient with an IV drip containing propranolol given at a rate that controls symptoms (usually 50–100 μg/min).

3. Institution of long-term thyroid suppression with propylthiouracil and iodide therapy. This will not be effective alone in the acute stage, but will allow orderly transfer to this regimen when acute symptoms subside, usually in 3–5 days.

4. Digitalization if symptoms are severe.

5. Both lithium acetate and plasmapheresis have been used to treat thyroid storm. Though promising, their efficacy is unproved.

Suggested Reading

Lee, T. C., Coffee, R. J., Mackin, J., Cobb, M., Routon, J., and Canary, J. J. The use of propranolol in the surgical treatment of thyrotoxic patients. *Ann. Surg.* 173:643, 1973.

Parsons, V., and Jewitt, D. Beta-adrenergic blockade in management of acute thyrotoxic crisis, tachycardia, and arrhythmia. *Postgrad. Med. J.* 43:756, 1967.

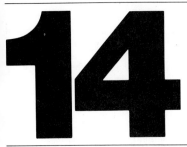

Surgical Infections

I. **Diagnosis.** The early and accurate diagnosis of surgical infection is essential, for delayed or inadequate therapy can result in overwhelming sepsis in an already stressed postoperative patient. Surgical infection usually can be treated successfully with specific antibiotics in conjunction with proper surgical care.

A. **History and physical examination** are still the surgeon's most important diagnostic tools. Although a number of serious infections are present prior to operation, most occur in the postoperative period. Directly related infectious complications include septicemia, intra-abdominal abscess, peritonitis, and wound infection. The infections that occur most frequently are those that involve the surgical wound and adjacent abdominal wall. These infections can be classified as **early** or **late,** based on their time of appearance. **Early wound infections** usually occur within 48 hr of operation and, in the majority of cases, are due either to **aerobic beta-hemolytic streptococcus** or to **anaerobic clostridia.** Diagnosis is based on clinical findings as well as on a Gram stain of needle-aspirated material. In these early infections, one should not wait for culture and sensitivity results before initiating treatment. Such delay would lead to massive tissue loss. **Late wound infections** usually occur between the fourth and seventh postoperative days. The cause of these infections is usually *Staphylococcus aureus* if the operation performed was classified as **clean.** Following gastrointestinal (GI) or gynecological surgical procedures, late infections usually are polymicrobial, the bacteria involved being representative of the endogenous microflora of the organ that has been surgically opened. These late infections manifest themselves by **induration** (the earliest sign), erythema, and pain. Excessive **wound pain** is a commonly overlooked early sign, particularly with wound infections caused by gram-negative organisms.

Auscultation of the chest may reveal the presence of pneumonia before it is evident on x-ray. **Rectal examination** may show tenderness and induration as signs of a developing pelvic abscess. Inspection of the calves and IV cannula dressings may reveal thrombophlebitis. In general, **fever occurring within the first 24 hr suggests pulmonary atelectasis; within 48 hr, a urinary tract infection; and after 72 hr, a wound infection.**

B. **Tests**

1. **Hematology and urinalysis.** Most bacterial infections produce an increase in the leukocyte count and a shift to the left in the differential count. This shift to the more immature forms of the polymorphonuclear leukocytes may signal infection before a rise in the total leukocyte count has occurred. The differential may also reveal lymphocytosis in viral infections, monocytosis in tuberculosis, eosinophilia in parasitic infections or hypersensitivity reactions (drug allergy), and toxic granulations of leukocytes in acute bacterial infections. A leukemoid response (total count over 25,000 cells/mm^3) may be seen in septicemia, pneumococcal infections, liver abscess or cholangitis, suppurative pancreatitis, necrotic bowel, and retroperitoneal phlegmon. Leukopenia is a sign of overwhelming bacterial infection, viral infection, or tuberculosis. Hemolytic anemia may be found with infections caused by *Clostridium perfringens* or group A streptococci.

2. **X-rays.** Routine chest x-rays may reveal generalized or focal atelectasis or may signal intra-abdominal infection or gastrointestinal leakage if air is identified under one of the diaphragms. In the workup of intra-abdominal sepsis, flat, upright, and decubitus x-rays may reveal a localized air-fluid level suggesting intra-abdominal abscess; or a spreading air pattern suggestive of a "gas-producing" infection may be seen. Specialized radiological procedures often are required in confirming a diagnosis of intra-abdominal sepsis. These studies include ultrasonography and computerized tomographic (CT) scanning; the choice of techniques depends primarily on the expertise of the local radiologist. Selective arteriography occasionally is of value. Gallium scans may also be helpful on occasion but are subject to an appreciable error rate and are difficult to interpret in the postoperative patient.

3. **Bacteriology**

   a. Observation of exudates and secretions (wound drainage, urine, sputum, etc.) for odor, color, and consistency may be helpful. Sweet, grapelike odors occur with *Pseudomonas,* urea odors with *Proteus,* and feculent odors with anaerobic organisms (*Bacteroides,* fusiforms, and clostridia).

   b. A **Gram stain** offers the earliest clues to the cause of an infection. Note should be taken of the polymorphonuclear leukocytes on the slide (few, many, loaded) and whether organisms can be seen inside them. Acid-fast and fungus stains can be used if these are in question.

   c. **Culture and sensitivity tests** are essential.. Both aerobic and anaerobic cultures should be requested. Ideally, anaerobic specimens should be transported immediately in a CO_2-filled tube and plated within 1 hr (otherwise, the organism will die, and the culture report will be negative). If the specimen must be held overnight, it should be placed in an anaerobic sterile vial or tube. Under no circumstances should an anaerobic specimen be refrigerated.

   d. **Blood cultures** are indicated in all serious infections. Careful cleaning of the venipuncture site with an iodine preparation should be followed by an alcohol swab. Blood should never be drawn for culture through an existing IV needle or catheter. It is important to obtain a number of blood cultures at different times. If possible, they should be obtained at the start of a chill or the beginning of a fever spike. Both aerobic and anaerobic cultures should be obtained.

   e. **Biopsy** of skin lesions and lymph nodes may be helpful. Avoid lymph node biopsy of the inguinal region. If no nodes are palpable, a scalene (fat-pad) node biopsy may be productive. Specimens should be sent for routine bacterial, acid-fast bacillus, and fungal cultures as well as to the pathology department for histological examination. Skin tests, except for tuberculosis tests, have limited usefulness. Serological tests are more reliable in the diagnosis of fungal diseases.

II. General principles of therapy

A. **Nosocomial infections.** Up to 15% of patients entering a general hospital will acquire an infection. Most of these will be caused by gram-negative bacilli. Even in units in which the risks of infection are stressed, breaks in technique occur.

   1. One third of **IV catheters** become colonized with bacteria within 2 days. Bacteremia will occur in 1% of patients with an IV catheter in place longer than 48 hr, and the risk of sepsis increases to 4–5% as the length of time the catheter remains in place increases. Since the advent of hyperalimentation, the figures are higher. IV catheters always should be removed and cultured, especially when bacteremia is suspected. Intra-arterial catheters may also be the site of sepsis and should be similarly handled.

2. **Foley catheters** should be connected to closed drainage systems and removed as soon as possible. Specimens of urine should be sent for culture and sensitivity testing at the time the catheter is removed.

3. **Breaks in technique** in the operating room also result in increased postoperative infection risk. Technical lapses most frequently involve improper ventilation, the surgical team's failure to cover all exposed hair, inadequate cleaning of the incision site, and failure to redrape and use a new set of instruments for closure of contaminated wounds.

4. **Improper preoperative management** also can increase the postoperative infection rate. Common errors include failure to employ preoperative baths with antiseptic soaps or solutions, and shaving of the operative site on the night before operation. Such shaving probably is not indicated in most patients. When practiced, it should be limited to the immediate preoperative period.

B. Treatment

1. Make a **diagnosis** (see I).

2. Select the proper **antibiotic,** as determined by the infecting organism and the following factors:

   a. **Effectiveness.** Gram-positive organisms are usually sensitive to penicillin and related compounds. Gram-negative aerobic organisms are likely to be sensitive to aminoglycosides or to second-generation cephalosporins, such as cefamandole or cefoxitin. Most anaerobic organisms are sensitive to penicillin. **Bacteroides fragilis** is the major exception; this organism usually responds to clindamycin, cefoxitin, chloramphenicol, metronidazole, carbenicillin, or ticarcillin. Other factors to consider are the penetration of the antibiotic into infected areas, whether the drug is bactericidal or bacteriostatic, and whether the antibiotic works in an acid environment. Erythromycin base taken orally is very effective in reducing *B. fragilis* organisms in the colonic lumen. However, because of the acid pH associated with tissue sepsis, this drug is often inactivated when used systemically.

   b. **Side effects and toxicity.**

   c. **Route of excretion.** The penicillins and aminoglycosides are excreted by the kidneys. Of the tetracyclines, chlortetracycline is the safest to use in the presence of renal failure. The drugs metabolized primarily by the liver include chloramphenicol, erythromycin, chlortetracycline, and clindamycin.

   d. In general, use **one antibiotic** rather than two when one microorganism is suspect in the infection.

   e. When there is no response to treatment by the end of 48 hr, the adequacy of antibiotic therapy should be **reevaluated.** Preliminary culture and disk sensitivities should be available by this time. In difficult cases, the bacteriology laboratory can provide precise antibiotic sensitivity levels by determining the minimal inhibitory concentration and the minimal bactericidal concentration. Serum antibiotic levels are indicated when aminoglycoside agents are employed.

C. Treatment of severe infection with unidentified bacteria

1. **No infection is so severe that it should be treated before culturing.** A Gram stain will prove especially useful in selecting the proper antibiotic. In patients with IV catheters, Gram stain and culture of the catheter tip can often provide an early diagnosis. Gram stains of an unspun urine specimen may give a clue to the presence of infecting organisms. In septicemia, microorganisms may be seen in gram-stained preparations of the buffy coat of centrifuged blood.

2. In critically ill patients with suspected sepsis, antibiotics have to be administered in advance of bacteriological confirmation. Many regimens are used, depending on the **most likely source of infection.** It is obvious that no combination will include all potential pathogens; therefore, some clinical judgment is necessary in selecting the most appropriate regimen.

D. **Gram-negative septicemia.** Clinical findings include disturbed sensorium, tachypnea, tachycardia, hypotension, fever, oliguria, and heart failure. In postoperative patients, the sudden appearance of tachypnea and hypotension suggests gram-negative septicemia. This condition has a 30–50% mortality; early diagnosis and treatment improve the chance of survival. **Important procedures in successful therapy** include:

1. Ensure an adequate airway.

2. Monitor **central venous pressure (CVP).**

3. Maintain adequate circulatory volume with **IV fluids and blood** on the basis of CVP values.

4. If CVP is elevated in the presence of hypotension, use **digitalis.** Give multiple small doses of digoxin or lanatoside C IV until the digitalizing dose is reached.

5. If there is no response to volume replacement and urine output is still diminished, use small doses of **isoproterenol.**

6. Avoid methoxamine and use only small doses of **norepinephrine** (Levophed) with adequate volume replacement.

7. Monitor **urine output** hourly.

8. The use of **corticosteroids** is controversial; however, a recent double-blind study has shown them to be efficacious in gram-negative sepsis. When employed, they should be given early as a single IV bolus of dexamethasone phosphate, 3–5 mg/kg, or methylprednisolone succinate, 15–30 mg/kg, over a 5- to 10-min period along with IV fluids.

9. If the identity of the organism is unknown, empirical treatment is begun until the results of the **blood cultures** are reported.

E. **Bacteriological versus clinical suprainfection.** Changes in the microbial flora of the skin, respiratory tract, and GI tract are seen in the most seriously ill patients, regardless of the underlying disease. Resistant gram-negative organisms, staphylococci, and fungi usually colonize such patients shortly after admission to the hospital. Factors increasing the incidence of colonization are antibiotic administration, use of inhalation therapy equipment, immunosuppressive or irradiation therapy, and depressed neurological status. The dilemma for the surgeon is to decide when bacteriological suprainfection becomes clinically significant or is associated with tissue-penetrating disease. One must use clinical variables, such as fever, leukocytosis, purulent sputum or wound discharge, deteriorating status, etc., to make this decision. However, it should be emphasized that **the bacteriology report must be judged in the total clinical setting;** reflex and uncritical use of antimicrobials on the basis of a positive sputum or wound culture is to be avoided.

III. **Specific microorganisms**

A. **Gram-positive cocci**

1. **Staphylococcal** infections are often localized **abscesses** containing creamy, yellow, odorless pus. This organism may also cause **cellulitis** with accompanying lymphangitis. Multiple small pustules suggest staphylococcal bacteremia.

a. Treatment of localized lesions consists of rest, heat, and elevation of the infected area. Incision and drainage are indicated in large localized abscesses or carbuncles.

b. Hospital-acquired staphylococci are almost invariably resistant to penicillin. Staphylococci outside the hospital also have a high incidence of resistance—in some series up to 70%. For this reason, **all staphylococcal infections must be treated with semisynthetic, penicillinase-resistant penicillins** (methicillin, oxacillin, nafcillin, cloxacillin) **or a cephalosporin** until antibiotic sensitivity is determined. Some hospitals have encountered virulent staphylococci resistant to all penicillins and cephalosporins; vancomycin may be useful in treatment of these organisms.

c. Clindamycin, erythromycin, or lincomycin can be employed in patients with penicillin allergy.

d. Pneumonia or septicemia resulting from staphylococci requires 4 wk of parenteral antibiotic therapy because of the high risk of coexisting endocarditis.

e. When prosthetic devices such as heart valves, neurosurgical drainage valves, or orthopedic pins become infected with staphylococci, antibiotics usually fail to cure the infection, and removal of the prosthesis is required.

2. Streptococci

a. Group A streptococci may cause **cellulitis** and erysipelas. Because of the involvement of lymphatics, there is often elevation and edema of the area, with red streaking of the skin.

b. **Fasciitis** involves the fascial tissue of wounds; the infection undermines the skin, often resulting in necrosis. These infections spead extremely rapidly and must be treated with large doses of parenteral penicillin (20 million units/day). Drainage and wide debridement also may be indicated.

c. **Burrowing ulcers** are caused by microaerophilic streptococci and coexisting staphylococci (Meleney's ulcer). Such lesions have a characteristic metallic sheen, cause necrosis of large areas of skin, and may produce sinus tracts in the underlying tissue. These should be incised, drained, and treated with large doses of penicillin.

d. **Subacute bacterial endocarditis** is usually caused by *streptococci* of the viridans group (70%) or *S. faecalis* and *S. bovis* (group D streptococci). All are sensitive to penicillin; 6 million units/24 hr given parenterally for 4 wk will usually be curative. *S. faecalis* organisms (enterococci) vary in their sensitivity patterns; most strains will be inhibited by penicillin (20 million units/24 hr) in combination with streptomycin (1–2 gm/24 hr) for 4–6 wk. *S. bovis* is usually susceptible to penicillin.

e. Anaerobic streptococci (*Peptostreptococci*) are normal flora in the mouth and GI tract. In contrast with other streptococcal wound infections, these organisms produce a thin brown discharge, often with crepitation in the infected tissues (**anaerobic cellulitis**). Treatment consists of appropriate incision and drainage and parenteral penicillin G, 10–20 million units/24 hr. Other antibiotics that are effective include cephalosporin, clindamycin, chloramphenicol, carbenicillin, ticarcillin, and metronidazole.

3. Pneumococci are the most common cause of bacterial pneumonia. A Gram stain of the sputum will show numerous gram-positive diplococci, often encapsulated or phagocytosed by polymorphonuclear leukocytes.

a. Pneumococci usually produce **lobar pneumonia,** although bronchopneumonia may occasionally be seen. Complications include empyema, lung abscess, endocarditis, and septic arthritis. **Septicemia** is seen in 25% of cases of pneumococcal pneumonia. Patients may develop toxic encephalitis or pancreatitis.

b. Most strains of pneumococci are sensitive to penicillin G. **Recommended therapy** for pneumonia is 1–2 million units of penicillin/24 hr parenterally in four divided doses. There is no evidence that larger doses of penicillin reduce mortality. Alternative agents are cephalosporin, erythromycin, lincomycin, and clindamycin. Tetracycline-resistant pneumococci have been reported, so this agent is not generally recommended.

   c. The outcome of pneumococcal infections depends on host factors. In many series, the mortality is still 30% despite antibiotic treatment.

B. Gram-positive rods

1. **Clostridia** are ubiquitous in nature and are present in the GI tract of humans and animals. Several species are associated with gas gangrene or anaerobic cellulitis. Clostridial septicemia or intra-abdominal abscess may be found with carcinoma of the large bowel or with traumatic injuries. Many clostridial septicemias are unexplained, and the disease may have a benign course even without therapy. Toxin production requires anaerobic conditions such as necrotic and devitalized tissue. All strains of clostridia are sensitive to penicillin. Tetracycline, chloramphenicol, and clindamycin are satisfactory alternative drugs. During treatment, attempt to alter the anaerobic environment necessary for the growth of these organisms, either by surgical debridement or by the use of a hyperbaric oxygen chamber.

2. **Diphtheroids** are the most common organisms present on skin. They are usually contaminants in wounds, but occasionally they may cause septicemia and infections of prosthetic cardiac valves.

3. *Listeria* may cause meningitis or septicemia in patients with cancer or those being treated with immunosuppressive drugs and in whom bacterial defense mechanisms are inhibited or compromised. Most strains of *Listeria monocytogenes* are sensitive to a variety of antibiotics; tetracyclines, penicillins, or aminoglycosides.

C. Gram-negative cocci

1. **Gonococci** most frequently cause genital infections, which are symptomatic in men, often asymptomatic in women. These organisms also may cause arthritis, meningitis, pharyngitis, ophthalmitis, and endocarditis. Septicemia is found more often with extragenital infections and may be associated with the finding of blood-filled vesicles in the skin. **Treatment** can be accomplished with penicillin, spectinomycin, ampicillin, or tetracycline. Penicillinase-producing organisms should be treated with spectinomycin.

2. **Meningococci** are introduced through the nasopharynx, producing initial septicemia and then lodging in the meninges, joints, or skin. The Waterhouse-Friderichsen syndrome is an overwhelming meningococcal infection presenting with shock. There is virtually a 100% mortality; patients show hemorrhage of the adrenal glands and evidence of a generalized Shwartzman reaction.

D. Gram-negative rods.
These organisms are widespread in the GI tract of man and animals and are present everywhere in the hospital environment. Some species are inherently pathogenic, such as *Salmonella* and *Pseudomonas,* while others have little potential for penetrating tissue. However, we have come to recognize that under appropriate circumstances any microorganism can cause disease in man.

1. *Escherichia coli* is the major coliform species in the GI tract. While most strains are sensitive to the majority of antibiotics, those associated with prolonged infections may become highly resistant. *E. coli* is the most common cause of acute urinary tract infections. It is also the major cause of septicemia.

2. *Klebsiella-Enterobacter* (*Aerobacter*) species are present in the GI tract, in contaminated food, and in the hospital environment. *Klebsiella* are generally sensitive to cephalosporin and resistant to carbenicillin, while *Enterobacter* species show the reverse pattern. Thickly encapsulated *Klebsiella* (types 1–6)

may cause Friedländer's pneumonia. Other strains cause urinary tract infections, intra-abdominal infections, and gram-negative pneumonia.

3. **Proteus** species may be inhabitants of the GI tract and are found in the hospital environment, especially in moist crevices. Indole-negative strains (*mirabilis*) are the most common cause of genitourinary infections and are usually sensitive to penicillins. Indole-positive strains (*rettgeri, morganii,* and *vulgaris*) cause more stubborn infections, resistant to many antimicrobial agents. Gentamicin and tobramycin may be effective antibiotics against these species. Because of the urea-splitting properties of *Proteus* strains, discharges from these infections are generally alkaline and have an ammonia smell.

4. **Pseudomonas** has become the most common gram-negative suprainfecting organism in many hospitals. These bacteria thrive in a moist environment and often contaminate respiratory equipment, soap dishes, and improperly dried instruments. *Pseudomonas* causes necrotizing wound and pulmonary infections, with invasion of blood vessels. Discharges are often green, with a distinctive odor from pyocyanin production. Most *Pseudomonas* strains currently are sensitive to gentamicin or tobramycin, but there has been an alarming increase in resistant strains. More resistance is seen to carbenicillin; strains may acquire resistance to this antibiotic during a single course of therapy. It is advisable to use an aminoglycoside and either carbenicillin or ticarcillin in combination for serious *Pseudomonas* infections. Resistant strains should be treated with amikacin.

5. **Serratia** species were formerly considered to be nonpathogenic. Recently, they have been associated with infections resulting from IV catheters. They may produce septicemia, endocarditis, and genitourinary infections. Approximately 20% of pathogenic strains are pigmented, and discharges may show a characteristic red color. *Serratia* are resistant to the majority of antibiotics; one of the aminoglycosides is recommended for these infections.

6. **Salmonellae** are present in animal or bird products or may be transmitted by human carriers. These organisms usually cause **mild gastroenteritis.**

   a. Antibiotic treatment of gastroenteritis is not advised, since it does not reduce the severity of clinical symptoms and may only prolong the carrier state. Antibiotic therapy is recommended for **septicemia, typhoidal symptoms, osteomyelitis, and localized abscesses.** For serious salmonellae infections, chloramphenicol is the drug of choice. Ampicillin may be used in milder cases.

   b. Antibiotics usually fail to eradicate the carrier state. In patients who are food handlers or who work in a hospital, cholecystectomy may be the only method of eradicating the carrier state of these organisms. Salmonellae may also cause food-borne epidemics within a hospital.

7. **Herellea-Mima** is a mixed group of gram-negative rods and cocci inhabiting the mouth and GI tract. They may cause infection in a compromised host. These organisms are generally resistant to penicillin but sensitive to most broad-spectrum antibiotics.

E. **Anaerobic bacteria.** This diverse group of fastidious microorganisms includes both gram-negative and gram-positive rods and cocci. They are the predominant members of the endogenous microflora of the human mouth, colon, and vagina and are found in high concentrations in other GI organs. Since the advent of improved anaerobic bacteriological collection and isolation techniques, obligate anaerobes have been isolated with increasing frequency from widely varied clinical infections. The critical factor necessary for the growth of anaerobes is an environment with decreased oxygen content, such as that found in abscesses, empyemas, and necrotizing infections.

   1. **Oral anaerobes** include *Bacteroides, Peptostreptococcus, Bifidobacteria, Fusobacterium,* and *Actinomyces.* The species of *Bacteroides* found here in-

cludes *B. oralis* and *B. melaninogenicus.* These anaerobes are isolated in high concentrations, particularly in dental plaque and around the periodontal membrane. They are noted to increase in patients with poor dental hygiene. These organisms result in local sepsis following head and neck surgery. If aspirated, they can result in lung abscess, putrid empyema, and necrotizing pneumonitis. They are generally highly sensitive to penicillin and the cephalosporins. Alternative agents include clindamycin, chloramphenicol, metronidazole, and carbenicillin. Treatment of actinomycosis requires long-term high-dose penicillin therapy.

2. **Intestinal anaerobes** include the oral anaerobes swallowed with saliva and food that transiently inhabit the upper GI tract in low numbers ($< 10^4$). In the distal ileum and colon, however, a resident anaerobic microflora is present in high concentrations (10^4–10^{10}). *B. fragilis* and *Clostridium* are major members of this flora, along with *Peptostreptococcus* and *Fusobacterium.* These colonic anaerobes frequently are associated with intra-abdominal and pelvic abscesses, wound abscesses, septicemia, and septic thrombophlebitis following colonic resection, penetrating traumatic colon injuries, or perforated appendicitis or diverticulitis. **Treatment** of these complications should include drainage where indicated, in addition to parenteral antibiotics.

   B. fragilis, the anaerobe most commonly implicated in these infections, is resistant to penicillin and should be treated parenterally with either clindamycin or metronidazole. Other useful agents include carbenicillin, ticarcillin, chloramphenicol, and cefoxitin. Currently, 30–40% of these organisms are resistant to tetracyclines.

3. **Vaginal anaerobes** include the same organisms mentioned in **2.** Vaginal cuff or pelvic abscess following hysterectomy and septic endometritis following childbirth or abortion are frequently due to these organisms, either alone or in combination with aerobic coliforms. When *B. fragilis* is suspected or isolated, **treatment** should include parenteral clindamycin or one of the other agents mentioned in **2.**

F. Fungi

1. *Candida albicans* is the most frequent fungus infection complicating surgical therapy. Oral thrush may be treated with general mouth care and nystatin gargles. Candidal septicemia usually is caused by an indwelling IV catheter, especially when the patient is receiving hyperalimentation. In most cases, removal of the catheter will abort the disease. Persistent fungemia or endocarditis requires intensive amphotericin B therapy. Compromised hosts are particularly susceptible to generalized candidiasis.

2. **Histoplasmosis, coccidioidomycosis, and blastomycosis** are generalized fungal infections less commonly seen in surgical practice. These infections are treated with amphotericin B and, in selected cases, with surgical excision of the infective focus. **Sporotrichosis** presents as a localized lesion of the extremity with lymphangitic spread; occasionally, generalized infections involving the lung and bone may occur. **Cryptococcus** usually causes meningitis or pulmonary infections.

G. Viruses

The role of viral infections in the surgical patient is generally not well understood, owing primarily to the difficulty of the techniques necessary for investigation of these organisms. Many types of viruses have been implicated in appendicitis and intussusception in children as well as in pancreatitis in adults. Viral infections due to cytomegalovirus have been observed in immunologically impaired patients with malignancy or after renal transplantation.

IV. Antibiotics

A. Penicillin

1. **Crystalline benzyl penicillin,** sodium or potassium salt, aqueous (penicillin G)

a. **Highly effective against many species of gram-positive and some gram-negative microorganisms.** All group A, beta-hemolytic streptococci, streptococci of the viridans group, and pneumococci are sensitive, but group D strains (enterococcus) are variably sensitive—first choice for sensitive staphylococci but ineffective against penicillinase-producing strains. Gonococci (except penicillinase-producing strains) and meningococci are sensitive, as are *Corynebacterium diphtheriae, Listeria monocytogenes, Treponema pallidum, Clostridium,* and *Actinomyces.* Some species of gram-negative enteric bacteria are affected by penicillin in high concentrations. This group includes *E. coli, P. mirabilis,* and many strains of salmonellae and shigellae. Oral anaerobes including *Peptostreptococcus, B. oralis,* and *B. melaninogenicus* are also usually sensitive.

b. **Mechanism of action.** Interferes with cell wall formation by inhibiting synthesis of muramic acid. Active mainly against rapidly growing organisms.

c. **Absorption.** One third to one half is absorbed orally; the drug is destroyed by gastric acid. The peak plasma level occurs in 1–2 hr. Parenterally, the peak blood level occurs in 15–30 min, with the effect lasting 3–4 hr, depending on renal function.

d. **Distribution.** Low concentrations (one tenth of serum) in meningeal, pericardial, and pleural spaces; significant concentrations in joints and bile; and very high concentrations in the kidney. When meninges are inflamed, penicillin penetrates into spinal fluid more readily.

e. **Excretion.** From 60–90% of the dose is excreted in urine, 90% by tubular excretion. Probenecid (0.5 gm/6 hr) will block tubular excretion and raise serum levels.

f. **Preparations**

   (1) **Aqueous (crystalline) penicillin**

   (a) **Oral** potassium penicillin G or sodium penicillin G in tablets of 50,000–500,000 units, given q6h, either a half hour before or 2 hr after meals.

   (b) **Parenteral.** Buffered or unbuffered potassium penicillin G in ampules of 1, 5, or 20 million units, given q4–6 hr by IM or IV injection. Available as a potassium or sodium salt (1.5 mEq/million units). Advantage: high peak levels. Disadvantages: rapid excretion, painful injection.

   (2) **Procaine penicillin** is for IM use only. Procaine penicillin and procaine penicillin with aluminum monostearate suspension are available in 1-ml cartridges and 10-ml vials, 300,000 units/ml. Limit the dose in a single site to 2 ml. Advantages: prolonged serum levels (24–36 hr), painless injections. Disadvantage: low serum (<1 mg/ml) and tissue levels.

   (3) **Benzathine penicillin G** (Bicillin) is for IM use only. It has the same spectrum and action as crystalline penicillin. Low concentrations in blood are present for 20–30 days. It is recommended for rheumatic fever prophylaxis.

2. **Phenoxymethyl penicillin** is more stable in gastric acid than is penicillin G and is better absorbed after an oral dose. It is available as Pen-Vee, Compocillin-VK, Pen-Vee K, and V-Cillin K in tablets of 125, 250, and 500 mg (125 mg equals 200,000 units). **Phenoxyethyl penicillin** may produce slightly higher blood levels than phenoxymethyl penicillin. It is available as Syncillin and Maxipen in 125-mg and 250-mg tablets.

3. **Ampicillin** is less effective than penicillin G against sensitive gram-positive cocci but more active against *Hemophilus influenzae, E. coli,* and some strains of *Proteus, Enterobacter, Salmonella,* and *Shigella.* It is ineffective against *Pseudomonas* species. It is destroyed by penicillinase. It is well absorbed after oral administration, with the peak blood level reached in 1–2 hr. It is excreted in urine and bile. Ampicillin (Penbritin, Polycillin) is available for PO use as 250- and 500-mg capsules; for parenteral use in vials of 250 mg–2 gm.

4. **Penicillinase-resistant penicillins**

   a. **Indicated** for treatment of infections caused by penicillinase-producing *Staphylococcus aureus.* These drugs are not as effective as penicillin G against other gram-positive organisms and have little effect on gram-negative bacteria. The mode of action is interference with cell wall synthesis.

   b. **Excreted** unchanged in the urine in the same manner as penicillin G.

   c. **Preparations**

      (1) Methicillin sodium (Staphcillin) is available in ampules of 1, 4, or 6 gm. It is inactivated by gastric acid and only available for parenteral use. The dose is 3–4 gm/6 hr IV or IM.

      (2) Oxacillin sodium (Prostaphlin) is available in 250- or 500-mg capsules, as well as in parenteral form.

      (3) Cloxacillin sodium (Tegopen). Resembles oxacillin.

      (4) Nafcillin sodium (Unipen) is available as 250-mg capsules or 500-mg ampules. Higher excretion in bile than other synthetic penicillins.

5. **Carbenicillin** is semisynthetic benzyl penicillin with good activity against gram-negative organisms but relatively poor activity against gram-positive strains. It is destroyed by penicillinase and should not be used in staphylococcal infections. Sensitive organisms include *Pseudomonas, Proteus* (both indole-positive and indole-negative), *Enterobacter* (but not *Klebsiella*), and *E. coli.* Doses of 1–2 gm/6 hr IV can be used in urinary tract infections. Carbenicillin is also active against the oral anaerobes as well as against *B. fragilis.* The dosage in severe infection should be in the range of 24–30 gm/day IV in divided doses. Oral preparations are available, but absorption is poor, resulting in low blood levels. Oral carbenicillin should not be used in serious infections.

6. **Ticarcillin** is a semisynthetic penicillin with a spectrum of activity similar to that of carbenicillin. It is given IV or IM.

7. **Reactions to penicillin and its analogues**

   a. **Hypersensitivity effects** include skin rashes, glossitis, stomatitis, fever, eosinophilia, angioneurotic edema, serum sickness, anaphylaxis, and Arthus reaction. These reactions may occur in 10–15% of patients treated with a penicillin preparation. However, a penicillin reaction does not necessarily render the patient sensitive to penicillin for life; most patients lose their hypersensitivity to the drug after some months or years. Before treating any patient with penicillin who has a questionable history of allergy, a skin test is mandatory. Penicillin G is diluted to a concentration of 1000 units/ml. A superficial scratch is made with a needle in the anterior forearm, and one drop of the penicillin solution is placed in the scratch. A positive wheal-flare reaction will occur within 15–20 min. If the scratch test is negative, an intradermal injection of the dilute penicillin solution should be attempted. Negative reactions to these tests give reasonable assurance that an anaphylactic reaction will not occur. It should be stressed that there is cross-sensitization among all penicillin preparations. The least sensitizing route is PO, followed by intradermal, IM, and the most challenging, IV.

b. **Renal insufficiency** has been reported with use of the semisynthetic compounds and rarely with penicillin G.

c. **Bone marrow depression** is a rare complication of therapy with semisynthetic penicillins. Some patients receiving high doses of carbenicillin or ticarcillin may develop hemorrhagic manifestations associated with abnormalities in coagulation test findings, such as in bleeding time and platelet aggregation. This complication is usually stopped by withdrawal of the drugs.

d. **Central nervous system (CNS) toxicity** is seen with all penicillins after very high doses, i.e., 40–80 million units of penicillin G, or with smaller doses of penicillins in the presence of renal insufficiency. The reaction begins with myoclonic twitching, proceeding to generalized seizures. Reducing the dose of penicillin will terminate the reaction; no sequelae have been reported.

e. **Irritative effects.** Epigastric distress and diarrhea may occur. The use of ampicillin has been associated with the development of antibiotic-induced colitis.

f. **Hemolytic anemia** of the Coombs'-positive type has been reported after large doses of penicillin.

B. **The first-generation cephalosporins have a structure similar to that of the penicillins;** hence, there is some cross-allergenicity. They are effective against gram-positive organisms, including penicillin-sensitive and penicillin-resistant staphylococci, streptococci, *Neisseria, Salmonella, P. mirabilis,* and most *E. coli* and *Klebsiella.* They are not effective against *Pseudomonas, Serratia,* indole-positive *Proteus,* enterococci, *Enterobacter,* or *B. fragilis.* They are active against most of the oral anaerobes.

1. **Mechanism of action.** Interference with cell-wall synthesis.

2. **Absorption.** IM or IV injection gives peak blood levels in 30 min. Cephalexin is 50% absorbed when given PO; low blood levels are achieved with oral preparations. Cephalosporins penetrate poorly into the meninges and should not be used in CNS infections.

3. **Excretion.** From 70–80% is excreted unchanged in the urine by glomerular filtration and some tubular excretion.

4. **Preparations.** Cephalothin (Keflin) is available as 10- and 50-ml ampules containing 1 and 4 gm of antibiotic respectively for IM or IV injection. Special IV ampules of 2 or 4 gm are available for dilution with 50–100 ml of 5% D/W. Cephaloridine (Loridine) is available for parenteral administration as a dry powder for reconstitution with sterile water in 5- and 10-ml ampules containing 0.5 and 1.0 gm of antibiotic respectively. Cephalexin (Keflex) is supplied in 250-mg capsules for oral administration.

5. **Reactions to the cephalosporins**

a. **Hypersensitivity effects.** Eosinophilia, fever, skin rashes, and serum sickness are reported. An increased incidence of reactions has occurred in penicillin-sensitive patients.

b. **Toxic effects.** Cases of neutropenia and depressed leukopoiesis have been reported. Cephaloridine is a frequent cause of renal insufficiency; the dose of this drug should never exceed 4 gm/24 hr.

c. **Irritative effects.** Thrombophlebitis and pain on IM injection are often seen with cephalothin. Infrequently, antibiotic-induced colitis has been reported.

C. **Second-generation cephalosporins** at present include cefamandole and cefoxitin. These drugs are similar to the first-generation cephalosporins in mechanism of action, basic pharmacokinetics, and drug toxicity. Their spectrum of activity differs from, and is more inclusive than, that of the older agent.

1. **Cefamandole** has a spectrum similar to that of the older agents against the gram-positive cocci and oral anaerobes, but activity against *E. coli, Klebsiella* species, and *Enterobacter* species is much greater.

2. **Cefoxitin,** derived from cephamycin C, is the most resistant of this antibiotic group to the effects of beta lactamases. It has a spectrum of activity similar to that of the first-generation cephalosporins against gram-positive cocci and oral anaerobes but greater activity against *E. coli* and *Klebsiella* species. Cefoxitin also has good activity against *B. fragilis.*

D. **Tetracyclines.** The first broad-spectrum antibiotics, the tetracyclines, are effective against many gram-positive and gram-negative organisms. They also inhibit the growth of rickettsiae, amebas, *Mycoplasma,* and agents of the psittacosis and lymphogranuloma venereum group. Nearly all strains of *Proteus* and *Pseudomonas* and many staphylococci and enterococci are resistant. Strains of *E. coli, Klebsiella,* and *Enterobacter* vary widely in sensitivity. Anaerobic streptococci and 30–50% of *B. fragilis* strains are resistant.

1. **Mechanism of action.** Inhibition of protein synthesis; these drugs are bacteriostatic.

2. **Absorption.** Incompletely absorbed after oral administration. Most active in the stomach and upper small bowel. Absorption is decreased by milk products and antacids as a result of a chelating effect. After oral doses, peak levels occur in 2–4 hr, lasting 6 hr or more. Demethylchlortetracycline and doxycycline produce significant blood levels for 12–24 hr.

3. The tetracyclines are **widely distributed** in tissues. Diffusion across the blood-brain barrier is good, even with noninflamed meninges. High concentrations are found in bile.

4. **Excretion.** From 20–60% of an IV dose is excreted in urine in the first 24 hr; a high proportion is protein-bound. Demethylchlortetracycline and doxycycline are longer-acting, owing to a decreased rate of renal excretion.

5. **Preparations**

   a. **Oral use.** Chlortetracycline hydrochloride, oxytetracycline, and tetracycline hydrochloride are available as 250-mg capsules. Demethylchlortetracycline is available as 75-, 150-, and 300-mg capsules. Doxycycline is prepared in 50-mg capsules.

   b. **Parenteral use.** Tetracycline preparations are supplied in 100-, 250-, or 500-mg vials. Parenteral doses are half those used orally.

   c. **Ophthalmic** preparations are available for local application.

6. **Reactions to tetracyclines**

   a. **Hypersensitivity effects.** Cheilosis, brown or black coating of the tongue, glossitis, vaginitis, and pruritus ani are relatively frequent side effects. Morbilliform rashes, dermatitis, angioneurotic edema, eosinophilia, and anaphylaxis occur but are rare.

   b. **Toxic effects.** Patients receiving large doses of tetracycline may develop jaundice and fatty liver. Pregnant women are especially prone to develop hepatotoxicity. Other effects include delay in blood coagulation, brown discoloration of teeth (in infants), increased intracranial pressure, and azotemia. Outdated drug may produce the Fanconi syndrome.

   c. **Irritative effects.** GI irritation is manifested by epigastric burning, nausea, emesis, and diarrhea. Pseudomembranous colitis has also been reported. IV administration is often followed by thrombophlebitis; IM use can lead to suppurative myositis. Photosensitivity of the skin occurs with demethyl-chlortetracycline.

   d. Suprainfection. Overgrowth of resistant microorganisms can cause staph-ylococcal enterocolitis and intestinal candidiasis.

E. Chloramphenicol. Primarily bacteriostatic, chloramphenicol has a wide spectrum of activity. It has an **inhibitory effect** against *E. coli, K. pneumoniae, H. influen-zae, Salmonella typhosa*, certain strains of *Proteus, Shigella*, and *Brucella*, some streptococci and staphylococci, the rickettsiae, and the psittacosis-lympho-granuloma groups of organisms. Most anaerobes (*Bacteroides*, fusiforms, strepto-cocci) are sensitive.

   1. Mechanism of action. Inhibition of protein synthesis.

   2. Absorption. Rapidly absorbed after oral administration.

   3. Distribution. Present in bile and cerebrospinal fluid (CSF) in high concentra-tion. Penetrates tissues in high levels.

   4. Excretion. Excreted in the urine (80–90%), but only 5–10% is in biologically active form.

   5. Preparation. Chloramphenicol is available as capsules of 50, 100, and 250 mg. Parenteral and ophthalmic forms are also available. The IM route should not be used because of poor absorption.

   6. Reactions to chloramphenicol

   a. Hypersensitivity effects. Agranulocytosis occurs in 1 in 30,000 adminis-trations of this drug. This reaction is not dose related. It usually follows a previous sensitizing dose. Most fatal cases are associated with inappropriate oral use for trivial viral infections. Bone marrow shows maturation arrest with vacuolization of granulocyte precursors. Skin rashes, fever, stomatitis, and anaphylaxis are rarely seen.

   b. Toxic effects. Anemia with a low reticulocyte count and increased serum iron is a dose-related, reversible effect. The "gray syndrome" is seen in premature infants and neonates who are unable to excrete chloram-phenicol, producing cyanosis, tachypnea, circulatory collapse, emesis, and diarrhea.

   c. Irritative effects. GI disturbances are seen with oral therapy including antibiotic-induced colitis.

   d. Suprainfection may occur, especially with *Candida* or staphylococci.

   7. Indications for chloramphenicol therapy. Typhoid fever, rickettsial infec-tions, and serious *Salmonella* infections should be treated with chloram-phenicol. Bacterial meningitis in a penicillin-sensitive patient can be treated with chloramphenicol. *Bacteroides* infections and anaerobic abscesses also are indications for use of this drug.

F. Erythromycin belongs to the macrolide class of antibiotics. It is effective against gram-positive cocci, i.e., group A streptococci, pneumococci, and 95% of staph-ylococci, including penicillinase producers. Some strains of *H. influenzae, Lis-teria, Brucella,* and *Treponema* are also sensitive. Anaerobic microorganisms, such as *Bacteroides, Peptostreptococci*, and *Clostridium*, also usually are sensitive, although this drug does not have a package insert recommendation for anaerobic infections. *Proteus, E. coli, Enterobacter, Klebsiella*, and *Pseudomonas* are resis-tant.

   1. Mechanism of action. Interferes with protein synthesis.

   2. Absorption. From 40–70% is absorbed in the upper small bowel. Peak plasma levels appear in 1–4 hr.

3. **Distribution.** Diffuses readily into body fluids. CSF levels are low.

4. **Excretion.** Excreted by the liver and pancreas. From 5–15% is excreted in the urine.

5. **Preparations**

   a. **Oral.** Erythromycin base, erythromycin stearate, and erythromycin estolate are available as 125- and 250-mg capsules and tablets. The dose is 250 mg–1 gm/6 hr. Where utilized in a preoperative bowel preparation, erythromycin base should be used because this drug is in the active form in the intestinal lumen, not first requiring biochemical alteration or absorption with biochemical alteration for its activity.

   b. **Parenteral** use is not recommended. IM injections are painful and cause myositis.

6. **Toxic effects**

   a. **Hypersensitivity effects.** Skin rashes, angioneurotic edema, serum sickness, and anaphylaxis. Cholestatic jaundice may occur with the estolate preparation. Liver biopsy shows periportal infiltration, mostly with eosinophils.

   b. **Irritative effects.** GI upset, vaginitis, and pruritus have been noted. Severe diarrhea may occur.

G. **Lincomycin** resembles erythromycin and can be used in place of it when parenteral therapy is needed in penicillin-sensitive patients who harbor grampositive coccal infections. It has **good activity** against group A streptococci, pneumococci, and 95% of staphylococci. Anaerobic infections with *Bacteroides* and anaerobic streptococci are successfully treated with lincomycin.

1. **Absorption.** Absorbed soon after oral administration; peak blood levels are obtained in 2–4 hr, with therapeutic levels lasting for 6–8 hr. IM and IV absorption is also good, with peak levels in 30 min, persisting for 8–12 hr. Therapeutic levels with IM dosage last for 24 hr.

2. **Distribution.** CSF penetration is up to 40% in the presence of meningeal infection; otherwise, it distributes readily in most body tissues.

3. **Excretion.** Up to 25% is excreted by the kidney in urine.

4. **Preparations.** Available in capsules of 250 and 500 mg and vials of 600 mg. The usual adult IV dose is 600 mg/6 hr; the usual IM dose is 600 mg/day.

5. **Side effects.** Diarrhea in most patients is a dose-related phenomenon with oral therapy. Diarrhea may be severe in 10% of patients, occasionally being associated with the passage of blood and on rare occasions leading to a clinical picture similar to that of ulcerative colitis. Skin rashes have been reported. Liver toxicity is occasionally seen with high doses.

H. **Clindamycin** is a derivative of lincomycin, differing only in the substitution of a chloride for a hydroxyl group on the lincomycin molecule. This change has resulted in better absorption and greater potency against anaerobic *B. fragilis* organisms. This drug also has increased activity against group A streptococci, pneumococci, and staphylococci.

1. **Absorption.** Absorbed rapidly after oral administration; peak blood levels are obtained within 1–2 hr. Parenteral absorption takes place rapidly, with peak serum levels occurring at about 10 min after IV administration and about 3 hr after IM administration.

2. **Distribution.** CSF penetration is poor; otherwise, this agent distributes readily in most body tissues.

3. **Excretion.** Mainly in the bile, with from 5–25% appearing in the urine.

4. **Preparations.** Available in 75- and 150-mg capsules and in vials of 300 and 600 mg. The usual adult IV dose is 600 mg q6–8h.

5. **Side effects.** Fewer GI complaints than with lincomycin; otherwise, very similar side effects. Diarrhea, occasionally severe, primarily follows oral administration. Discontinuing this agent usually results in alleviation of diarrheal symptoms. Diarrhea can progress to severe pseudomembranous colitis in about 1 in 53,000 patients. Antidiarrheal medications should be avoided lest this toxicity be increased.

I. **Streptomycin.** Because of the high incidence of bacterial resistance, the indications for streptomycin are relatively limited. It is combined with penicillin in treating *S. faecalis* or *H. influenzae* infections, brucellosis, tularemia, and plague, and it is combined with isoniazid (INH) in treating tuberculosis.

1. **Resistant bacteria.** Exposure to the drug may convert highly sensitive strains to resistant ones in as short a time as 48 hr. Delay in emergence of bacterial resistance is achieved by combination with other antibiotics.

2. **Mechanism of action.** Interferes with protein synthesis.

3. **Absorption.** Poorly absorbed PO; IM and subcutaneous injections are well absorbed.

4. **Distribution.** Streptomycin is distributed in the extracellular fluids, especially in the pericardial and peritoneal cavities. Pleural and synovial fluids also contain appreciable drug activity. With normal meninges, CSF penetration is poor.

5. **Excretion.** From 50–60% is excreted unchanged in urine in the first 24 hr. A small portion is excreted in the bile. The feces contain a small amount.

6. **Preparation.** Streptomycin sulfate is available for parenteral injection in vials containing 0.5, 1, or 5 gm. A dose of 1 gm/24 hr IM may be given for 30–45 days. For tuberculosis therapy, 1 gm three times a week is used.

7. **Reactions to streptomycin**

   a. **Hypersensitivity effects.** Skin rashes, fever, blood dyscrasia, stomatitis, anaphylaxis, exfoliative dermatitis, and eosinophilia.

   b. **Toxic effects.** Most important effects involve the eighth nerve. Patients receiving 2 gm or more/24 hr for more than 1–2 wk may manifest vestibular disturbances; recovery may require 12–18 mo. Neural disturbances in hearing also occur; a high-pitched tinnitus is often the first sign of toxicity; nerve deafness often is not reversible. Scotomas, peripheral neuritis, apnea, and encephalopathy are also reported. Toxic renal effects are manifested by proteinuria and reduced volume of urine flow.

   c. **Irritative effects.** Pain at the site of injection; sterile abscesses.

J. **Kanamycin** is effective against *E. coli, Enterobacter, Klebsiella, Salmonella, Shigella, Neisseria,* and *S. aureus.* Most strains of *Proteus, Pseudomonas,* and anaerobes are resistant.

1. **Mechanism of action.** Causes incorrect transcription of messenger RNA within bacteria.

2. **Absorption.** Poorly absorbed PO. IM injection produces peak levels in 1 hr.

3. **Distribution.** Diffuses into most body fluids in significant concentrations. CSF penetration is poor.

4. **Excretion.** From 50–80% is recovered in the urine.

5. **Preparation.** Kanamycin sulfate (Kantrex) is available in vials of 250 and 500 mg and as 0.5 gm oral capsules. The IM or IV dosage in adults with normal renal function is 15 mg/kg/24 hr in two divided doses.

6. **Side effects**

  a. **Hypersensitivity effects** include eosinophilia, fever, rashes, and pruritus.

  b. **Toxic effects.** Ototoxicity (damage to both the cochlear and vestibular parts) and nephrotoxicity (hematuria, proteinuria, and cylindruria) are the most important effects. Nephrotoxicity is reversible on cessation of treatment. Kanamycin has a curarelike action on neuromuscular transmission; paralysis of respiration has been reported following intraperitoneal instillation of the drug.

  c. **Irritative effects** include GI distress, stomatitis, and proctitis.

K. **Amikacin** is a semisynthetic aminoglycoside derived from kanamycin. It is effective against a wide range of gram-negative organisms, including *Pseudomonas*, *E. coli*, *Proteus*, *Providencia*, and the *Klebsiella-Enterobacter-Serratia* group. Amikacin is the drug of choice in strains of *Pseudomonas* that are resistant to gentamicin and tobramycin.

  1. **Mechanism of action.** Interferes with protein synthesis.

  2. **Absorption.** Poorly absorbed PO. An IM injection produces peak serum levels in 1 hr, with significant serum levels persisting for 8–10 hr.

  3. **Distribution.** CNS penetration may reach 40–50% of the serum concentration when the meninges are inflamed. Otherwise, it diffuses well into other tissues.

  4. **Excretion** is primarily through renal mechanisms.

  5. **Preparations.** Amikacin sulfate (Amikin) is available in 2-ml vials of 100 mg and 500 mg and in a 4-ml vial of 1 gm. The recommended IM and IV dosage in adults with normal renal function is 15 mg/kg/day in two or three equally divided doses. Serum antibiotic assays should be employed in monitoring the seriously ill patient.

  6. **Side effects** include ototoxicity, nephrotoxicity, and neurotoxicity (described in **J.6.b**).

L. **Gentamicin** is an aminoglycoside with good activity against *Pseudomonas*, indole-positive *Proteus, Enterobacter, Klebsiella, E. coli, Serratia*, and *Staphylococcus*. It is the preferred treatment for *Pseudomonas* infections and severe or resistant gram-negative infections acquired in the hospital. However, *Pseudomonas*-resistant strains are reported, but infrequently.

  1. **Mechanism of action.** Interferes with protein synthesis.

  2. **Absorption.** Poorly absorbed PO. An IM injection gives peak levels in 30–60 min, which persist for 8–12 hr.

  3. **Excretion** is mainly by glomerular filtration.

  4. **Preparation.** Gentamicin is available in single-use vials (40 mg/ml) or in multiple-dose vials. Approved for IM and IV use. The initial dose in serious infections is 5 mg/kg/24 hr in three divided doses; thereafter, 1–3 mg/kg/24 hr in three divided doses. In renal insufficiency the same initial 24-hr dose is used, but subsequent dosage is reduced (see Chap. 11). Serum antibiotic assays should be employed in monitoring the seriously ill patient.

  5. **Toxic effects** occur primarily in the renal systems and the eighth nerve (usually vestibular). The renal deficits are usually reversible; auditory losses are usually permanent. The toxicity of gentamicin is similar to that of other aminoglycosides, and the effects are additive.

M. **Tobramycin** is an aminoglycoside with good activity against *Pseudomonas, Proteus, Klebsiella, Enterobacter, Serratia, Providencia*, and *E. coli*. Strains of *Pseudomonas* resistant to gentamicin are frequently also resistant to tobramycin.

1. **Mechanism of action.** Inhibits the synthesis of protein.

2. **Absorption.** Poorly absorbed PO. Peak serum levels occur 30–90 min after IM administration and last for about 8 hr.

3. **Distribution.** Low penetration into bile and CSF. Diffuses well into tissues.

4. **Excretion.** Eliminated almost exclusively by glomerular filtration.

5. **Preparations.** Tobramycin sulfate (Nebcin) is available in 2-ml ampules of 20 mg and 80 mg and in disposable syringes with 60 and 80 mg. The recommended IM or IV dosage in adults with normal renal function is 3 mg/kg/day in three equally divided doses. Serum antibiotic assays should be used in monitoring the seriously ill patient.

6. **Side effects.** Nephrotoxicity and eighth nerve toxicity (similar to gentamicin).

N. The **polymyxins** are bactericidal against gram-negative bacteria, including many strains of *Pseudomonas*. *Proteus* species are usually resistant.

1. **Mechanism of action.** Interferes with lipoprotein in cell membranes, causing permeability changes in bacterial cell wall.

2. **Absorption.** Not absorbed PO. After parenteral administration, peak levels are reached in 1–2 hr.

3. **Distribution.** CSF penetration is poor, even in the presence of meningitis.

4. **Excretion** is via the kidney, although excretion is delayed.

5. **Preparations.** Polymyxin B (Aerosporin) is available in vials of 20 and 50 mg for parenteral injection; the usual adult dose is 2.5 mg/kg/24 hr in four divided doses. Colistin (Coly-Mycin) (polymyxin E) is marketed for IM use in vials of 150 mg. The average adult dose is 5 mg/kg/24 hr in three divided doses. The dose of either drug should be reduced in the presence of renal insufficiency.

6. **Reactions to the polymyxins**

   a. **Hypersensitivity effects** include drug fever, skin rashes, pruritus, dizziness, and transient paresthesias.

   b. **Toxic effects** include severe ataxia, leukopenia, and granulocytopenia. A curarelike effect leading to respiratory arrest has been found with colistin.

   c. **Irritative effects** include GI disturbances and pain at injection sites.

O. **Metronidazole,** a synthetic antibacterial compound, is active in vitro against most obligate anaerobes including *Bacteroides fragilis*. It does not appear to possess any clinical relevant activity against facultative anaerobes or obligate aerobes.

1. **Mechanism of action.** Intracellular alteration and activation of metronidazole occurs with the elaboration of bactericidal metabolites which destroy both duriding and nonduriding cells.

2. **Absorption.** Excellent absorption following PO dose. Disposition of metronidazole in the body for both PO and IV dosage forms, with an average elimination half-life in healthy humans of eight hours.

3. **Distribution.** Good CNS penetration as well as other areas including saliva and breast milk.

4. **Excretion.** Primarily (60–90%) renal mechanisms.

5. **Preparations.** Metronidazole hydrochloride (Flagyl) is the IV preparation used in anaerobic bacterial infections. Each single-dose vial contains 500 mg metronidazole and 415 mg mannitol. The usual dosage regimen of 15 mg/hg loading dose followed six hours later by 7.5 mg/hg and repeated every six hours at the same dosage. Oral metronidazole is available for the treatment of trichomonisis or amebiasis in addition to anaerobic infections.

Table 14-1. Prophylactic Antibiotics

Procedure	Organism Usually Causing Infection	Recommended Drug	Adult Dose Beginning 1 Hour before Surgery
Clean surgery with prosthesis			
Heart valve	*Staphylococcus aureus*	Cephalosporin[a]	1 gm q4h IV
Hip replacement	*Staphylococcus epidermidis*		
Vascular graft	Streptococci		
Clean contaminated surgery			
Biliary tract	Enteric gram-negative bacilli	Cephalosporin[b]	1 gm q4h IV
Gastroduodenum	Enteric gram-negative bacilli	Cephalosporin[b]	1 gm q4h IV
	Streptococci		
	Oral anaerobes		
Colonic resection	Enteric gram-negative bacilli	Oral neomycin plus erythromycin base with or without a parenteral cephalosporin[c]	See schedule in text
	Bacteroides fragilis		1 gm q4h IV
Vaginal hysterectomy	Enteric gram-negative bacilli	Gentamicin	1.5 mg/kg q8h IM
	Bacteroides fragilis	plus clindamycin,	600 mg q6h IV
		or a cephalosporin[c]	1 gm q4h IV

[a]First-generation agents preferred.
[b]Cefamandole or cefoxitin preferred because of better coverage against enteric gram-negative bacilli.
[c]Cefoxitin preferred because of better coverage against *B. fragilis.*

6. **Toxic effects** include convulsive seizures and peripheral neuropathy which are reversible. Oral administration of metronidazole in rodents has shown mutagenic and carcinogenic activity.

V. Prophylactic use of antibiotics

A. Parenteral preoperative antibiotics

1. Much controversy exists concerning the use and value of prophylactic parenteral antibiotics. There appears to be no value in their use in clean operative procedures such as hernia repair or thyroidectomy. The use of antibiotic prophylaxis in the patient who undergoes a clean surgical procedure in the presence of **decreased host resistance** (e.g., metabolic derangements, agammaglobulinemia, corticosteroid or immunosuppressive therapy) is generally not indicated. This view is based on the failure of commonly utilized prophylactic antibiotics to cover the relatively rare and dissimilar organisms that cause infections in this clinical setting. In **clean-contaminated and contaminated wounds**, antibiotics appear to be of value if appropriate agents are started early and continued only for short periods of time (1–2 days).

2. Experimental and clinical studies have shown that if antibiotics are to prevent formation of a primary infection, they must be given within 3 hr of tissue contamination. Practically speaking, this means that antibiotics should be started during the immediate preoperative period in patients in whom bacterial contamination is highly likely or known to be present. This will provide tissue levels of the antibiotic at the time the bacterial invasion occurs.

3. The choice of antibiotics depends on a knowledge of the nature of the offending microflora and on the expected antibiotic sensitivities of these microorganisms. When the GI tract is the source of the bacterial contamination, antibiotics that suppress both the aerobic coliforms and anaerobic *Bacteroides* should be given. When the operating room environment and the patient's skin are the source of contamination, as in most cardiovascular and orthopedic patients, antibiotics active against aerobic streptococci and staphylococci should be employed.

4. The **prophylactic use of antibiotics appears to be indicated** in the following types of operative procedures (recommended drugs are listed in Table 14-1):

   a. **Gastroduodenal operations** done in the presence of compromised normal bacterial inhibitory factors (secretion of gastric acid, normal gastric motility). These cases include bleeding or obstructing duodenal ulcer, gastric ulcer, and gastric malignancy.

   b. Orthopedic procedures involving **fixation of open fractures** or **implantation of large foreign bodies,** such as total hip replacement.

   c. Operative procedures (including dental work) done on **patients with valvular heart disease or indwelling cardiac prosthetic valves.** Procedures done with **extracorporeal heart-lung bypass.**

   d. Peripheral vascular procedures that include the use of **prosthetic grafts.**

   e. Repair of **soft tissue traumatic injuries** when there has been a delay in surgical debridement or when tissue of questionable viability has been left behind.

   f. **Cholecystectomy** for chronic calculus cholecystitis done in a patient at increased risk (age > 70, jaundice, fever, acute symptoms, previous biliary tract operation) or in patients in whom bacteria are seen on a Gram stain of bile done during the operation.

   g. **Vaginal hysterectomy** in premenopausal women.

B. Patients in whom **antibiotics are indicated as therapy** include all patients who have intra-abdominal sepsis, whether following penetrating abdominal trauma or disease states in which organ inflammation or perforation has occurred. The drugs used should be effective against the predominant members of the endogenous microflora of the diseased organ. Therapeutic antibiotics are generally continued for a 5- to 7-day period or as long as the clinical course dictates.

C. Preoperative bowel preparation

1. **Nonintestinal operations.** If a patient is to have a general anesthetic, the colon should be evacuated the night before the operation. An empty colon may be an aid in exposure, but the principal reason for emptying the colon is to avert uncontrolled defecation with its hazard of contamination. Colonic evacuation is promoted by enemas in patients who cannot defecate spontaneously.

2. **Small-bowel operations.** As the small-bowel content is liquid and transit time is rapid, preparation usually is unnecessary. Restricting alimentation 8–12 hr prior to operation usually will suffice. Preoperative antibiotic preparation should be employed when distal ileal operations are planned because of the resident bacterial microflora present at this level of the intestine.

3. **Colon operations**

   a. The **objectives** of preparation of the large bowel are removal of the feces from the bowel lumen and reduction of the bacterial population.

   b. **Methods** used to accomplish preparation of the colon are (1) reduction in residue content of the diet, (2) chemical and mechanical stimulation and evacuation of the bowel, and (3) administration of antibiotics.

   c. **Mechanical cleaning of the colon is the most important single element in preparation.** It will remove all gross feces and reduce aerobic coliforms.

   d. **Antibiotic bowel preparation is ineffective if mechanical cleaning has not been accomplished.**

   e. **Stimulant cathartics** act by increasing peristalsis, either by irritating the mucosa or by acting on the autonomic intramural plexuses in the bowel wall. Bisacodyl (Dulcolax) or dioctyl calcium sulfosuccinate (Surfak) is preferred. Do not use castor oil; it is unnecessarily unpleasant.

   f. **Saline cathartics** are slowly absorbed salts that act osmotically to increase the volume of bowel content and stimulate peristalsis. Because they bring fluid into the bowel lumen, saline cathartics help keep feces in a more fluid state, thereby promoting evacuation. In this group of agents, magnesium sulfate is the agent of choice.

   g. Nonabsorbable sulfonamides require several days to accomplish a maximal reduction in colonic bacterial flora. During this period, overgrowth of yeasts and other organisms causes diarrhea, which is undesirable. Therefore, sulfonamides are not used in antibiotic preparation of the colon.

   h. Neomycin and kanamycin are effective within 18 hr in reducing the aerobic colonic microflora. Both agents afford only irregular suppression of the fecal anaerobes, including *Bacteroides*, the most numerous fecal bacteria.

   i. **Neomycin in combination with erythromycin base** has been found to suppress the entire colonic microflora adequately and is the combination of choice for bowel preparation. Erythromycin base with a pH-dependent coating is used because this form of the drug is protected from gastric acidity and is released in the intestinal lumen as an active drug. It does not have to be biochemically altered, or absorbed and biochemically altered, for activity. The activity of erythromycin against the anaerobes in the intestinal lumen is probably dependent on the local neutral-to-alkaline pH. The following is recommended for **colon preparation:**

   Day 1: Low-residue diet. Bisacodyl, 1 capsule at 6 P.M.

   Day 2: Continue low-residue diet. Magnesium sulfate, 30 ml of 50% solution (15 gm) at 10 A.M., 2 P.M., and 6 P.M. Saline enemas until the return is clear during the early evening.

   Day 3: Clear liquid diet. Neomycin, 1 gm, and erythromycin base, 1 gm,

PO at 1 P.M., 2 P.M., and 11 P.M. Magnesium sulfate, 30 ml of 50% solution at 10 A.M. and 2 P.M. No enemas. IV maintenance fluids started if clinically indicated.

Day 4: Operation at 8 A.M.

j. Complications

(1) Dehydration can be prevented by maintaining PO or IV fluid intake at 3000 ml/day during the mechanical and antibiotic preparation of the colon.

(2) Enterocolitis resulting from overgrowth of yeasts or resistant staphylococci is now uncommon because of the short duration of oral antibiotic intake (20 hr). The first clue is passage of a small diarrheal stool through the anus or colostomy early in the postoperative period. Gram-stain a smear of the first postoperative stool; if predominant gram-positive cocci are seen, start treatment. Staphylococcal overgrowth requires a systemic antibiotic such as dimethoxyphenyl penicillin (methicillin), 1 gm q4h IM or IV. In addition, give vancomycin, 2 gm stat, then 1 gm q6h PO, which will be effective against staphylococci within the bowel. If the overgrowth is of yeasts, resumption of oral intake is the best measure; repopulation of the bowel with *Lactobacillus acidophilus* (Bacid or Lactinex, 2 capsules bid) may be of limited help.

D. Prevention of bacterial endocarditis in patients with valvular disease or prosthetic heart valves.

1. Dental and upper respiratory procedures Aqueous penicillin G, 1–2 million units IM or IV, plus procaine penicillin, 600,000 units IM, 30–60 min before the procedure. Follow with penicillin V, 500 mg PO q6h for four to eight doses. In penicillin-allergic patients, vancomycin, 1 gm IV infused over 30 min, beginning 1 hr before the procedure; follow with erythromycin, 500 mg PO q6h for four to eight doses.

2. Gastrointestinal and genitourinary procedures Aqueous penicillin G, 2 million units IM or IV (or ampicillin, 1–2 gm IM or IV), plus gentamicin, 1.5 mg/kg IM, 30–60 min before the procedure. Repeat both drugs q8h for two more doses. In penicillin-allergic patients, give vancomycin, 1 gm IV infused over 30 min, plus gentamicin, 1.5 mg/kg IM, starting 1 hr before the procedure and repeated q8h for two postprocedure doses.

Suggested Reading

Fullen, W. D., Hunt, J., and Altemeier, W. A. Prophylactic antibiotics in penetrating wounds of the abdomen. *J. Trauma* 12:282, 1972.

Kaplan, E. L., Anthony, B. F., Bisno, A., Durack, D., Houser, H., Millard, H. D., Sanford, J., Shulman, S. T., Stillerman, M., Taranta, A., and Wenger, N. Prevention of bacterial endocarditis. *Circulation* 56:139A, 1977.

Nichols, R. L., Broido, P., Condon, R. E., Gorbach, S. L., and Nyhus, L. M. Effect of preoperative neomycin-erythromycin intestinal preparation on the incidence of infectious complications following colon surgery. *Ann Surg.* 178:453, 1973.

VI. Wound and soft tissue infections

A. Prevention

1. All wounds including those made at the operating table as well as those resulting from trauma, provide a perfect environment for bacterial growth.

2. Infections can be minimized if wound management follows these principles:

a. Minimize contamination by use of aseptic techniques.

b. Remove all debris, devitalized tissue, and foreign bodies.

c. Achieve complete hemostasis.

   d. Preserve the blood supply.

   e. Handle tissue gently to keep operative trauma at a minimum.

   f. Avoid and eliminate dead space during closure.

   g. Close the wound with careful layer-to-layer approximation without tension.

   h. Keep operative time at a minimum to reduce the numbers of bacteria in the wound.

   i. Lavage the wound with liberal amounts of sterile saline before closure of the skin and subcutaneous tissue.

3. Do not depend on antibiotics to make up for errors or carelessness in wound management.

B. Therapy of established infections

1. Treatment measures available

   a. Local moist heat relieves pain and increases blood and lymph flow. Heat is best applied by intermittent moist compresses; this hastens localization whereas prolonged heat encourages edema and satellite infection.

   b. Incision and drainage are indicated whenever infection is localized or occurs in a closed space or viscus. Fluctuance signals the appropriate time for drainage of most superficial abscesses. When in doubt, needle aspiration may be diagnostic, especially in deeper infections. The incision must be large and must be in the most dependent area of the wound. Superficial wound abscesses should be packed lightly with gauze after drainage, while deeper abscesses are kept open by the use of rubber drains or sump tubes.

   c. Systemic antibiotics usually are not indicated for uncomplicated wound abscesses. Incision and drainage are the essential treatment.

   d. Appropriate parenteral antibiotics are required, in addition to incision and drainage, when there is evidence of **septicemia** (systemic toxicity, high fever) or **progression of infection** despite adequate drainage. Systemic antibiotics also are indicated in conjunction with surgical drainage in all cases of intra-abdominal abscess. Choose antibiotics initially on the basis of the Gram stain and clinical information.

   Purulent material from the deepest aspect of the wound should be sent for aerobic and anaerobic culture and sensitivity studies. Generally speaking *E. coli* (aerobe) and *B. fragilis* (anaerobe) are the usual causes of wound sepsis following GI or gynecological surgery, while *Staphylococcus* and *Pseudomonas* are the usual causative organisms when intra-abdominal viscera have not been resected or opened. The organisms causing surgical infections, as well as the antibiotics that prove most effective, are listed in Table 14-2.

2. General guidelines for the management of soft tissue infections

   a. Unlocalized infections. No pus under pressure (cellulitis, lymphangitis) Treat with antibiotics, local heat, rest, and elevation. Surgical incision and drainage are not indicated.

   b. Unlocalized early infection in closed space. Pus under pressure (tendon sheath, fascial space, hollow viscus infections). Treat with antibiotics; incise and drain. Follow with rest, elevation, and local heat.

   c. Localized acute infection (abscess). Incise and drain; give antibiotics only if the patient has systemic symptoms or there are local signs of progression of the bacterial invasion.

C. Special types of surgical infections

1. Necrotizing fasciitis is a serious infection caused by hemolytic streptococci or staphylococci. It involves the epifascial tissues of an operative wound, laceration, abrasion, or puncture. It may be fulminant or remain dormant 6 or more

days before beginning its rapid spread. Subcutaneous and fascial necrosis accompanies extensive undermining of the skin and results in gangrene. Treatment is excision of the entire area of fascial involvement, administration of large doses of penicillin (12–20 million units/day), and appropriate systemic support.

2. **Chronic progressive bacterial synergistic gangrene** (Meleney's synergistic gangrene) is caused by the synergistic action of microaerophilic nonhemolytic streptococci and aerobic hemolytic staphylococci. The incubation period is 7–14 days. Cellulitis is followed by gangrenous ulceration that is progressive unless treated. Radical excision of the ulcerated lesion and its gangrenous borders is imperative, along with large systemic doses of penicillin.

3. **Human bite wounds** are contaminated with a combination of aerobic nonhemolytic streptococci, anaerobic streptococci, *B. melaninogenicus,* spirochetes, and staphylococci. The original wound must be treated by debridement, thorough cleaning with irrigation, and immobilization; systemic antibiotics, usually penicillin, must be used. When infection has become established, radical debridement of the infected area is imperative and must be accompanied by antibiotic therapy.

4. **Nonclostridial gangrenous cellulitis** caused by *B. melaninogenicus* and anaerobic streptococci is typified by a progressive gangrenous infection of the skin and areolar and fascial tissues. Prompt incision and drainage and large doses of penicillin are necessary. Supportive treatment is imperative, since toxemia with dehydration, fever, and prostration rapidly develops.

5. **Clostridial cellulitis** is a serosanguineous, crepitant, septic process of subcutaneous, retroperitoneal, or other areolar tissue caused principally by *C. perfringens* (also known as *C. welchii*). It differs from gas gangrene in that the infection does not involve muscle. The infection spreads rapidly via fascial planes. Extensive gangrene results from vascular thrombosis. Systemic effects are moderate if the infection is treated promptly. Early surgical debridement and penicillin therapy are necessary.

6. **Clostridial myonecrosis (gas gangrene)** is an anaerobic infection of muscle characterized by profound toxemia, extensive local edema, massive necrosis of tissue, and a variable degree of gas production. The causative organisms are the clostridia, which abound in soil, dust, and the alimentary tract of most animals and which usually are saprophytic. *C. perfringens* is the most common organism causing gas gangrene. All clostridia owe their pathogenicity to soluble exotoxins that destroy tissue and blood cells. Clostridia enter a wound, multiply in the presence of devitalized muscle, and elaborate necrotizing exotoxins. Disruption and fragmentation of normal nontraumatized muscle cells and capillaries result in massive necrosis, hemorrhage, and edema. There is no fibrin formation or polymorphonuclear leukocytic reaction. The affected muscles are first red and friable but progress to a purplish black, stringy, pulpy mass. The presence of gas is variable. The affected area swells and discharges a brownish, malodorous fluid. The overlying skin initially shows blotchy ecchymoses (marbling), then blackens, and finally sloughs. The diagnosis of gas gangrene is based on typical clinical findings as well as on the presence of large gram-positive rods on stain of the wound fluid. Delays in diagnosis, even for just a few hours, will greatly increase the mortality.

   Treatment of gas gangrene. Immediate removal of involved muscle groups is necessary. Amputation is employed if the remaining muscles are insufficient for useful function. High doses of IV penicillin and whole blood are given preoperatively and postoperatively. Multiple treatments with hyperbaric oxygen (oxygen at three times atmospheric pressure) may reduce the amount of debridement necessary and lower the mortality. Untreated gas gangrene is fatal in all cases. The fatality rate in treated patients ranges from 25–40%.

7. **Tetanus** is caused by a spore-forming obligate anaerobe, *Clostridium tetani,* occurring in the feces of humans and animals and capable of long survival in

Table 14-2. Antibiotic Treatment of Common Organisms Causing Wound or Intra-abdominal Infections

Organism	Drug(s) of Choice	Daily Dose and Route (Adult)	Alternative Drugs
AEROBES			
Enterobacter	Gentamicin[a-c] *or* Tobramycin[a-c] *or* Amikacin[a-c]	240–300 mg IM or IV 240–300 mg IM or IV 900–1100 mg IM or IV	Cefamandole
Escherichia coli	As for *Enterobacter*	As for *Enterobacter*	Cefamandole or cefoxitin
Klebsiella	As for *Enterobacter*	As for *Enterobacter*	Cefamandole or cefoxitin
Proteus mirabilis	Ampicillin	2–4 gm IV or IM	First-generation cephalosporin
Proteus, indole-positive	As for *Enterobacter*	As for *Enterobacter*	. . .[e]
Pseudomonas[d]	As for *Enterobacter*	As for *Enterobacter*	. . .[e]
Serratia	Gentamicin[e]	240–300 mg IM or IV	Tobramycin,[e] amikacin,[e] or cefoxitin[e]
Staphylococcus aureus	Oxacillin *or* Methicillin[f]	4 gm PO 4 gm IM or IV	First-generation cephalosporin
Staphylococcus epidermidis	First-generation cephalosporin	4–6 gm IM or IV	. . .[e]

Streptococcus			
Group A	Penicillin	2.4 million units IM or IV	Erythromycin or first-generation cephalosporin
Group D (*S. faecalis*)	Ampicillin *and* Gentamicin[a-c]	2–4 gm IM or IV 240–300 mg IM or IV	...
ANAEROBES			
Bacteroides, oral strains	Penicillin	6.0 million units IM or IV	First-generation cephalosporin carbenicillin, ticarcillin, clindamycin, or metronidazole
Bacteroides fragilis	Clindamycin	2400 mg IV	Carbenicillin, chloramphenicol, cefoxitin, ticarcillin, or metronidazole
Clostridium	Penicillin	20 million units IV	Tetracycline, chloramphenicol
Peptostreptococcus	Penicillin	6.0 million units IM or IV	First-generation cephalosporin or clindamycin
Actinomyces	Penicillin	20 million units IM or IV	...

[a] Usually divided into three equal doses administered q8h.
[b] Dose is usually calculated according to body weight.
[c] Monitor dose with serum antibiotic level, and modify dose in renal insufficiency
[d] Drug of choice in resistant strains is amikacin.
[e] Choose drug according to sensitivity tests.
[f] Methicillin-resistant strains should be treated with vancomycin.

soil. Two **exotoxins** are produced: tetanospasmin, a neurotoxin, and tetanolysin, a hemolysin. The optimal culture medium for germination of tetanus spores is provided by dead muscle and clotted blood. Traumatic injuries with compound fractures and devitalization of muscle are very susceptible to tetanus infection. Equally vulnerable are small puncture wounds harboring a clot deep in the tissues.

a. Locally produced tetanolysin contributes to optimal growth conditions through its lecithinase, gelatinase, esterase, and lipase activity. Tetanospasmin, the neurotoxin responsible for the clinical features of the disease, does not act peripherally or locally but is carried to the CNS and acts centrally. In order to neutralize blood-borne toxin, antitoxin must be present before tetanospasmin becomes fixed by nerve cells. Hence, antitoxin therapy given at the time symptoms are apparent only limits further intoxication of nerve cells and cannot reverse developing symptoms.

b. There is considerable variability in progression of the disease from onset. There may be a prodromal period of headache, stiff jaw muscles, restlessness, yawning, and wound pain beginning 6–15 days after a traumatic wound. The active stage follows in 12–24 hr, with trismus, facial distortion, opisthotonos, pain, clonic spasms, and seizures. Acute asphyxia is a major hazard and may result from either spasm of the respiratory muscles or aspiration. The shorter the incubation period, the poorer the prognosis.

c. Treatment of established tetanus is as follows:

(1) Give tetanus human immune globulin (Hyper-Tet), 3000 units IM, immediately to neutralize circulating toxins. An additional 1000 units can be injected into and immediately proximal to the wound. Widely debride and drain the contaminated wound at least 1 hr after administration of immune globulin. Then give 500 units immune globulin IM daily. If symptoms persist longer than 2 wk, repeat administration of the large initial doses of the immune globulin.

(2) Establish and maintain an airway; use respirator support and oxygen as needed. Tracheostomy will be needed in every patient with more than prodromal symptoms and should be done before the situation becomes urgent.

(3) Control muscle spasms with IM meprobamate or chlorpromazine. If spasms persist, curare should be given.

(4) Maintain sedation with IM barbiturate. Place the patient in a quiet, dark room and keep environmental stimulation at a minimum to avoid triggering seizures. Control convulsions with IV thiopental (Pentothal).

(5) Give penicillin in high doses.

(6) Maintain nutrition parenterally or feed via a gastrostomy.

(7) Sphincter spasm will prevent voluntary urination; drain the bladder via an indwelling catheter to a closed system.

(8) Actively immunize with tetanus toxoid after the patient has recovered. With appropriate early care, 75% of patients survive. There is no neurological residual in patients who survive.

d. Tetanus prophylaxis principles are:

(1) Tetanus is absolutely preventable by prior active immunization. Effective active immunization (not associated with a fresh wound) is accomplished by injection of alum-precipitated toxoid, 0.5 ml; repeat this dose at 1 and 6 mo.

(2) Immediate meticulous surgical care of the fresh wound is of prime importance. Removal of devitalized tissue, blood clots, and foreign bodies obliteration of dead space, and prevention of tissue ischemia in the wound are the objectives of initial treatment. Wounds that are seen late or that are grossly contaminated may be left unsutured after debridement, protected by a sterile dressing for 3–5 days, and then closed by delayed primary suture if the tissues appear clean and healthy.

(3) Patients previously immunized (including reinforcing doses) within the past 10 yr should be given 0.5 ml fluid tetanus toxoid booster.

(4) Patients immunized more than 10 years previously should be treated as follows:

(a) Uncontaminated wound: 0.5 ml fluid tetanus toxoid.

(b) Grossly contaminated wound: 0.5 ml fluid tetanus toxoid and 250 units tetanus human immune globulin; start penicillin therapy.

(5) Patients not previously immunized should be treated as follows:

(a) Clean minor wounds: Immunize with alum-precipitated tetanus toxoid; give 0.5 ml alum-precipitated toxoid at once, and repeat at 1, 2, and 6 mo.

(b) Contaminated wound: Start active immunization with 0.5 ml alum-precipitated toxoid, and repeat at 1, 2, and 6 mo in addition to passive immunization with 250 units human immune globulin; start penicillin therapy.

VII. Septicemia is a severe form of infection characterized by invasion and multiplication in the bloodstream of large numbers of bacteria. Fever usually is high, spiking, and accompanied by chills. Tachycardia accompanies or precedes fever and is proportional to it. Leukocyte counts may not show much abnormality in sepsis; the differential count is more reliable. Nearly always there is a shift to the left. Petechial-like lesions may be seen in the skin or conjunctivas in septicemia caused by streptococci, meningococci, or *Pseudomonas*. Anemia secondary to hemolysis may appear rapidly in septicemia due to staphylococci, *Pseudomonas*, *E. coli*, and *Clostridium*. Shock is frequent in gram-negative septicemia but occurs less often with gram-positive sepsis. Metastatic abscesses, especially involving bone, brain, or spleen, are not unusual after septicemia. Any injured tissue is easily infected during septicemia. Diagnosis is aided by a high index of suspicion.

A. The **cause of septicemia** is an infection somewhere in the body that is seeding the bloodstream. The type of bacteria causing sepsis usually can be identified from the source of the infection:

1. Wound or intra-abdominal infection: coliforms, *Bacteroides*, or *Staphylococcus*.

2. Burns: *Pseudomonas, Serratia,* or *Staphylococcus*.

3. IV site: *Serratia, Klebsiella, Bacteroides,* or *Staphylococcus*.

4. Lung: pneumococcus, *Streptococcus, Staphylococcus, Klebsiella,* or *Pseudomonas*.

5. Urinary tract: usually, *E. coli* or *Proteus*.

6. CNS: pneumococcus or meningococcus.

B. Management of septicemia

1. Establish an etiological diagnosis

a. Septicemia rarely develops early in the postoperative period unless the operation was in or through infected tissues or the patient had a preexisting infection.

b. Examine the patient for clues to the source of infection. Is there pain or redness in the surgical wound or at an IV infusion site? Does the patient have purulent sputum, cough, pleuritic pain, rales, or dullness? Is there diarrhea? Is there dysuria or flank pain? Are there pain in the shoulder and an immobile diaphragm, suggesting a subphrenic abscess? Is there a pelvic or prostatic mass on rectal examination? Is there headache or nuchal rigidity?

  c. Carry out appropriate laboratory studies: blood count; urinalysis; Gram stain of any discharge or of sputum or urine; chest x-ray; and fluoroscopy for diaphragm motion.

2. Take appropriate cultures: blood (50 ml from single or multiple sites), urine, sputum, wound or other drainage, stool if diarrhea is present, and CSF if there is headache or nuchal rigidity. **Always obtain cultures prior to starting antibiotics.**

3. Antibiotics should be started immediately after the physical examination has been completed and cultures have been taken. Antibiotics are given in high doses by the IV route and, when possible, should be bactericidal in action and as specific as possible. The choice of antibiotic is based on the probable source of infection, the most likely bacteria found in that area, and information gained from Gram stains of material obtained from the infected area (see Table 14-1). If the infection is not responding readily to the agents being used, the antibiotics should be changed in accordance with the results of cultures and sensitivity studies when these become available.

4. Drainage. When a collection of pus is sealed off, forming an abscess, it is difficult for antibiotics to penetrate the area. An abscess should be drained as soon as its presence and location are determined and the patient's overall condition permits. Drainage is done only after large doses of antibiotics have been given.

VIII. Treatment of antibiotic-induced colitis

A. General comments

1. Many commonly employed antibiotic agents can cause diarrhea and subsequent pseudomembranous colitis.

2. These agents include ampicillin, cephalosporins, lincomycin, clindamycin, and the tetracyclines.

3. Studies have shown that most cases of antibiotic-induced colitis occur due to an overgrowth of *Clostridium difficile* within the colonic lumen. This microorganism elaborates exotoxins that, when in contact with the colonic mucosa, cause the characteristic changes.

4. *C. difficile* is extremely resistant to most antibiotics.

B. Treatment of suspected cases

1. When diarrhea occurs in a patient who has received any of the antibiotics mentioned in **A**, the agent should be discontinued.

2. IV fluids and electrolytes should be given to cover the losses from the diarrhea.

3. Avoid the use of narcotic antidiarrheals, which, when used, will intensify the syndrome.

4. Give vancomycin PO, 150 mg q6h, to those patients who do not respond to the preceding measures. Therapy is usually continued 5 days.

IX. Isolation procedures

A. General comments

1. Isolation procedures are a prime source of frustration, wasted time, and wasted facilities in most hospitals.

2. The unnecessary use of strict isolation procedures is harmful, since an unneeded barrier is placed between the patient and the nurses and physicians. The isolation barrier tends to interfere with observation and care of the patient and is damaging to patient morale.

3. Failure to use appropriate isolation procedures also is harmful, since a patient with a communicable infection then may become a threat to all patients and staff in the hospital.

4. Reasonable isolation procedures have as their objective the **interruption of pathways of transmission of communicable infections** either from an infected patient to others or from the environment to a highly susceptible patient.

5. Isolation should be discontinued as soon as the infection hazard is minimal.

6. To isolate a patient, all that is required is a room containing a sink and a closed soap dispenser. **Outside** the room place a table or cart containing gowns, masks, gloves, dressings, and any other materials needed repeatedly. **Inside** the room place a commode for the patient's use if the room has no bathroom, a linen hamper to receive contaminated linen, and plastic bags in which to discard disposable items.

7. Hand washing before and after attending each patient is professionally proper behavior. As a matter of isolation technique, however, thorough hand washing is carried out either on leaving or on entering the isolation room, depending on the objectives being sought by isolation. Hands are washed on leaving in most isolation situations but are washed on entering the room of a patient in protective isolation.

8. It is pointless to isolate patients with minor wound infections caused by common fecal organisms, since these organisms are ubiquitous in the hospital. This does not mean that careless dressing technique is condoned; such wounds must always be covered with an adequate dry dressing.

B. Strict isolation

1. **Indications.** Infections at any site with staphylococci, group A streptococci, meningococci; open cavitary tuberculosis; clostridial myonecrosis; "traditional" communicable infections, such as smallpox and diphtheria, and hepatitis.

2. **Technique**

   a. **Gown.** Put on outside the room on entering, and discard inside the room when leaving.

   b. **Mask.** Put on when entering the room, and discard when leaving.

   c. **Gloves.** Wear if in contact with the patient.

   d. **Hand washing.** On leaving the room.

   e. **Linen, equipment.** Discard when possible; place linen in marked bags and autoclave before routine laundering, or use an inner plastic bag that is soluble in hot water; dressings should be placed in impenetrable bags for incineration; disinfect equipment before removing from the room, or remove wrapped for autoclaving.

   f. **Terminal cleaning.** Air the room for 2 hr with the windows open and the doors closed. Furniture, floors, and soiled walls then should be washed with a germicidal solution.

C. Wound isolation

1. **Indications.** Grossly infected or copiously draining wounds infected with organisms other than those requiring strict isolation.

2. Technique

a. Gown. Wear if in direct contact with the patient.

b. Mask. Wear if in close contact with the patient.

c. Gloves. Wear if in direct contact with the patient during dressing changes.

d. Hand washing. On leaving the room.

e. Linen, equipment. Discard when possible; place linen in marked bags for routine laundering, contaminated dressings in an impenetrable bag for incineration; disinfect equipment before removing from the room, or remove wrapped for autoclaving.

D. Stool precautions

1. Indications. Patients with enteric infections in which viable organisms are passed in the feces (amebiasis, salmonellosis, shigellosis, and similar infections).

2. Technique

a. Gown. Wear if in direct contact with the patient.

b. Mask. Not necessary.

c. Gloves. Wear if in direct contact with the patient or when handling material contaminated by feces.

d. Hand washing. On leaving the room.

e. Linen, equipment. Discard when possible; place linen in marked bags for routine laundering; disinfect equipment before removing from the room, or remove wrapped for autoclaving.

f. Stools are passed or discarded directly into the sewage system; if the patient uses a bedpan, or if a laboratory stool specimen is removed from the room, wrap and treat the containers as contaminated.

E. Urine precautions

1. Indications. Patients with infections in which viable organisms are passed in the urine (leptospirosis, certain cases of genitourinary tuberculosis).

2. Technique

a. Gown. Wear if in direct contact with the patient.

b. Mask. Not necessary.

c. Gloves. Wear if in direct contact with the patient.

d. Hand washing. On leaving the room.

e. Linen, equipment. No special precautions unless the patient is incontinent.

f. Urine is passed or discarded directly into the sewage system; if the patient uses a bed urinal or bedpan, or if the laboratory urine specimen is removed from the room, wrap and treat the containers as contaminated.

F. Protective (reverse) isolation

1. Indications. Premature and newborn infants, patients with reduced resistance to bacterial infections—acute burns, exfoliative dermatitis, agranulocytosis, and similar acute illnesses.

2. Technique

a. Gown. Put on outside the room on entering, and discard outside the room on leaving.

   b. Mask. Put on when entering the room, discard after leaving.

   c. Gloves. Not necessary.

   d. Hand washing. On entering the room.

   e. Linen, equipment. No special precautions.

G. Infections not requiring isolation

1. Peritonitis or empyema.

2. Wound infections that are not draining copiously.

3. Pneumonia.

4. Tetanus.

5. Animal bites.

6. Food poisoning.

7. Any infection requiring an animal or arthropod vector or intermediate host, if the vector or host can be excluded.

8. Infections limited to the bloodstream, such as subacute bacterial endocarditis or septicemia.

I. **Available blood components,** and indications for their use, are listed in Table 15-1. A brief review of each of these components will emphasize the important therapeutic considerations.

A. **Whole blood, citrate-phosphate-dextrose.** Whole blood, because of reactions and the serum hepatitis risk, should be used only when blood loss exceeds 20–30% of the patient's normal circulating blood volume (1000–1500 ml in average-sized adults). Packed cells, reconstituted with Ringer's lactate or serum albumin, represent a safer material and should always be used in preference to whole blood if availability is not a problem. Lesser hemorrhage is better treated with colloid (serum albumin) or crystalloid (Ringer's lactate, saline) in appropriate amounts. With chronic hemorrhage or hemorrhage lasting more than 24 hr, hemodilution has usually occurred, and other components are more appropriate. When large volumes (more than 5 units) of whole blood are to be infused, central venous pressure (CVP) or pulmonary capillary wedge pressure monitoring is necessary to avoid circulatory overload.

B. **Packed cells, washed cells, frozen cells.** It is important to keep the hematocrit at or above 30% in patients with acute and subacute hemorrhage. If fluid resuscitation is accomplished with asanguineous fluids, the hematocrit should be checked after every 3 liters of fluid infused, so that the red cell mass is kept at a proper level, If the hematocrit falls below 30% (hematocrit is accurate to ±3%), packed or frozen cells should be given. One unit of packed cells will increase the hematocrit 4% if bleeding has stopped. Frozen cells are superior to packed or washed red cells, as they present an extremely low risk of serum hepatitis. Further, frozen cells have been demonstrated to have excellent oxygen-dissociating characteristics, with an oxyhemoglobin dissociation curve identical to that of the cells in the fresh state.

C. **Serum albumin.** Plasma has been replaced by 5% serum albumin in treating patients with fluid sequestration (third-space effect) or moderate degrees of blood loss. A great deal of controversy exists as to the merits of serum albumin (colloid) versus crystalloid; if the patient can tolerate sodium loading (no cardiac, pulmonary, or renal disease), crystalloid may be advantageous. More concentrated albumin solution (25%) is used to replenish the protein pool in patients who cannot generate endogenous protein or who have suffered excessive protein losses. Administration of large volumes of plasma protein fraction has been reported to result in moderate to severe hypotension in a few patients; the precise nature of the vasodepressor (vasodilator) material is not known, but may be bradykinin, prekallikrein activator, or acetate buffer. Similar large volumes of plasma, the source material of serum protein, do not precipitate similar hypotensive episodes, nor does fractionated serum albumin ("salt poor"). Incidentally, concentrations of sodium in serum albumin range from 120 to 160 mEq/liter, which is hardly "salt poor." Compared with equivalent intravascular volumes of crystalloid, at 390–500 mEq/three liters, the amount of sodium infused is certainly less.

D. **Plasma (single unit).** Prolonged IV hyperalimentation requires the addition of trace elements not readily obtainable in IV preparations (e.g., cobalt, copper,

Table 15-1. Available Blood Components

Component	Major Therapeutic Effect	Indications
Whole blood, CPD	Volume, RBC mass	Acute, severe hemorrhage (no packed cells available)

Packed RBCs
  Washed RBCs
  Frozen RBCs
	RBC mass	Acute hemorrhage
		Chronic anemia,
		acute anemia

Serum albumin, 5%	Plasma volume	Burns, peritonitis, intestinal obstruction, hemorrhage
Serum albumin, 25%	Albumin pool	Nephrotic syndrome, liver failure, hypoproteinemia(?)
Plasma	Plasma volume	Trace elements (see text) (hyperalimentation)
Ultrafresh whole blood	Platelets, factor V, fibrinogen	Thrombocytopenia with hemorrhage; factor V, fibrinogen deficits; DIC
Platelet-rich plasma	Platelets	Thrombocytopenia without hemorrhage
Fresh-frozen plasma	Plasma prothrombin precursors	Massive transfusional therapy, liver disease, von Willebrand's disease
Cryoprecipitate	Factor VIII, fibrinogen	Hemophilia
Factor concentrates (factor IX complexes)	Factors VII, VIII, IX, X	Specific factor deficits

manganese, zinc). The simplest, although not necessarily the safest, way to provide these is to add 250 ml of plasma to the IV fluid schedule once or twice weekly. In the last 2 years, commercial preparations of intravenous zinc chloride and of cobalt have become available. These have largely eliminated the necessity for single-unit plasma administration for the purpose of providing trace elements.

E. Ultrafresh whole blood, platelet-rich. Platelet counts above 75,000/mm^3 allow for normal hemostasis and do not require treatment. If an operation is necessary, and the platelet count is less than 75,000/mm^3, abnormal bleeding during and after operation may occur. If platelet counts are below 30,000/mm^3, spontaneous bleeding can occur at any time. In either event, platelets can be increased by administration of ultrafresh whole blood (if blood volume is low), given within 36 hr of withdrawal from the donor. If blood volume is normal, volumes of ultrafresh whole blood required to raise platelets will cause circulatory overload, but platelet-rich plasma or platelet concentrates are used. If thrombocytopenia is a result of disseminated intravascular coagulation (DIC), platelets should *not* be given until heparin is administered, the cause of DIC is eliminated, or both.

F. Fresh frozen plasma. This component provides all clotting factors, labile and stable, in one preparation: There are no platelets, and the concentration of fibrinogen is low. Previously used to treat hemophilia, fresh frozen plasma is now used in massive whole-blood transfusions, liver disease, von Willebrand's disease, and any state in which prothrombin precursors are required. Fresh-frozen plasma can be used to provide trace elements in lieu of single unit plasma but with a hepatitis risk essentially identical to that of whole blood.

G. Cryoprecipitate. Hemophilia is best treated with cryoprecipitate, which is antihemophilic factor (factor VIII), with some fibrinogen and other clotting factors in lower concentration. Large volumes of cryoprecipitate may be required to control

Table 15-2. Acute Transfusion Reactions

Reaction	Frequency	Components Involved
Allergic reaction	4% of all recipients; 50% of recipients with prior history of atopy	Whole blood, packed cells, occasionally plasma
Febrile (minor) reaction	2% of recipients	Whole blood, occasionally packed cells or plasma
Acute hemolytic reaction	0.03% of recipients	Whole blood, packed cells
Bacteremia (severe febrile reaction)	0.01% (or less) of recipients	Usually whole blood
Circulatory overload	Unknown	Any
Delayed hemolysis	Unknown, probably frequent	Whole blood, packed cells

bleeding in severe hemophilia or to permit elective surgery in the patient with hemophilia. Cryoprecipitate is the safest and most effective form of human fibrinogen currently available since the hepatitis risk from cryoprecipitate is relatively low and the fibrinogen content is satisfactory. It may be required in a large amount to treat patients with known DIC. Only after adequate heparin therapy and/or removal of the cause of DIC should this material be infused. Both cryoprecipitate and fresh-frozen plasma are delivered from the blood bank in a frozen state and should be thawed in a water bath at or below 37°C (98.6°F). If hot water is used, thermolability causes a serious decrease in factor VIII activity. One half of the contents of the unit should be rendered liquid by the thawing process and the unit then hung, allowing the remainder to thaw at room temperature.

H. Fibrinogen. Because of the extraordinary risk of serum hepatitis with lyophilized human fibrinogen it has been withdrawn from the list of components that are available in practice. In the extremely rare instances of congenital hypofibrinogenemia or afibrinogenemia, cryoprecipitate is currently the agent of choice.

I. Specific coagulation factors. In the past few years, antihemophilic factor has become commercially available, as well as have various and sundry mixtures of factors II, VII, VIII, IX, and X. These are provided in a lyophilized state, as a rule, requiring reconstitution with crystalloid. These concentrates are designed to provide large amounts of the component clotting factors in a small volume of fluid. However, the risk of serum hepatitis with their use—since they are produced from large plasma pools—is astronomical. It is frequently safer to administer fresh-frozen plasma rather than to assume the severe hepatitis risk with these concentrates. Even with the administration of hepatitis B immune globulin to modify or prevent serum hepatitis in recipients of these materials, the risks remain prohibitive.

II. Immediate transfusion reactions (Table 15-2). Transfusion should be stopped by clamping the IV tubing at the first sign of any untoward reaction, so that the nature of the transfusion reaction can be determined. In most cases, the transfusion reaction will be found to be minor and will subside spontaneously or with specific treatment. In such cases, administration of the involved unit of blood may be continued, or it may be discarded. Reactions due to bacterial contamination or to incompatible blood make mandatory not only cessation of transfusion of that unit of blood but also investigation of the source of the problem, as well as the immediate treatment outlined in **A** and **B**.

A. Reactions in which blood may be continued

1. **Allergic reactions** have been reported in 4% of recipients of whole blood, packed cells, or, less often, fresh-frozen plasma. Rarely, severe reactions may involve bronchospasm or laryngospasm.

   a. Usual **symptoms** are flushing, chills, fever, and urticaria, with or without subjective complaints of itching. **Itching and hives occur only in allergic reactions, not in other varieties of transfusion reaction.**

   b. The **cause** of allergic transfusion reactions is passive transfer of donor antigen to the sensitive recipient. The antigen generally has been ingested by the donor just prior to donation of the unit of blood.

   c. Allergic reactions may occur in at least 50% of patients with a previous history of atopy, hay fever, or bronchial asthma. Such patients should be transfused with packed, washed plasma-free erythrocytes, if possible. Patients who have been previously transfused and have had allergic or febrile reactions have at least a 65% of chance of having another, similar reaction. Again, washed erythrocytes can significantly diminish the incidence of these reactions and should always be used in patients with a history of previous allergic reactions.

   d. **Allergic reactions do not occur until the patient has received ½ unit of whole blood (250 ml) or ½ unit of packed cells (125 ml).** If chills and fever develop in a patient early in the course of transfusion (less than 50 ml), the reaction is more likely a hemolytic reaction or due to bacterial contamination than an allergic reaction. It is imperative that the volume of blood, packed cells, or plasma already infused be documented at the time of onset of symptoms.

   e. As a rule, it is not desirable to stop the transfusion if a patient has an allergic reaction, unless symptoms fail to respond to treatment. In some instances, symptoms do not develop until after the transfusion has been completed.

   f. In most circumstances, administration of an **antihistaminic,** diphenhydramine (Benadryl), 50 mg, is the treatment for patients who develop symptoms of allergic reaction. Prophylactic administration of an antihistaminic should be reserved for patients with known allergies or those who have had previous transfusion reactions of the allergic type.

2. **Febrile reactions.** In some instances during a transfusion, a patient will experience fever, sometimes accompanied by flushing, headache, or chills. The fever rarely exceeds 39.4°C (103°F); the patient is not toxic and may be unaware of any untoward happening. Febrile reactions usually are caused by leukoagglutinins or platelet agglutinins present in the recipient; less often, they are due to transfusion of antibody. **Transfusion of more than ½ unit of infused blood or cells is required to cause symptoms. Aspirin** may be administered PO or rectally to reduce the fever; diphenhydramine is of some benefit if fever persists longer than 2–3 hr. Febrile reactions are usually preventable by the administration of washed or frozen erythrocytes, since these processes effectively rid the suspending plasma of granulocytes and platelets.

3. **Circulatory overload** is not really a transfusion reaction but is an error in administering an excessive volume of blood or other colloid at a more rapid rate than the circulatory system can tolerate. CVP or pulmonary artery wedge pressure always should be monitored if the patient has a history of heart disease. As with major hemorrhage, it is important to keep CVP below 15 cm H_2O during the course of rapid transfusion (pulmonary artery wedge pressure below 16 mm Hg). If the patient continues to have a volume or red cell deficit, circulatory overload frequently can be handled by reducing the rate of infusion,

administering rapid-acting digitalis IV and, if necessary, giving 60 mg of furosemide IV.

B. Reactions in which blood must be stopped

1. **Severe febrile reactions, bacterial contamination.** Approximately 0.1% of all units of whole blood are contaminated with **cold-growing organisms.** Transfusion of the bacteria and toxins in the blood results in a temperature over 39.4°C (103°F), intense flushing, headache, vomiting, diarrhea, and hypotension. The rapidity of onset and the severity of the reaction vary considerably, but typically, the patient appears acutely ill and frequently will develop shock. The bacteria usually are gram-negative (occasionally gram-positive) facultatively anaerobic, cold-growing organisms.

   a. Contamination of a unit of blood by bacteria can be suspected if the **supernatant plasma is turbid,** has a brownish or brownish purple discoloration, or does not display a sharp line of demarcation at the interface between red cells and plasma following 12–18 hr of refrigeration in an undisturbed state.

   b. **Whenever bacterial contamination is suspected, the transfusion must be stopped;** samples of the donor unit and of the recipient's blood are incubated at incubator temperature, at refrigerator temperature, and at room temperature in both aerobic and anaerobic environments. Septicemia is treated, as in any such instance, with **IV fluids, antibiotics, corticosteroids and transfusion of fresh uncontaminated blood,** if indicated.

2. **Hemolytic transfusion reactions.** Administration of grossly incompatible blood occurs once in 3000 transfusions. In order for this reaction to occur, whole blood or packed cells must be administered; major hemolytic reactions do not occur when plasma, platelet-rich plasma, or similar blood components are given.

   a. The mismatch resulting in these reactions may be a result of faulty bloodbank technique or, equally, the result of an error by the treating physician in failing to identify correctly the patient and the unit of blood. It should be routine practice to match the label on the unit with the patient's wrist identification tag; the name and hospital number on both must be identical.

   b. When a hemolytic reaction occurs, the incompatible donor cells are agglutinated by preexisting antibodies in the recipient's plasma. Much less commonly, donor plasma antibody may react with the cells of the recipient; such plasma incompatibility rarely results in a serious reaction.

   c. A hemolytic transfusion reaction may be characterized as either the **slowly developing type,** with jaundice appearing hours or days after the transfusion, or the much more dramatic but less common **fulminant type,** with immediate appearance of symptoms due to rapid cell agglutination in the recipient. The symptoms of the fulminant reaction are the result of DIC and consist of chills and fever, tachypnea, tachycardia, flank pain, constriction in the chest or back, pain in the extremities, and occipital headache. The patient may vomit. Symptoms progress to oliguria, hemoglobinuria, and jaundice. If the reaction occurs during operation, the patient exhibits sudden unexpected bleeding and severe hypotension leading to shock.

   d. **The signs of a serious hemolytic transfusion reaction always occur during transfusion of the first 100 ml of blood or cells.** The patient always should be under close observation during the early part of a transfusion of whole blood or packed cells. It is helpful to monitor the pulse rate, to observe any wounds or incisions for signs of abnormal bleeding, and to watch both blood pressure and respiration to detect transfusion reaction in the sedated or anesthetized patient.

   e. **If a hemolytic transfusion reaction is suspected, the transfusion must be stopped at once.** Residual donor blood, together with a sample of recipient blood and urine, is sent to the laboratory. Regrouping of the donor and recipient blood, repeat cross matching, and an indirect Coombs' test should reveal any significant incompatibility. It is also necessary to check the recipient's blood sample for irregular antibodies; a cell panel is used for this purpose. Increased free plasma hemoglobin, methemoglobinemia, and hemoglobinuria will help to confirm the diagnosis. Schumm's test for methemoglobin is helpful if the investigation is delayed for more than 6 hr.

   Blood also should be drawn for a platelet count and for measurement of fibrinogen and fibrin split products. If platelets are below 75,000/mm^3, fibrinogen is below 100 mg/100 ml, and fibrin split products are markedly elevated, the patient should receive **IV heparin** immediately. The patients are usually given 20 mg (2000 IU) as an initial bolus, and then 500–800/mg/hr is given by continuous pump infusion. Hypotension also must be treated; if it is the result of hypovolemia, another transfusion of compatible (freshly cross-matched) blood or serum albumin must be administered rapidly. If blood volume is deemed to be normal and hypotension persists, vasopressors may be required. Oxygen administration is useful support. *Fibrinogen and ϵ-amino-caproic acid (EACA) should not be given to a patient with a hemolytic transfusion reaction.*

   Corticosteroids have been advocated, and it is not harmful to administer 100 mg of hydrocortisone IV. Attempt to promote **diuresis** by rapid infusion of 100 ml of 20% mannitol. At the same time, an infusion of 40 mEq of **sodium bicarbonate** is given along with rapid administration of 1000 ml of Ringer's lactate solution. The purpose of the Ringer's lactate infusion and the alkalization of the urine with bicarbonate is to attempt to wash through any free hemoglobin present in the tubules and to reduce the degree of tubular damage. The patient should be observed carefully for development of acute renal failure. Depending on the degree of tubular damage, hemolytic transfusion reactions are followed either by frank renal failure or by a diuretic episode.

3. **Delayed hemolytic reactions** occur from one to several days after transfusion of apparently compatible blood and are characterized by the appearance of jaundice and hemoglobinuria. They are considered to be caused by an anamnestic response to a previous transfusion or pregnancy. The patient is treated as described for immediate hemolytic reactions.

III. Late transfusion reactions

A. **Isosensitization** is not strictly a transfusion reaction but a consequence of the infusion of large numbers of unidentified antigens attached to red cells. When a patient is given a unit of blood or a unit of packed cells, there is a possibility that a factor carried on the red cells will sensitize the recipient whose red cells do not contain such a factor. From 10–21 days is required for antibody to develop to the infused antigen or antigens. Thus, the possibility of an isosensitization reaction is not of consequence until after 2 wk following transfusion. However, if such a patient later were to be given universal donor blood (type O, Rh-negative) or were to become pregnant, the possibility exists that a serious recipient reaction to the newly transfused blood, or even erythroblastosis in the pregnant female, could occur. Unfortunately, there is no way to predict the occurrence of isosensitization, nor can it be prevented. The occurrence of such incidents reemphasizes the need to be circumspect about administering the whole blood or packed cells, using these materials only when they are necessary.

B. **Disease transmission.** Four diseases may be transmitted by blood transfusion: serum hepatitis, brucellosis, malaria, and cytomegalovirus inclusion disease. Syphilis will not be transmitted in bank blood that has been cooled to refrigerator temperature 4–7°C (39–45°F) for 12 hr or longer.

Table 15-3. Incidence of Serum Hepatitis B
Transmission by Type of Blood Component

Component	Hepatitis Risk (%)
Whole blood	0.2–0.7
Packed, washed red cells	<0.1
Frozen red cells	<0.1
Serum albumin	0
Platelet pack	0.1–0.2
Fresh-frozen plasma	0.1–0.2
Cryoprecipitate	0.1–0.2
Fibrinogen	10–20
Factor IX concentrates	10–20

1. **Serum hepatitis.** The incidence of serum hepatitis varies according to the source of donor blood and the number of units transfused, but occurs in 0.1–0.3% of patients receiving blood. If blood is obtained from voluntary or "family" donors, the incidence is lower. If the blood is commercially purchased from "professionals" paid for their donation, the risk is much greater. Testing of bank blood for hepatitis antigen has decreased the frequency of serum hepatitis transmission, although it has not eliminated this possibility. The incidence with packed, washed, or frozen cells is considerably less (Table 15-3).

   a. The mortality of serum hepatitis in a transfusion recipient is 12%, the majority of patients succumbing being under age 5 or over age 65. The incubation period of serum hepatitis is 35–120 days. Some recipients undoubtedly have anicteric hepatitis and only mild or transient hepatic dysfunction. In others, the disease may be extremely severe; it is rare for very elderly patients to survive an attack of serum hepatitis. The use of hyperimmune globulin may modify the disease in susceptible patients but probably does not prevent infection. Within 1 wk of transfusion, 3 ml can be given IM, and a similar dose should be administered 1 and 3 mo later.

   b. Serum hepatitis (hepatitis B) has yielded, under investigation, viruslike particles, called Dane particles. The outer shell of the Dane particles contain an antigen, as do some smaller particles, designated HB_sAg, or hepatitis B surface antigen. The core of the Dane particle contains HB_cAg, or hepatitis B core antigen. Antibodies are known as anti-HB_s and anti-HB_c. HB_sAg is discovered by immunofluorescence during the attack of hepatitis B and disappears when the patient recovers, following which anti-HB_s can be found. Anti-HB_s does not indicate active infection but, rather, may signify resolution of the carrier state. Anti-HB_c is found in all carriers of HB_sAg, and may have something to do with replication of hepatitis B virus. Furthermore, in the absence of detectable HB_sAg, potentially infective blood may be indicated by the presence of anti-HB_c. All blood to be transfused is tested for HB_sAg, and positively removes that unit from the donor pool. Practically speaking, approximately 80% of bloods infective for hepatitis B prove to be positive for HB_sAg.

   c. Evidence is accumulating that a recently described form of hepatitis (non-A, non-B) may also occur and is a relatively frequent occurrence following transfusion. This is often anicteric, probably viral, and tends to be less severe than hepatitis B.

   d. The use of frozen red blood cells has been shown to diminish the incidence of serum hepatitis. The use of packed cells, especially washed cells, also has been associated with a decrease in the incidence of serum hepatitis. It is not clear why freezing cells or washing cells diminishes the incidence of hepatitis, but it is assumed that the concentration of virus in the plasma of transfused material is diminished.

2. **Brucellosis.** Although rarely transmitted by transfusion, brucellosis may occur if a person donates blood during the 10-day prodromal stage of clinical infection, thus transmitting viable *Brucella* organisms to the recipient. Chills, fever, myalgia, and an erythematous skin eruption are common symptoms, ordinarily occurring 7–14 days after the transfusion. **Treatment** with tetracycline or chloramphenicol is specific.

3. **Malaria** is a rare complication of blood transfusion. The occurrence of a spiking fever 1–10 days after transfusion always should arouse a suspicion that *Plasmodium* organisms have been transmitted by transfusion. Blood smears should be done on repeated occasions to detect the infecting organisms. **Treatment** with antimalarial drugs should be started promptly.

4. **Cytomegalovirus inclusion disease,** formerly considered uniquely a complication of extracorporeal bypass for cardiac surgery, is now known to occur under other circumstances, with either large or small volumes of blood. Spiking fever, few symptoms, atypical lymphocytes in the peripheral smear, altered liver function tests, and positive cold agglutinins are characteristic. The incubation period is 1–6 wk, and the process is self-limited except in immunosuppressed patients, in whom the disease may be fatal. Other viruses (rubeola, Epstein-Barr, infectious mononucleosis) are rarely transmitted to normal recipients.

IV. Complications of massive transfusion

A. **The rapid administration of large quantities** of acid-citrate-dextrose or citrate-phosphate-dextrose preserved banked blood (one half of the circulating blood volume or more) is likely to result in one or several problems unless the patient is carefully monitored and certain preventive measures are undertaken.

1. **Hypothermia** is common if blood is administered rapidly through a central venous catheter or through a peripheral vein under pressure. Transfusion within 1–2 hr of 3–5 units of bank blood at refrigerator temperature may lower the recipient's body temperature by 3–4°C (5–7°F), resulting in diminished cardiac output and metabolic acidosis. In this state, certain drugs, a change in ventilation, or other usual pathophysiological phenomena may trigger cardiac arrest.

Blood should be prewarmed when it has to be given rapidly in large volume. Warming should never be attempted by placing the blood container in warm water; rather, a long coil of tubing in the infusion line is immersed in a water bath at 35°C (95°F). These devices are commercially available and should always be employed in patients undergoing major intra-abdominal or intrathoracic surgery or subjected to trauma in whom major bleeding has occurred or is anticipated during operative repair.

2. **Citrate intoxication, fall in ionized calcium.** Citrate is present in excess in both ACD- and CPD-preserved bank blood. When citrate is infused into a normal recipient, binding of ionized calcium is not important, since there is rapid mobilization of calcium from bone. Previously, it was thought that an adult could tolerate the excess citrate in a unit of blood given as rapidly as 1 unit q10min (6 units/hr). However, recent data indicate that patients with preexisting myocardial disease may experience a considerable fall in cardiac output with depression of ionized calcium by transfused citrate. For every 3–5 units of whole blood, or every 5–8 units of packed cells, 1 gm of calcium chloride, or 4 gm of calcium gluconate, should be given, assuming that the transfusion rate is such that the whole blood or packed cell volume is administered in 4 hr or less. The calcium atom in calcium gluconate represents 9% of the molecule by weight; the calcium in calcium chloride, on the other hand, is 37% of the molecule by weight. For this reason, to administer an equivalent amount of

calcium as calcium gluconate requires giving four times as much as when calcium chloride is used.

a. Patients in whom inadequate stores of bone calcium may permit a citrate-induced ionized calcium deficit to develop during massive transfusion include small children, elderly or osteoporotic patients, especially if there is metastatic replacement of bone by tumor, and patients who have been bedridden for 8–10 wk or more.

b. **When citrate intoxication occurs, it does not lead to abnormal bleeding as is commonly supposed but, rather, affects myocardial function,** causing bradycardia, arrhythmias, and hypotension.

c. If the possible development of citrate intoxication is suspected, give the patient 1 gm of calcium chloride IV prior to infusion of every 3–5 units of whole blood. Excess citrate infusion initially results in acidosis, but as the liver metabolizes the citrate to bicarbonate, metabolic alkalosis develops. It is rarely necessary to treat either the acidosis or the alkalosis, assuming no other cause of either derangement.

The full role of ionized calcium, aside from that in augmenting myocardial contractility, is not well delineated. Preliminary evidence, for example, indicates that ionized calcium is responsible for binding together the subcomponents of C1 complement, allowing the complexing subcomponents to form C3. This complexing may be interfered with by such agents as edetate (EDTA) or citrate, which bind ionized calcium.

As has been noted, when calcium gluconate is used, the dose of the material must be four times greater than when calcium chloride is used. For this reason, calcium overdosage—and cardiac arrest—can occur with the administration of calcium chloride, unless one is cognizant of the greater amount of calcium in each molecule of calcium chloride.

3. Hyperkalemia. When blood is banked, potassium continuously leaks from the erythrocytes into the surrounding plasma. The plasma potassium concentration may approach 25 mEq/liter after 21 days. This leakage of potassium is related to loss of cell membrane integrity resulting from hypoxia, as well as to phosphate enzyme deterioration during storage.

When the cells are infused into the recipient and are reoxygenated, the leaked potassium is taken up again, reducing the plasma concentration of potassium in the recipient. However, hyperkalemia can be a problem if extremely rapid transfusion transiently raises the plasma concentration of potassium. Although rare, this factor has been implicated in sudden cardiac arrest and should be kept in mind if the blood administered is more than 10 days old. It is always wise to intersperse fresh units of blood with others during transfusion of large volumes.

4. Acidosis. The pH of 2-week-old bank blood is 6.5 owing to leakage of lactate and pyruvate into the surrounding plasma due to red cell hypoxia during storage. If aged blood is transfused rapidly, development of acidosis is theoretically possible. However, plasma buffers will handle large amounts of hydrogen ion provided the patient was not acidotic prior to transfusion.

a. Effective treatment of shock with transfused blood usually results in clearing of the associated acidosis when shock is the only cause of acidosis; administration of buffers such as sodium bicarbonate or tris (hydroxymethyl) aminomethane (THAM) may not be necessary. Sodium bicarbonate is customarily transfused at a rate of 40 mEq for every 3–5 units of blood transfused: if THAM is required because of severe hyponatremia or congestive heart failure in the transfused person, a 0.3-molar solution is made by dissolving 36 gm of THAM in 1000 ml of dextrose and water. This material is normally administered at 1–3 ml/min (36–108 mg), with frequent monitoring of arterial pH to prevent overtreatment. The major disadvantage of THAM is that it binds bicarbonate, precipitiously drops plasma carbon dioxide tension, and may cause respiratory arrest. To use THAM safely, the patient should be on a ventilator, or a ventilator should be present at the bedside, and personnel should closely monitor the patient so that intubation and initiation of mechanical ventilatory support can be provided if necessary.

b. In patients with preexisting acidosis who are to receive 1 unit of blood q20min or more rapidly, transfused blood should be buffered with IV sodium bicarconate, 20 mEq for each unit transfused.

5. Hyperammonemia. The concentration of ammonia in bank blood begins to rise after 5–7 days and reaches high levels after 2–3 wk of storage. In normal patients, this is unimportant, but in patients with severe liver disease, especially those with preexisting hyperammonemia, it is important that administered blood not be more than 5–7 days old, or that red cells be resuspended in serum albumin or Ringer's acetate solution.

6. Coagulation defects. When massive transfusions are given, representing half the patient's blood volume or more (roughly 2500 ml) in 12 hr or less, bleeding may occur. Bleeding is said to be the result of dilutional decreases in platelets and other labile clotting factors. In most patients, however, platelet counts are not reduced to critically low levels (less than $75,000/mm^3$), since marrow replacement of platelets is extremely rapid. Unless the volume transfused in a 12-hr period exceeds the patient's own blood volume, some explanation other than dilution must account for rare true coagulation defects. Coagulation defects can be prevented if every fifth unit transfused is less than 36 hr old. In addition, if more than 10 units of whole blood is given in a 24-hr period, it is probably wise to administer 1 unit of fresh-frozen plasma for every 3 units of whole blood.

B. Post-transfusion lung syndrome and other pulmonary complications. Most lung problems (hypoxia) that develop following transfusion are caused by circulatory overload or by reactions to transfusion of multiple units. The administration of large volumes of bank blood through a standard nylon mesh filter permits enormous amounts of microaggregated cells and fibrin to enter the pulmonary and other circuits, causing respiratory insufficiency and DIC. To prevent this complication, whenever more than 4 units of whole blood is to be administered in 1 day, the blood is given through a micropore filter effective in removing microaggregates (Pall or Swank).

Suggested Reading

Baker, R. J., and Nyhus, L. M.   Diagnosis and treatment of immediate transfusion reaction. *Surg. Gynecol. Obstet.* 130:665, 1970.

DeVenuto, F., Friedman, H. I., Neville, J. R., and Peck, C. C.   Appraisal of hemoglobin solution as a blood substitute. *Surg. Gynecol. Obstet.* 149:417, 1979.

Medical Letter.   Blood products. *Med. Lett. Drugs Ther.* Vol. 21, No. 23 (Nov. 16, 1979).

Mollison, P. L.   *Blood Transfusion in Clinical Medicine* (6th ed.). Oxford: Blackwell, 1979.

Olinger, G. N., Hottenrott, C., Mulder, D. G., Maloney, J. V., Jr., Miller, J., Patterson, R. W., Sullivan, S. F., and Buckberg, G. D.   Acute clinical hypocalcemic myocardial depression during rapid blood transfusion and postoperative hemodialysis. *J. Thorac. Cardiovasc. Surg.* 72:503, 1976.

Olinger, G. N., Werner, P. H., Bonchek, L. I., and Boerboom, L. E.   Vasodilator effects of the sodium acetate in pooled protein fraction. *Ann. Surg.* 190:305, 1979.

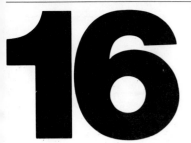

I. Mechanisms of hemostasis

A. Hemostasis involves a series of reactions that serve to prevent excessive blood loss following injury to blood vessels and also to maintain the fluid state of intravascular blood. **Normal intima prevents fibrin clot formation** and probably is essential in keeping the blood fluid. If fibrin forms intravascularly, the partially occluded vessel endothelium secretes fibrinolytic activator. When activator permeates the clot, entrapped plasminogen is converted to plasmin, and fibrinolysis occurs.

B. Following **injury**, a series of reactions (Fig. 16-1) occur rapidly.

1. Vascular response. Reflex contraction of smooth muscle of the blood vessel wall occurs in the region of injury. Smaller blood vessels may close completely.

2. Platelet response. Platelets adhere to exposed collagen at the point of endothelial injury. Contact with collagen activates a series of biochemical reactions in the platelets, starting with the release of arachidonic acid, which forms prostaglandins, endoperoxides, and thromboxanes. Under the influence of thromboxane A_2, the platelet releases material such as adenosine diphosphate and serotonin, which causes further aggregation and results in the formation of a firm platelet plug. **Aspirin** inhibits the cyclo-oxygenase of platelets, preventing the formation of prostaglandin G_2, a precursor of thromboxane A_2.

3. Formation of fibrin (intrinsic system). For maintenance of vessel closure, a series of protein and phospholipid reactions leading to thrombin and fibrin formation occur. Most of the required proteins are adsorbed to the platelet surface and are readily available for the required interaction at the site of vessel injury.

4. Formation of fibrin (extrinsic system). At the site of vascular injury, the tissues supply a thromboplastic material that interacts with coagulation factor VII to initiate further fibrin formation. Both the extrinsic and the intrinsic pathways are required for adequate fibrin formation. Deficiency of proteins in either pathway, or of lipoprotein for platelets, can result in excessive blood loss.

II. Diagnosis of abnormal bleeding

A. History and physical examination

1. Bleeding after dental extractions or previous operations is suggestive of a hemostatic defect but is not specific.

2. Sudden onset of bleeding from multiple sites suggests disseminated intravascular coagulation (DIC).

3. Epistaxis suggests abnormal capillaries, as in hereditary telangiectasia, but can also be seen with platelet disorders and in von Willebrand's disease.

4. Petechiae indicate a possible platelet disorder or, less frequently, the presence of acute, severe stasis.

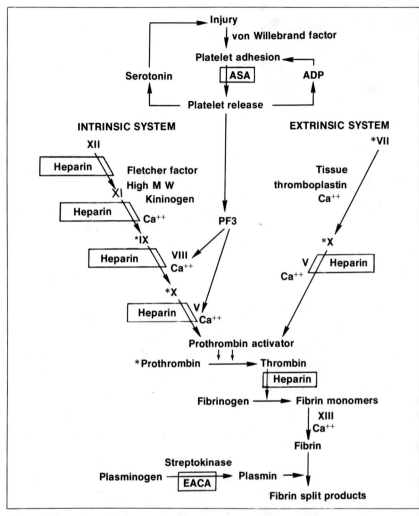

Figure 16-1. The clotting reactions. Asterisk (*) indicates vitamin K–dependent factor whose synthesis is impaired by warfarin. Boxed items denote inhibitors.

5. Purpura and menorrhagia suggest von Willebrand's disease, platelet decrease or dysfunction, or sensitivity to aspirin or another medication.

6. Hemarthrosis and deep muscle hematomas suggest hemophilia.

7. The inheritance history can be helpful, as follows:

   a. Sex-linked recessive inheritance is seen with hemophilia A and B (factors VIII and IX) and with a rare form of thrombocytopenia.

   b. Autosomal dominant inheritance characterizes the most common bleeding disorders: von Willebrand's disease, thrombopathy (platelet dysfunction), thrombocytopenia, and hereditary telangiectasia.

Table 16-1. Clinical Setting of Coagulopathy

Clinical Setting	Platelet Disorder	Plasma Factor Deficiency*	Disseminated Intravascular Coagulation	Primary Fibrinolysis
Acute problem				
Multiple transfusions	X	X		
Incompatible transfusion			X	
Shock			X	
Cardiac arrest			X	
Multiple trauma			X	
Chronic disease				
Liver disease	X	X	X	X
Renal disease	X	X		
Collagen disease	X	X	X	
Polycythemia	X			
Leukemia	X		X	X
Chronic idiopathic thrombocytopenic purpura	X			
Metastatic cancer	X	X	X	X
Surgery				
Open-heart	X	X	X	X
Vascular	X		X	
Prostatic				X
Medication				
Warfarin (Coumadin)		X		
Long-term antibiotics		X		
Aspirin	X			

*Plasma factor deficiency without DIC or primary fibrinolysis.

    c. Autosomal recessive inheritance is seen with plasma coagulation factor abnormalities other than factors VIII and IX. These conditions are rare.

B. Types of acute coagulation disorders. The acquired coagulopathies most frequently encountered in surgical patients are (1) platelet disorders, (2) plasma factor deficiencies, (3) DIC, (4) primary fibrinolysis, (5) exogenous anticoagulants, and (6) incomplete surgical control (i.e., bleeders). The clinical situations commonly associated with acute coagulation disorders are listed in Table 16-1.

1. Platelet disorders

    a. Thrombocytopenia can occur in the following circumstances:

        (1) From "washout" when multiple transfusions of bank blood are required.

        (2) From excess protamine sulfate administered to neutralize heparin.

        (3) With post-transfusion purpura.

        (4) With drug-induced thrombocytopenia.

        (5) During DIC.

        (6) From decreased marrow production as a consequence of replacement by tumor cells, radiotherapy, or chemotherapy.

        (7) In chronic idiopathic thrombocytopenic purpura.

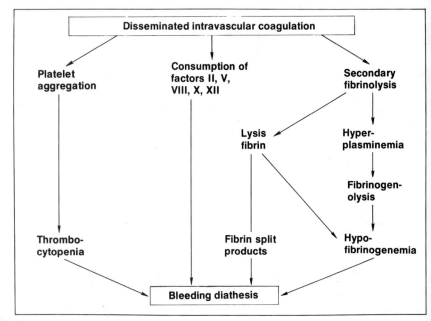

Figure 16-2. Pathophysiological mechanisms in DIC.

    b. Thrombopathy, or abnormal platelet function, is most often seen in acute or chronic renal disease in which the platelet surface becomes coated with metabolic waste products. Its occurrence cannot be predicted on the basis of serum creatinine levels, since major constituents of the adherent waste are phenolic acids and succinic acid derivatives. Thrombopathy can also occur in hepatic disease and as an idiopathic disorder.

    c. Thrombocythemia is present when the platelet count exceeds 1,000,000/mm^3. The most common cause is iron-deficiency anemia; platelet function is normal. Myeloproliferative disorders (e.g., polycythemia vera, essential thrombocythemia) frequently are associated with thrombocythemia. Finally, transient thrombocythemia characterized by normal platelet function is frequent after splenectomy.

2. Plasma factor deficiencies

    a. With increasing frequency, patients in the postoperative period develop **deficiencies of vitamin K** and subsequently, of the K-dependent coagulation proteins (II, VII, IX, and X). Contributing factors are antibiotic therapy, poor nutritional status, and biliary diversion or obstruction.

    b. Liver disease results in **deficiency of factor V** as well as of the vitamin K–dependent factors. Thus, a factor V level will often distinguish between liver disease and vitamin K deficiency.

3. DIC is characterized by thrombocytopenia, multiple plasma coagulation factor deficiencies, and secondary fibrinolysis as a result of intravascular fibrin formation (Fig. 16-2). Causes include:

    a. Hypoxia with endothelial damage (shock, cardiac arrest, septicemia, viremia, and heat stroke).

    b. Multiple trauma (fat emboli, crush injuries, tissue necrosis, and burns).

c. Intravascular hemolysis (extracorporeal circulation, incompatible blood transfusion, acquired hemolytic anemia, sickle cell anemia, and paroxysmal nocturnal hemoglobinuria).

d. Metastatic carcinoma.

e. Obstetrical problems (abruptio placentae, amniotic fluid embolus, and retained dead fetus).

f. Giant hemangioma.

g. Antigen-antibody reactions.

4. Generalized primary fibrinolysis of clinical significance is rarely encountered. It must be carefully distinguished from the secondary fibrinolysis of DIC, because the therapies are different and **not interchangeable.**

a. Primary fibrinolysis can be seen in liver disease, in metastatic carcinoma, in association with open-heart surgery, in prostatic surgery, and in oral surgery.

b. Hyperfibrinolysis usually results from the release or production of an excess of plasminogen activators. The activators may result in generalized (liver disease) or localized (prostatic surgery) fibrinolysis and hemorrhage.

5. Exogenous anticoagulants

a. Heparin. Unless the clotting time is markedly prolonged, bleeding in the presence of heparin is caused by some other abnormality. Thrombocytopenia, with or without new thromboses, can occur with heparin administration. In the absence of thrombocytopenia, bleeding is most commonly associated with an underlying disorder, such as malignancy, ulcer, or surgical trauma.

b. Warfarin (Coumadin). In the therapeutic range (prothrombin time up to 2.5 times the control), bleeding may be enhanced following trauma or when medications such as aspirin have been used. With warfarin excess, deficiencies of factors II, VII, IX, and X are extreme. Bleeding can be spontaneous or can follow minimal trauma.

c. Antiplatelet drugs (aspirin, sulfinpyrazone, dipyridamole, butazolidin, benzodiazepines, antihistamines). Response to these drugs is extremely variable, but in many cases their use can result in clinically significant bleeding.

C. Coagulation tests and their interpretation The values given in Tables 16-2 and 16-3 for "normals" are only approximate. Patient results must always be compared with the specific laboratory's "normals."

1. Bleeding time

a. This test measures the time necessary for bleeding from a standardized cut made in the forearm to stop.

b. The normal value for the Ivy bleeding time done with a proximal pressure cuff maintained at 40 mm Hg is 2–6 min. The Simplate (template) bleeding time is normally between 3 and 10 min.

c. Normal results depend on adequate numbers of platelets, adequate platelet function, and normal reflex vascular contraction.

d. Since access to the patient's forearm is required, this test cannot be done conveniently in the operating room.

e. A prolonged bleeding time may occur with thrombocytopenia, von Willebrand's disease, and following the ingestion of antiplatelet drugs. However, in the last case, there usually is some underlying coagulation disorder.

Table 16-2. Differential Diagnosis of Acute Coagulation Disorders

Disorder	Bleeding Time	Platelet Count	Prothrombin Time	Thrombin Time	Factor V Assay	Partial Thromboplastin Time	Fibrinogen	Fibrin Split Products	Prothrombin Consumption Time
Platelet disorders									
Thrombocytopenia	Long	Low	Normal			Normal			Abnormal
Thrombopathy	Normal or long	Normal	Normal			Normal			Abnormal
Thrombocythemia		Increased	Normal			Normal			
Disseminated intravascular coagulation	Long	Low	Long	Long	Low	Long	Low	Increased	
Primary fibrinolysis		Normal	Normal or long	Normal or long	Normal or low		Low	Slight increase	
Anticoagulants									
Heparin			Normal	Long	Normal	Long			
Warfarin (Coumadin)			Long			Long			
Medications									
Antibiotics			Normal or Long		Normal or Long				
Aspirin	Long		Normal or Long		Normal or Long				

Table 16-3. Coagulation Tests in Plasma Factor Deficiency

Factor Deficiency	Coagulation Test[a]				
	Prothrombin Time	Partial Thrombo-plastin Time	Prothrombin Consumption Time	Factor V Assay	Fibrinogen
I	A	A	N	. . .[c]	A
II	A	A	. . .[c]	N	
V	A	A	A	A	
VII	A	N	N	N	
VIII[b]	N	A	A		
IX	N	A	A		
X	A	A	A	N	
XI	N	A	A		
XII	N	A	A		

N = normal; A = abnormal.
[a]Results indicated are for single-deficiency states; with multiple abnormalities, individual assays may be required.
[b]Factor VIII deficiency occurs in both hemophilia A and von Willebrand's disease.
[c]Uninterpretable for technical reasons.

2. Platelet count

a. A normal quantitative platelet count is 150,000–350,000/mm³.

b. A quantitative count is preferable, but examination of a blood smear allows an estimate of platelet numbers. The presence of five or more platelets/high-power field (approximately 75,000/mm³) in a blood smear indicates that adequate numbers of platelets are present for hemostasis if their function is normal.

c. Thrombocytopenia can result in abnormal surgical hemorrhage if the platelet count is 50,000/mm³ or less. Spontaneous hemorrhage is not usually a problem until the platelet count falls to about 20,000/mm³ or less.

3. Prothrombin time (PT)

a. The normal PT is 12 ± 0.5 sec.

b. The PT is influenced by plasma factors I, II, V, VII, and X.

c. Vitamin K deficiency or administration of vitamin K antagonist drugs results in a prolonged PT owing to deficiencies of factors II, VII and X. Factor IX deficiency also occurs but is not detectable by the PT.

d. In liver disease, the PT is prolonged owing to deficiencies of factors II, V, VII, and X. The deficiency of factor V differentiates liver disease from vitamin K deficiency in the absence of DIC. Normal factor V is 80–100%.

4. Partial thromboplastin time (PTT)

a. The normal value is less than 45 sec.

b. Normal results are obtained with levels of factors I, II, V, VIII, IX, X, XI, and XII above 30% of normal, which also approximates the hemostatic level.

c. If the PT is normal but the PTT is abnormal, the deficiency is limited to factors VIII, IX, XI, and XII.

d. The PTT is totally insensitive to qualitative and quantitative platelet defects.

5. Fibrinogen (factor I)

a. The normal range is 150–400 mg/100 ml.

b. Mild deficiency, in the range of 100–150 mg/100 ml, occurs in liver disease and with primary fibrinolysis.

c. Levels of less than 100 mg/100 ml are seen in DIC.

d. If DIC occurs in patients with septicemia but without the stress of operation, fibrinogen levels usually are above 100 mg/100 ml.

e. Because of its "stress protein" nature, fibrinogen may be deceptively high with infections and obstetrical problems.

6. Fibrin split products

a. Fibrin split products result from the action of plasmin on fibrin and sometimes on fibrinogen.

b. Fibrin split products contain many of the same antigenic sites as fibrinogen and thus may be assayed with fibrinogen antiserum. Using a tanned red cell hemagglutination inhibition immunoassay, the normal range is 0–10 μg/ml.

c. Increased fibrin split products are routinely observed in the absence of DIC or hyperfibrinolysis following surgery and in cases of multiple trauma.

d. With primary fibrinolysis, fibrin split product levels are usually 0–50 μg/mg.

e. In DIC, fibrin split products levels over 80 μg/ml are often seen.

7. Thrombin time (TT)

a. The TT is a measure of the rate of fibrin formation when thrombin is added to plasma.

b. The normal TT is within 10 sec of the control using 1 unit/ml of thrombin.

c. The TT is abnormal in the presence of heparin, low concentrations of fibrinogen and/or certain fibrin split products. The presence of heparin can be differentiated from fibrin split products by substituting a snake venom extract (Reptilase) for thrombin in the TT. Unlike thrombin, the action of Reptilase is not affected by heparin.

8. Prothrombin consumption time (PCT)

a. The PCT measures factors XII, XI, X, IX, VIII, V and platelets but is most sensitive to platelet defects. The normal range is 17–35 sec.

b. With platelets numbering less than 70,000/mm³, or adequate numbers of poorly functioning platelets, the PCT is abnormal (in the range of 8–15 sec).

c. An abnormal PCT can be anticipated when the levels of factors XII, XI, X, IX, VIII, or V fall below 5–10%.

d. By adding sources of various factors, the deficient factor can be identified. For platelet abnormalities, an abnormal PCT will be corrected only by platelets or a platelet substitute, such as hemolysate. Factor V and VIII deficiencies will be corrected with adsorbed plasma, factor IX and X deficiencies will be corrected with aged serum, and factor XI and XII deficiencies will be corrected with both adsorbed plasma and aged serum.

Table 16-4. Treatment of Acute Coagulation Disorders

Abnormality	Diagnostic Features	Specific Therapy
Thrombocytopenia	Platelets < 50,000/mm	Platelet concentrate infusions
Thrombopathy	Abnormal platelet aggregation studies Abnormal PCT corrected with platelet substitute Clinical setting (drugs, history etc.)	Platelet concentrate infusions
DIC	Platelets < 50,000/mm³ Factor V < 30% PT > 16 sec PTT > 50 sec Fibrinogen < 100 mg/100 ml Elevated FSPs	Supportive measures, including restoration of blood volume, red cell mass, etc. Definitive therapy of underlying cause, e.g., antibiotics for sepsis, uterine evacuation for abruptio placentae Heparin, 2000 units q4h, if DIC not controlled by above Fresh frozen plasma and platelets as required
Plasma factor deficiency	History of known factor deficiency Demonstrable factor deficiency	Cryoprecipitate: contains fibrinogen, factor VIII, VW factor Commercial factor IX concentrate: factors II, VII, IX, X Commercial Factor VIII concentrate FFP: essentially all coagulation factors
Anticoagulants		
Antiplatelet drugs	Clinical situation	Discontinue drug. Platelet concentrates if not controlled by the above
Warfarin (Coumadin)	Clinical situation	Fresh frozen plasma. IV vitamin K (takes at least 18 hr to reverse warfarin)
Heparin	Clinical situation	Protamine sulfate, 25–50 mg/Volutrol. (If TT is still prolonged, repeat the initial dose.)
Primary fibrinolysis	**Absence of DIC** Increased plasminogen activator	ε-Aminocaproic acid (Amicar) 5 gm IV, followed by 1 gm/hr IV for 2–3 hr, then 1 gm/2 hr PO or IV **Caution:** Amicar is absolutely contraindicated in DIC

III. Managing the surgical patient with suspected acute coagulopathy

A. General approach

1. Draw blood for platelet count, fibrinogen, PT, factor V, PTT, and TT.

2. Until laboratory results are obtained, use fresh-frozen plasma and packed red cells.

3. On the basis of laboratory results, give definitive treatment as outlined in Table 16-4.

B. Therapy for specific factor deficiencies

Levels of specific coagulation factors are specified in percent of normal activity (e.g., a hemophiliac patient with a factor VIII level of 10%). In general, coagulation factor levels of 30% or greater are hemostatic. However, in treating the bleeding patient, one must raise the factor activity much higher than 30% to assure that the level remains above 30% until the next dose is given. Coagulation factor concentrates are measured in "units"; for example, 1 unit of factor VIII is the amount of factor VIII present in 1 ml of plasma containing 100% activity. The total units required are given by the following **formula**: Units to be transfused = patient weight (kg) × 60 (ml plasma/kg body weight) × increment of factor desired (units/ml plasma).

For example, a bleeding hemophilia A patient can be assumed to have a factor VIII level of 0%. The loading dose should be sufficient to raise the deficient factor to twice the desired minimum level (usually 60%). Maintenance therapy consists of one half the loading dose given every half-life, which for factor VIII is 12 hr. Assuming a weight of 70 kg. yields: Units required = 70 kg × 60 ml/kg. × 0.6 units/ml = 2520 units of factor VIII. Thus, the loading dose would be 2500 units followed by 1250 units q12h.

Finally, when confronted by a bleeding hemophiliac patient with a known factor deficiency, assume a factor VIII level of 0. *Do not delay therapy while trying to obtain a factor VIII level!*

Factor IX has a half-life of 24 hr; the maintenance regimen would be given on a q24h schedule. Half-lives for other factors can usually be obtained from your hospital blood bank.

IV. Monitoring anticoagulant therapy

A. Warfarin
affects the intrinsic, extrinsic, and common pathways. However, the PT is the test of choice because of its simplicity, sensitivity, and reproducibility. General therapeutic anticoagulation is achieved with PTs between 20 and 30 sec.

B. Heparin.
Many tests are used to monitor heparin, including the PTT, Lee-White clotting time, the thrombin time, and the activated recalcification time. All these tests have their advantages and disadvantages. The proper test to use is that which your hospital's coagulation laboratory has selected for monitoring heparin, since it is the test in which your laboratory has the most confidence.

C. Antiplatelet drugs
are usually not monitored.

Suggested Reading

Mielke, C. H., and Rodvien, R. (eds.).   *Mechanisms of Hemostasis and Thrombosis.* Miami, Fla. Symposia Specialists, 1978.

Quick, A. J.   *The Hemorrhagic Diseases and the Pathology of Hemostasis.* Springfield, Ill.: Thomas, 1974.

Rossi, E. C. (ed.).   Symposium on hemorrhagic disorders. *Med. Clin. North Am.* 56:1, 1972.

Silver, D., and McGregor, F. H.   Non-mechanical causes of surgical bleeding. *Curr. Probl. Surg.* January, 1970.

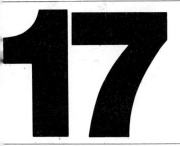

Pulmonary Embolus

Pulmonary emboli usually originate from occult thrombi in the venous circulation. The less common varieties of pulmonary emboli—septic and fat emboli—are discussed separately.

I. Causes and effects

A. Factors predisposing to pulmonary emboli include lower extremity trauma, visceral cancer, heart failure, immobility, obesity, advanced (+70) age, and a history of venous thrombosis or pulmonary embolism.

B. Sources of fatal pulmonary emboli are indicated in Table 17-1. **In surgical patients, most emboli originate in the legs or pelvis**, while on a medical service, the heart also is an important source of emboli.

C. The immediate consequences of a pulmonary embolus are related to both mechanical effects and humoral reflex effects.

1. **Mechanical effects** resulting from passage and lodgment of the clot are relatively insignificant until more than 25% of the pulmonary artery circulation is occluded. With 25–30% blockage, **pulmonary artery mean pressure begins to rise**. As pulmonary artery occlusion approaches 35%, the pulmonary artery mean pressure exceeds 30 mm Hg, and right atrial mean pressure also rises. Cardiac output remains normal or increased until pulmonary artery occlusion exceeds 50% (massive embolism). Underlying cardiac or respiratory insufficiency contributes significantly to premature failure of cardiac output. The mechanical effects of a pulmonary embolus also result in:

   a. Arrhythmia, as the clot traverses the right atrium and ventricle.

   b. Dilation of bronchial arteries, which serve as collateral vessels to the distal pulmonary arterial tree.

   c. Decreased pulmonary blood flow, which results in:

      (1) Decreased cardiac output, systemic hypotension, and shock.

      (2) High ventilation-perfusion ratio caused by decreased pulmonary arteriolar circulation in areas of normal alveolar ventilation and leading to arterial hypoxemia and a high arterial-alveolar gradient for carbon dioxide.

      (3) Myocardial hypoxia, ectopic irritable foci, and arrhythmia.

   d. Infarction, only with less than 10% of pulmonary emboli. The development of an infarct depends on:

      (1) Completeness of occlusion.

      (2) Effectiveness of collateral circulation.

      (3) Condition of the lung; congestion or infection increases the likelihood of infarction.

Table 17-1. Sources of Fatal Pulmonary Emboli

Source	Surgical Service (%)	Medical Service (%)
Right side of heart	0	25
Inferior vena cava	10	18
Pelvic veins	15	15
Iliofemoral and leg veins	40	0
Calf veins	17	42

Surgical service data from C. Crane, *N. Engl. J. Med.* 257:147, 1957. Medical service data from G. T. Smith, L. Dexter, and G. J. Dammin. In A. A. Sasahara and M. Stein (Eds.), *Pulmonary Embolic Disease.* New York: Grune & Stratton, 1965. P. 126.

    2. Humoral reflex effects, although less significant than mechanical effects, probably are due in most instances to the release of biologically active amines (e.g., histamine and serotonin) from platelets. Humoral reflex effects include:

      a. Increased pulmonary artery resistance and pressure; decreased pulmonary blood flow.

      b. Bronchoconstriction, causing increased airway resistance and resulting in decreased compliance, decreased alveolar ventilation, hypoxemia, and tachypnea.

      c. Systemic hypotension not related to alterations in pulmonary blood flow.

II. Clinical features

  A. The first sign of pulmonary embolus in 70% of patients is the embolus itself. Less than one third of patients exhibit even minimal clinical signs of venous disease before the embolus. But, of patients with fatal pulmonary embolus, 85% have had some warning sign—a prior minor embolus or symptomatic venous disease.

  B. Signs and symptoms are listed in Table 17-2. Note that dyspnea, tachypnea, and a loud second pulmonic sound are common. The "classic" signs of pleuritis, hemoptysis, and a pleural friction rub are not common; they are not really signs of pulmonary embolus but of infarction.

  C. Unexplained asthma or heart failure appearing in a hospitalized patient is very suggestive of pulmonary embolus.

  D. The most common incorrect diagnoses in patients having pulmonary emboli are congestive heart failure, pneumonia, and myocardial infarction.

  E. Leukocytosis of greater than 15,000/mm^3 is unusual with pulmonary embolus; if the leukocyte count is high, pneumonia is more likely.

  F. The **"diagnostic enzyme pattern"** of elevated lactic dehydrogenase and bilirubin with normal serum glutamic-oxaloacetic transaminase values is found in only 12% of patients. Although elevation of lactic dehydrogenase is common (>80%), it is of no value in differentiating pulmonary embolus from pneumonia. Elevation of bilirubin is related to heart failure resulting from the pulmonary embolus, rather than to any direct effect of the embolus.

  G. Blood gases. The most consistent finding is PaO$_2$ less than 80 mm Hg; PaCO$_2$ values remain normal or, with tachypnea, may decrease.

  H. The **electrocardiogram (ECG) is neither a sensitive nor a specific diagnostic aid** in cases of pulmonary embolus. Many patients have a preexisting abnormal ECG, and most of these show no change. Only one fourth of patients with a

Table 17-2. Clinical Signs and Symptoms of Pulmonary Embolus

Signs and Symptoms	Frequency (%)
Dyspnea	100
Tachypnea (+20/min)	95
Loud P_2	95
Tachycardia (+90/min)	70
Fever	55
Rales	55
Cough	50
Pleuritic pain	35
Phlebitis	30
Hemoptysis	25
Pleural friction rub	20
Cyanosis	15
Gallop rhythm	15
X-ray infiltrate	15
Substernal pain	10
Syncope	5
Shock	5

pulmonary embolus will show abnormal ECG changes; 80% of these changes will be rhythm disturbances. The classic ECG changes of pulmonary embolus (large P waves, right axis deviation, S–T segment depression, T wave inversion, etc.) are uncommon, found in only 5% of all patients with a proved pulmonary embolus. The major value of an ECG is differentiation of a pulmonary embolus from a myocardial infarction.

I. Tests designed to **detect occult deep venous thrombosis** may be helpful. These are phlebography, impedance plethysmography, Doppler ultrasound, and ^{125}I-fibrinogen scans.

1. Phlebography and iliofemoral venography are excellent methods of visualizing clots in the deep venous system, but they fail to demonstrate the age of the clot, adherence of the clot, and, indeed, the clinical significance of these thrombi.

2. Impedance plethysmography is a rapid, noninvasive method for detecting deep venous thrombosis. However, the test is less accurate than venography, and there are significant numbers of false-negative tests.

3. Doppler ultrasound flow studies accurately detect femoral and popliteal thromboses but cannot be used to detect infrapopliteal venous thrombosis.

4. ^{125}I-fibrinogen uptake studies are very sensitive and probably detect clinically insignificant thrombi as well as significant ones. To be positive, the test must be performed while the thrombi are developing.

J. **Chest x-rays** may be entirely normal (50%) or may show the following:

1. Prominent pulmonary artery (hilar) shadows.

2. Diminished vascular markings in the area of embolization.

3. Enlarged right ventricle or widening of the superior mediastinum.

4. Small pleural effusion or elevation of the diaphragm.

5. Cone, hump-shaped, or other nondescript densities based on the pleural surface, usually in the lower lobes, and suggestive of pulmonary infarction (15% of patients).

K. Pulmonary angiography is the definitive diagnostic examination in patients with suspected pulmonary embolus. Visualization of **an intraluminal filling defect, an abrupt vessel cutoff, or loss of side branches (pruning) is a diagnostic sign.** Delayed filling of the pulmonary artery and a delayed venous phase are suggestive angiographic signs but are not diagnostic of pulmonary embolus.

1. **Contrast media** should be injected through a catheter selectively placed into the main pulmonary artery; this catheter subsequently can be retracted and used to measure right ventricular pressure (see **M**).

2. **Pulmonary cineangiography** details flow and vascular motion and is a valuable study if the results of routine pulmonary angiography are equivocal.

3. Pulmonary angiography is dangerous if the patient is in shock or in marked heart failure; if the examination is to be done in such patients, partial bypass should be established first.

4. Although formal pulmonary angiograms are desirable, acceptable substitutes may be obtained by rapid injection of 50 ml of contrast medium from a hand-held syringe. The injection is made through a large-bore (16-gauge) catheter, placed in the right side of the heart, during exposure of a chest film. This method will demonstrate only large emboli, but those are the only ones likely to require this emergency procedure.

5. **The major complications** of angiography include transient hypotension and arrhythmias, which can be reduced by avoiding injections directly into the right heart. Vessels 2 mm or smaller cannot be visualized on angiography, so microemboli may be overlooked with this technique.

L. Pulmonary scanning following injection of radioiodinated macroaggregated serum albumin, ^{51}Cr, or ^{99m}Tc also is an excellent diagnostic measure and is simple to perform. The lung scan is **particularly useful in differentiating a major pulmonary embolus from acute myocardial infarction.** A lung scan is not as specific as an angiogram in the diagnosis of a pulmonary embolus. The scan really demonstrates diminished blood flow in the lung; a picture similar to that of pulmonary embolus also can be produced by neoplasms, atelectasis, pneumonia, and emphysematous bullae. In the case of neoplasms, atelectasis, or pneumonia, the chest x-ray will be grossly abnormal, whereas with pulmonary embolus, the chest x-ray is likely to be normal or to show only subtle changes. The differentiation between an emphysematous bleb and a pulmonary embolus can be made with the addition of a ^{133}Xe ventilation scan; an emphysematous bulla produces a hypoventilated area, as opposed to the normally ventilated area seen in pulmonary embolism.

M. Catheterization of the right side of the heart and measurement of pulmonary artery and right ventricular end diastolic pressure are important adjuncts to pulmonary angiography and provide useful prognostic data that aid in making critical therapeutic decisions.

III. Therapeutic measures

A. Anticoagulation

1. Indications

a. **Prophylactic.** Anticoagulants may be used prophylactically in any patient who has a high risk of developing a pulmonary embolus. This indication for anticoagulation is controversial except in patients with a history of venous disease or pulmonary embolism.

b. **Therapeutic.** Patients with suspected or proven pulmonary embolus, or deep venous thrombosis, should receive anticoagulants as prophylaxis against further thrombosis or embolism.

2. Contraindications

a. Absolute

(a) Trauma to, or recent operation on, the brain or spinal cord.

(2) Clotting disorder (blood dyscrasia, liver disease).

(3) Septic phlebitis.

(4) Subacute or acute bacterial endocarditis.

b. Relative

(1) Major visceral injury.

(2) Acute fractures.

(3) Recent operation on the thorax, abdomen, or retroperitoneum that could lead to concealed bleeding.

(4) History of cerebral hemorrhage.

(5) Hypertension (diastolic >120 mm Hg).

(6) Gross hematuria, melena, or other present evidence of bleeding.

(7) History of the presence of gastrointestinal cancer, ulcer, or other bleeding lesions.

3. Heparin schedule

a. Heparin may be given either by intermittent IV injection or continuous IV infusion. The latter method requires closer supervision and the use of a constant controlled infusion pump.

(1) **Intermittent method** 10,000–15,000 units of sodium heparin initially, followed by 5000–10,000 units q4h thereafter (minimal dose 60,000 units in first 24 hr).

(2) **Continuous method** 5000-unit bolus, followed by 1000 units/hr thereafter.

b. Heparin therapy should be monitored by partial thromboplastin time (PTT). Careful monitoring to assure a heparin effect will not decrease the incidence of bleeding (8%) but will reduce the incidence of recurrent thromboembolism during anticoagulation. PTT is more reproducible than clotting time and is therefore preferred.

c. Blood for PTT is drawn prior to therapy and redrawn 30 min prior to the next heparin dose (twice on day 1, daily thereafter). PTT should be maintained at 1–1½ times normal (50–80 sec).

d. Continue therapy unless major bleeding occurs. Heparin treatment is not interrupted because of microscopic hematuria, minor epistaxis, appearance of guaiac-positive stools, or similar evidence of minor and tolerable blood loss.

e. Heparin is usually continued for 8–10 days (the approximate time for venous thrombi to become firmly adherent to the vein wall) or until all acute symptoms have subsided and the patient is fully ambulatory.

4. Warfarin (Coumadin) schedule (oral or parenteral)

a. The antithrombin effect of warfarin is negligible until after 5–7 days of therapy. Therefore, warfarin is started 2–3 days after the onset of heparin therapy, continued concomitantly with heparin for 5–7 days, and then continued after heparin has been discontinued.

b. Blood samples for prothrombin time are obtained immediately prior to the next heparin dose, to minimize the effect of heparin on that determination. Prothrombin time should be obtained daily during the first week, twice weekly during the second week, and weekly to twice monthly thereafter.

c. When warfarin is given along with heparin for 5–7 days, a loading dose of warfarin is unnecessary; simply give 10–15 mg daily, adjusting the dose subsequently according to the prothrombin values. Prothrombin time should be kept at two to three times normal.

d. Following a documented episode of pulmonary embolism, oral anticoagulation should be continued for a minimum of 4 mo—longer if the threat of recurrent embolism is great.

e. **Warfarin should be avoided in pregnant patients** since it crosses the placental barrier and may cause cerebral hemorrhage in the infant. Heparin, which does not cross the placenta, is used in place of warfarin and, if being used at the time of delivery, can be reversed with protamine sulfate and reinstituted 4 days later.

f. When the patient has been maintained within the therapeutic range for 1 wk, total the week's dose of warfarin, and divide by 7; the result is a satisfactory daily dose for future maintenance.

5. Management of bleeding in anticoagulated patients

a. If bleeding is minimal, simply reduce the amount of anticoagulant given.

b. If bleeding is massive during heparin anticoagulation, the heparin effect can be neutralized rapidly with protamine sulfate (each mg of protamine sulfate neutralizes approximately 100 USP units of sodium heparin). Protamine is itself an anticoagulant, and further bleeding will occur with larger doses. Transfusion does not correct the clotting abnormality produced by heparin.

c. If bleeding is massive during warfarin anticoagulation, this can be reversed with vitamin K_1, 10–25 mg parenterally, as well as by transfusion of fresh frozen plasma or whole blood. Some effect of vitamin K_1 is noted at 2 hr, but complete warfarin reversal takes 6–24 hr.

B. Venous interruption operations

1. Objective. Immediate prevention of recurrent pulmonary embolus. Because collateral circulation develops around any venous obstruction, late recurrence of emboli from or via collateral venous channels still may occur after venous interruption.

2. Indications

a. When anticoagulant therapy is contraindicated.

b. When anticoagulant therapy fails (major bleeding complication, recurrent pulmonary embolus).

c. First pulmonary embolus in a high-risk patient.

d. History of recurrent pulmonary emboli.

e. Septic phlebitis.

f. Septic pulmonary embolus.

g. Following pulmonary embolectomy.

3. **Contraindications.** In the presence of marked heart failure (pulmonary artery pressure >35 mm Hg), the mortality of caval ligation approaches 50%.

4. **Complications**

   a. Acute volume sequestration in the legs, with transient decreased cardiac output.

   b. Acute and chronic venous insufficiency of the legs.

   c. Recurrent pulmonary emboli via large collateral veins (in 10–20%).

   d. Specific complications attend the use of an intracaval umbrella, i.e., caval thrombosis, erosion into the intestine or aorta, retroperitoneal bleeding, and umbrella embolus.

5. **Choice of operation**

   a. Insertion below the renal veins via the internal jugular vein of an **intracaval umbrella balloon** or **wire filter** is the method of choice in high-risk patients who are in need of caval interruption.

   b. **Caval interruption** may be accomplished by ligation, plication, silk screen, plastic clip, or stapling techniques. Caval interruption usually is performed through a retroperitoneal approach. The vena cava is ligated just below the left renal vein. If gonadal vein ligation seems advisable as well, an intraperitoneal approach is used.

   c. Significant differences between caval ligation and caval plication with respect to the incidence of recurrent embolus or leg sequelae have not been demonstrated. Caval plication frequently results in complete interruption, since the channels through the plication or umbrella quickly occlude with either newly formed thrombus or small recurrent emboli.

   d. Femoral vein ligation is indicated only when the source of embolus clearly has been demonstrated by phlebography and iliofemoral venography to arise from the lower extremity. This may be the procedure of choice in high-risk patients, but the incidence of recurrent embolism is greater than that following caval ligation.

   e. Anticoagulation should be instituted or reinstituted 24 hr postoperatively after caval interruption and continued for 4–6 mo.

   f. Routine use of elevation and elastic stockings will reduce the degree of postoperative edema of the legs. Edema eventually will clear completely in half these patients as venous collaterals develop. Persisting edema probably is due to underlying venous disease in the legs.

C. Thrombolytic agents

1. **Objective.** To speed the natural processes of clot dissolution. Two thrombolysins, urokinase and streptokinase, have been studied extensively. Both act by enhancing the fibrinolytic system.

2. **Indication.** Massive pulmonary embolism that initially appears to require pulmonary embolectomy.

3. **Choice of agent**

   a. **Urokinase** is a natural fibrinolysin recovered from human urine. Administration is not associated with fever or allergic reactions, and effective blood levels can be achieved. The chief objection to urokinase is its great expense and the high incidence of abnormal bleeding attending its use. The drug has been extensively investigated and, although it is theoretically advantageous, improvement in mortality from pulmonary embolism with its use has not been demonstrated.

b. Streptolysin is unsatisfactory because administration produces fever and is associated with a high incidence of allergic reactions. Also, it is difficult to maintain blood concentrations that are high enough to alter the rate of clot lysis.

D. Pulmonary embolectomy

1. **Objective.** Mechanical removal of clot from the pulmonary arteries.

2. **Indications**

    a. Persistent and progressive shock in a patient with massive pulmonary embolism documented by angiography.

    b. Chronic pulmonary hypertension in a patient with angiographic evidence of right or left main pulmonary artery occlusion.

3. **Techniques**

    a. Pulmonary embolectomy under direct vision through **pulmonary arteriotomy** accompanied by cardiopulmonary bypass. This is the usual method and carries a 33% mortality risk.

    b. Pulmonary embolectomy without cardiopulmonary bypass using temporary inflow (caval) occlusion. This method is used when bypass is not available. It is associated with a 50% mortality risk.

    c. Transvenous pulmonary embolectomy using a vacuum-cup catheter. This newer method holds promise and can be done at the time of partial cardiopulmonary bypass using the femoral vein. It is difficult to remove all the clot by this method. However, if major occlusive clots are removed, the patient's condition will improve.

IV. Prophylaxis of pulmonary embolus This involves reducing those elements that promote venous thrombosis.

A. Reduce intimal injury

1. No infusions should be made into lower extremity veins.

2. Only buffered, isosmolar solutions should be infused into peripheral veins; hypertonic or nonneutral solutions should be administered slowly via a catheter inserted into a central vein.

B. Reduce stasis

1. Encourage early postoperative walking. Getting the patient up to sit in a chair is of no value and actually promotes stasis; the patient must walk.

2. Maintain activity in bed with calf and patellar setting exercises and changes in position.

3. Elevate the patient's legs 15 degrees when the patient is supine. Wrapping the legs with elastic bandages is not effective in increasing venous flow at rest.

4. **Elastic below-knee stockings** provide support for the calf musculature and prevent stasis in subcutaneous veins. Elastic stockings do not promote venous flow at rest but enhance the beneficial effects of leg exercise. Wrapping the legs with elastic bandages should achieve the same effect as elastic stockings. However, the bandages slip, often acting as a tourniquet and promoting venous stasis, so bandage wrapping should not be used.

C. Reduce hypercoagulability. Prophylactic anticoagulation of patients with lower extremity fractures and similar high-risk patients (see **III. A. 1**) reduces the risk of pulmonary embolus. Warfarin is the drug of choice for prophylactic anticoagulation and should be continued for a minimum of 3 mo or until the patient is fully active.

V. Management of pulmonary embolus

A. Initial treatment in any suspected pulmonary embolus includes:

1. Immediate **anticoagulation with heparin** to reduce distal propagation of thrombus beyond the embolus.

2. Administration of **oxygen** to increase blood PO_2 and reduce pulmonary artery pressure.

B. Classify patients for further management into three groups on the basis of clinical findings.

1. **Group I.** No shock or heart failure.

2. **Group II.** No shock, but heart failure is present.

3. **Group III.** Patient is in shock, but no vasoactive drugs are being given.

C. Treatment of group I patients: no shock or heart failure

1. Confirm the diagnosis with a lung scan or angiogram.

2. High-risk patients need inferior vena cava interruption. Ligation or umbrella placement is performed because these patients have a high risk of recurrent pulmonary emboli and a high mortality with recurrent embolization. Follow with anticoagulation, beginning 24 hr postoperatively.

D. Treatment of group II patients: heart failure, no shock

1. Catheterize. Confirm the diagnosis with an angiogram. Measure pulmonary artery or right ventricular end diastolic pressure.

2. Pressure less than 35 mm Hg: anticoagulation with heparin; treat heart failure. When failure clears, perform inferior vena cava interruption.

3. Pressure more than 35 Hg: embolectomy may be needed; administer anticoagulants, and observe carefully for 2–3 hr; if the patient is not improving, proceed with embolectomy.

E. Treatment of group III patients: in shock

1. If shock does not persist or if it responds readily to minimal doses of vasopressors, treat as group II: administer heparin, treat shock and heart failure; when shock and failure clear, perform inferior vena cava interruption.

2. If shock persists with or without vasopressors:

   a. Perform partial cardiopulmonary bypass.

   b. Catheterize, and confirm the diagnosis with an angiogram. Measure pulmonary artery or right ventricular end diastolic pressure.

   c. If the diagnosis is confirmed, perform transvenous embolectomy or convert to total bypass and perform pulmonary embolectomy.

VI. Septic pulmonary emboli

A. The embolus originates from septic thrombophlebitis.

B. Emboli tend to be small and multiple and to produce multiple foci of infection in the lungs.

C. Anticoagulants are contraindicated, since they tend to promote hemorrhage into infected pulmonary foci and rupture of mycotic aneurysms.

D. Treatment involves three essential steps:

1. **Proximal venous ligation.** There is no indication for plication or other partial venous interruption procedures. A pelvic focus of infection is frequent; in this situation, gonadal veins also must be ligated.

2. **Antibiotics** in high doses.

3. **Drainage** of any closed infection. If the embolus originated in a septic superficial thrombophlebitis, the involved vein segment should be stripped. Hysterectomy and bilateral salpingo-oophorectomy may be indicated for septic abortion or tubo-ovarian abscesses.

VII. Bone marrow and fat emboli

A. Ninety-five percent of fat emboli are associated with fractures, which disrupt venous channels in the bone marrow and allow fat particles to enter the venous circulation. Embolization of bone marrow occasionally occurs following fracture of a major long bone, the pelvis or sternum, or following median sternotomy or multiple soft tissue injuries.

B. Seventy-five percent of the fat emboli are trapped in the pulmonary circulation. Depending on their number, they may produce no symptoms or only respiratory symptoms. If the emboli pass on into the systemic circulation, a variety of symptoms may appear, primarily due to cerebral embolization.

C. The fat embolus lodged in the pulmonary capillaries is acted on by lipase to produce free fatty acids. These fatty acids are toxic and produce disruption of the alveolar capillary membrane and destruction of surfactant, leading to pulmonary edema, pulmonary hemorrhage, and alveolar collapse.

D. Clinical manifestations usually begin 12–96 hr after injury and consist of:

1. **Dyspnea and tachypnea**, occasionally associated with cyanosis, rales, or a pleural friction rub.

2. **Cerebral symptoms**, such as confusion, delirium, or coma.

3. **Petechial hemorrhages** found primarily on the chest wall, axillae, flanks, and subconjunctivas. Retinal petechiae also may be seen on fundoscopic examination.

4. **Temperature** usually up to 38.8°C (102°F).

E. Laboratory findings:

1. **Lipuria.** Fat in the urine is seen in 60% of cases of fat embolism, usually within the first 3 days.

2. Elevated serum lipase is found in 50% of cases of fat embolism, usually after 3 days.

3. Chest x-rays are either normal or reveal bilateral stippled or fluffy pulmonary infiltrates.

4. The ECG occasionally may show evidence of right heart strain.

5. Hematocrit fall is common and is thought to be related to pulmonary hemorrhage.

6. Low PaO_2 with compensatory respiratory alkalosis is a consistent finding in fat embolism.

F. Treatment consists of:

1. Correction of hypovolemia.

2. Gentle splinting and immobilization of fractures.

3. Respiratory support with oxygen.

4. Parenteral corticosteroids. Methylprednisolone, 125 mg IV, follow. . y 80 mg q6h for 3 days. Antacids are given concomitantly to help avert ga . .ntestinal bleeding.

5. Alcohol and heparin also may be given IV, but their use is controversial. Heparin promotes lipase activity, whereas alcohol inhibits lipase.

Suggested Reading

Hume, M., Sevitt, S., and Thomas, D. P. *Venous Thrombosis and Pulmonary Embolism.* Cambridge: Harvard University Press, 1970.

Hunter, J. A., Dye, W. S., Javid, H., Najafi, H., and Goldin, M. D. Permanent transvenous balloon occlusion of the inferior vena cava: Experience with 60 patients. *Ann. Surg.* 186:491, 1977.

McIntyre, K. M., Sasahara, A. A., and Sharma, G. V. R. K. Pulmonary thromboembolism: current concepts. *Adv. Intern Med.* 18:199, 1972.

A significant improvement in burn care has been made in recent years. Advancement in the field of critical care medicine has contributed to more adequate resuscitation and monitoring of extensively burned patients in the period immediately after the burn. Because of a better understanding of altered metabolism, more adequate nutritional care can be given. Surgical excisional therapy has become a clinical reality.

I. Emergent phase (0–72 hr post burn)

A. Initial assessment

1. **History.** A complete history should be obtained simultaneously while performing the physical examination and giving initial treatment.

   a. **History related to the burn.** The following should be ascertained: **when** (the time of burn); **where** (open or closed space; if in a closed space, **how long**); **what** (e.g., hot water, flame, chemical, electrical)

   b. **General history.** Any preexisting diseases and/or previous operations, allergies, and medications are important, as are a family history and a review of systems.

2. **Physical examination**

   a. **General examination.** A complete physical examination is essential.

   b. **Assessment of the burn.** This is a most important factor in planning of appropriate fluid therapy and surgical intervention. It is also a good prognostic indicator.

      (1) **The Rule of Nines** is the easiest way to estimate the extent of burn in adults: The head and neck constitute 9% of the total body surface area; each upper extremity constitutes 9%; the anterior trunk, 18%; the posterior trunk, 18%; each lower extremity, 18%; and the genitalia, 1%. Children have a proportionally larger head and smaller lower extremities. A burn diagram (Fig. 18-1) can be used to obtain a more accurate estimate of the burn size.

      (2) **Depth of burn wounds.** The wound can be classified as partial thickness or full thickness. Partial-thickness (intradermal) injuries appear red or pink, often with blister formation. They heal spontaneously by reepithelialization from the intact skin appendages (hair follicles, sebaceous and sweat glands) if these are not destroyed by subsequent infection. Full-thickness injuries may be charred, or marble gray in color, dry, and anesthetic. Partial-thickness injuries also may be anesthetic because of neuropraxis of nerve endings in the skin after the burn. Thus, the pain response is useful only when it is positive, indicating the presence of a partial-thickness burn.

      (3) **Unburned areas** of the body surface should also be mapped and the extent of the intact skin estimated for two purposes: First, it will serve to check the accuracy of the extent of the burn (The sum of the burned and unburned area should be 100% of the total body surface.) Second, it

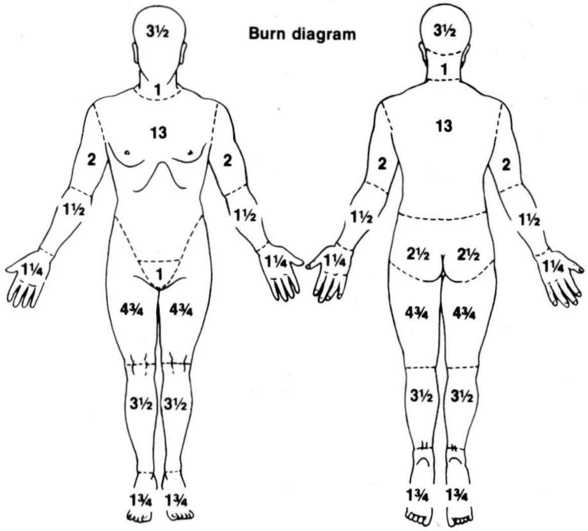

Area	Infant	1-4	5-9	10-14	15	Adult
Head	19	17	13	11	9	7
Neck	2	2	2	2	2	2
A-Trunk	13	13	13	13	13	13
P-Trunk	13	13	13	13	13	13
R-Butt	2½	2½	2½	2½	2½	2½
L-Butt	2½	2½	2½	2½	2½	2½
Genital	1	1	1	1	1	1
R-U-Arm	4	4	4	4	4	4
L-U-Arm	4	4	4	4	4	4
R-L-Arm	3	3	3	3	3	3
L-L-Arm	3	3	3	3	3	3
R-Hand	2½	2½	2½	2½	2½	2½
L-Hand	2½	2½	2½	2½	2½	2½
R-Thigh	5½	6½	8	8½	9	9½
L-Thigh	5½	6½	8	8½	9	9½
R-Leg	5	5	5½	6	6½	7
L-Leg	5	5	5½	6	6½	7
R-Foot	3½	3½	3½	3½	3½	3½
L-Foot	3½	3½	3½	3½	3½	3½

Figure 18-1. Using both the diagram and table, one can estimate the extent of the burn. The table allows for surface area adjustments in younger children.

will help in the planning of staged operations involving multiple auto-grafts.

3. Initial management (in emergency room)

a. Secure the airway.

b. Measure vital signs.

c. Remove the patient's clothing.

d. Start a large-bore intravenous line(s).

e. Start infusing Ringer's lactate.

f. Estimate the extent of the burn.

g. Calculate the fluid requirements.

h. Insert a nasogastric tube (for burns over 25%).

i. Sedate by intravenous medication.

j. Immunize against tetanus.

k. Cover with a clean sheet.

l. Admit or transfer to a burn care facility.

4. Criteria for hospital admission

a. Adults with partial-thickness burns of more than 15% of the total body surface.

b. Children with partial-thickness burns of more than 10% of the total body surface.

c. Adults or children with full-thickness burns of more than 2% of the total body surface.

d. Smoke inhalation with or without cutaneous burns.

e. Burns of the face, both hands, perineum, or both feet.

f. Electrical burns of any size.

B. Fluid resuscitation. There are many options for fluid resuscitation available: crystalloid (Parkland formula), hypertonic saline, and colloid-containing solutions (Brook formula). The most widely accepted of these is the Parkland formula. Since the response of each patient is different, and any formula is only a rough guideline in initiating the resuscitation process, it is more important to monitor the response properly and adjust fluid administration than it is to select any particular formula.

1. Crystalloid resuscitation (Parkland formula)

a. First 24 hr

(1) Ringer's lactate solution (without dextrose): for adults, 4 ml/body weight (kg)/% burn; for children, 3 ml/body weight(kg)/%burn.

(2) Provide 24-hr metabolic water needs as 5% D/W.

(3) Rate of infusion: **first 8 hr**, 50% of the total amount; **second 8 hr**, 25% of the total amount; **third 8 hr**, 25% of the total amount.

(4) No colloid in the first 16–24 hr.

b. Second 24 hr

(1) No sodium-containing solutions if the response has been satisfactory.

(2) Maintenance dose of 5% D/W (metabolic water needs).

(3) Colloid (fresh-frozen plasma or human albumin) to bring the serum albumin level above 3 gm/100 ml

    (4) In children, colloid can be started after 16 hr if the response has not been totally satisfactory.

  c. Third day and thereafter

    (1) As soon as the gastrointestinal (GI) tract has resumed peristaltic activity, oral or tube feedings should be started.

    (2) After capillary permeability returns to normal, edema fluid is reabsorbed by the high oncotic pressure of plasma.

2. Monitoring. The following should be measured repetitively and treatment directed to achieving the goals indicated:

  a. Sensorium: clear.

  b. Vital signs

    (1) Systolic blood pressure above 120 mm Hg in adults.

    (2) Heart rate below 120/min in adults.

    (3) Temperature below 38°C (100.4F).

    (4) Respiratory rate between 12–20/min.

  c. Hourly urinary output above 0.5 ml/kg/hr.

  d. Central venous pressure about 10 cm saline (trend is more important than absolute value).

  e. Blood chemistry (electrolytes, albumin, sugar, blood urea nitrogen, creatinine, etc.) all in normal range.

  f. Arterial blood gases and hemoglobin or hematocrit all in normal range.

  g. With a Swan-Ganz catheter, more sophisticated measurement of pulmonary capillary wedge pressure and cardiac output can be obtained, and more precise fluid titration can be performed. The objective is to optimize oxygen availability to the tissues (see Chap. 12).

  h. Prophylactic digitalization should not be used. Dopamine or other short-acting drugs should be given only after inadequate cardiac contractility is demonstrated with adequate preload (measured by pulmonary capillary wedge pressure).

C. Smoke inhalation

1. Assessment

  a. History of closed-space fire.

  b. Facial burns.

  c. Singed nasal hairs.

  d. Carbonaceous material in the oropharynx.

  e. Signs of acute respiratory distress (stridor, wheezing, etc.).

  f. Measurement of carboxyhemoglobin.

  g. Arterial blood gases.

  h. Chest x-ray.

2. Pathophysiology

  a. Acute functional anemia (excessive carboxyhemoglobin).

  b. Acute upper airway obstruction (edema of oropharyngolarynx).

  c. Early ventilatory support for oxygenation failure.

  d. Vigorous chest physiotherapy.

3. Management

  a. Administration of 100% oxygen for 3 hr or until carboxyhemoglobin is known to be in the safe range.

  b. Careful observation and early intubation to prevent disastrous upper airway obstruction (blood gases and the chest x-ray may be normal!).

  c. Early ventilatory support for oxygenation failure.

  d. Vigorous chest physiotherapy.

D. Escharotomy. Full-thickness burns produce obligatory edema in the subcutaneous tissues, the eschar being nonpermeable to water. Thus, circumferential full-thickness burns can cause vascular compromise with distal gangrene of extremities, or chest wall constriction with impaired ventilation.

  1. Extremities. The color, capillary blanching, and pulses should be carefully followed. Ultrasonic Doppler flow measurements are useful. If there is evidence of impaired blood flow, escharotomy is indicated; it should be performed along the medial and lateral aspects of the extremity (and fingers, if needed).

  2. Chest. If chest wall movement becomes restricted, escharotomy should be done to allow completely unrestricted motion of all portions of the chest wall. All the following incisions must be made: over the clavicles, sternum, bilaterally in the anterior axillary line, and bilaterally along the costal margins (Fig. 18-2).

II. Acute phase This covers the period from resuscitation to completion of wound healing.

A. Wound care

  1. Topical antibacterial agents

    a. Silver sulfadiazine cream

      (1) Broad antimicrobial activity against gram-negative and gram-positive bacteria, as well as yeasts.

      (2) Penetration through eschar is fairly good; eschar separation is somewhat delayed.

      (3) Application is painless, and the patient is soothed.

      (4) Can be used with dressings that then will not adhere and are easily changed without hemorrhage or pain.

      (5) There are no side effects, such as electrolyte imbalance or metabolic acidosis.

      (6) Absolute contraindications

        (a) Term pregnancy, premature infants, newborn infants during the first month of life (because of the possibility of kernicterus).

        (b) Hypersensitivity to silver sulfadiazine.

        (c) Glucose 6-phosphate dehydrogenase deficiency (possible hemolysis).

      (7) Relative contraindications

        (a) It is not known whether or not there is a cross-sensitivity to other sulfonamides.

        (b) Safe use during pregnancy has not been established (can be used if the need for therapeutic benefit is greater than the possible risk to the fetus).

      (8) Apply to a thickness of about $1/16$ in. bid after cleaning the wound.

      (9) In extensive burns, it is advisable to monitor serum sulfur concentrations and renal function and to look for sulfur crystals in the urine.

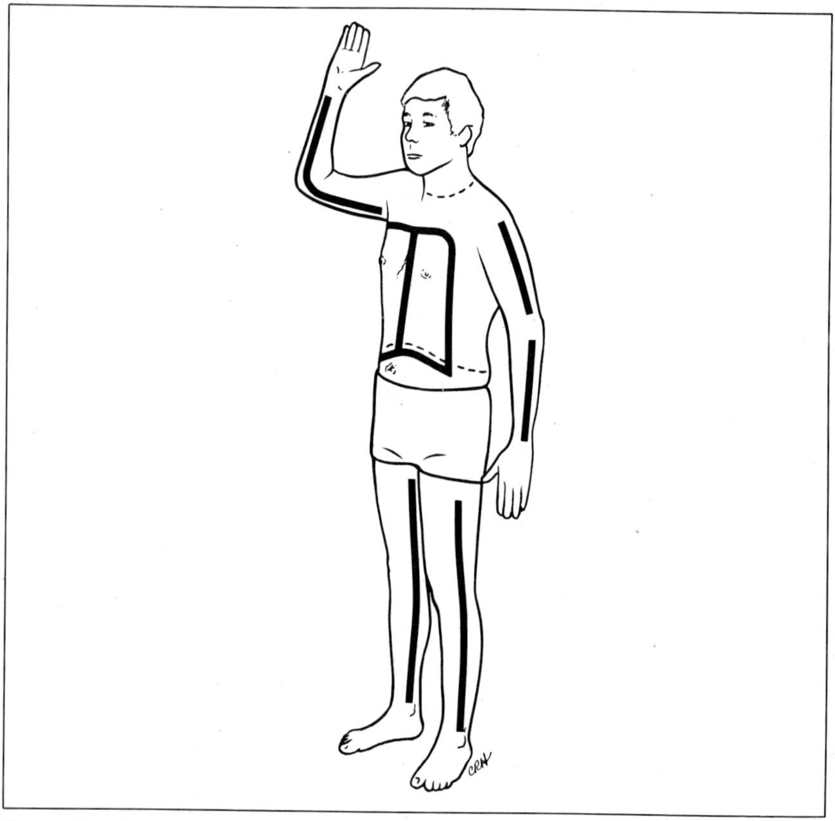

Figure 18-2. Locations for incisions needed to provide adequate decompression of the extremities and adequate expansion of the chest.

    b. Silver nitrate solution (0.5%)

        (1) Broad-spectrum bacteriostatic agent (all the usual pathogens are sensitive in vitro, although some strains of *Enterobacter* and *Klebsiella* require a 1% concentration).

        (2) Penetration through eschar is poor.

        (3) Requires a bulky dressing and continuous (q2h) soaking.

        (4) Electrolyte imbalance (hyponatremia) must be monitored and corrected.

        (5) Methemoglobinemia (usual complication) is dependent on the coexistence of a rare strain of *Enterobacter cloacae*, which converts nitrate to nitrite on the burn wound.

        (6) Elemental silver is not absorbed.

        (7) Discoloration (brown to black staining) of the patient's skin as well as the bed, floor, wall, etc. (silver chloride deposition and exposure to light) is a disadvantage.

2. Initial wound care

    a. On admission, clean the wound with bland soap and water, removing all dirt and loose devitalized tissues.

b. Blisters may be left intact if they are smaller than 5 cm in diameter.

c. Copious amounts of water should be used to clean and irrigate chemical burns. Do not waste time looking for an antidote.

d. In case of chemical burns involving the eyes, irrigate with copious amounts of sterile normal saline (water will increase conjunctival edema because of hypotonicity).

e. When burns involve the scalp, axilla, and pubic area, the hair should be shaved until an adequate margin of unburned skin is obtained.

f. After cleaning and initial debridement, apply a topical agent and bulky dressing.

g. Suspend the upper extremity with an IV pole. The elbow should rest on pillows.

h. In hand burns, apply silver sulfadiazine cream and a coarse mesh gauze dressing to each finger individually, with the thumb in abduction.

3. Management of partial-thickness burns

a. If a dry, thick scab has formed without maceration, fluid collection, or hemorrhage underneath, it should be left alone. It serves as a natural protective layer, prevents water evaporation and desiccation of underlying healthy tissue, and retards bacterial seeding. When epithelial healing has taken place underneath, the scab will fall off by itself. A shower or quick tub bath once a day is sufficient for general hygiene and wound-cleaning purposes.

b. When the intermediate-to-deep partial-thickness wound starts separating, the slough can be removed by twice-daily saline or silver sulfadiazine coarse mesh dressings, with or without a brief shower or quick tub bath.

c. Partial-thickness wounds should heal without grafting in about 3 wks.

d. In case of a very deep partial-thickness burn that has not healed by the end of 3 wks, autografting should be performed by the end of the fourth week.

e. For extensive, deep partial-thickness wounds, superficial excision may be performed with a dermatome or free-hand knife (Watson or Goulian) down to the zone of marginal viability. The procedure will not cause significant blood loss if carefully performed. It may be performed at the bedside if general anesthesia is contraindicated. It will remove the bulk of culture media for bacteria, and topical agents then do not have to penetrate through a thick layer of dead tissue.

f. For deep partial-thickness wounds of the dorsum of the hands, primary tangential excision and immediate autografting may be the treatment of choice. This procedure may shorten the time to complete wound healing, and a functionally better result may be obtained.

4. Management of full-thickness wounds

a. Conservative approach

(1) Silvadene occlusive dressings and daily dressing changes in the hydrotherapy tank until the eschar separates.

(2) As the eschar separates, debridement is performed daily.

(3) Split-thickness autografting when the wounds are well granulated.

(4) Disadvantages

(a) Prolonged preoperative period (3–6 wks).

(b) In small (less than 10%) full-thickness burns, the total hospitalization is prolonged.

(c) In larger burns, the patient may develop invasive burn wound sepsis, which carries a high mortality risk.

b. Early excisional approach

(1) As soon as the general condition is stabilized, full-thickness burn wounds may be excised sequentially down to healthy tissue, with immediate autografting.

(2) The amount of excision at one sitting depends on the availability of an experienced surgical team, facility, blood, and other factors.

(3) Advantages

(a) Eliminates the phase of eschar separation, which carries the risk of invasive burn wound sepsis

(b) Shortens the hospitalization for smaller burns.

(4) Disadvantages

(a) Large blood loss.

(b) Additional stress of surgery and anesthesia.

5. Biological and synthetic dressings

a. Advantages

(1) Reduction in evaporative water loss.

(2) Reduction in electrolyte and protein losses.

(3) Prevention of desiccation of underlying tissue.

(4) Suppression of bacterial proliferation.

(5) Stimulation of healing (reepithelialization) of partial-thickness burns.

(6) Reduction of wound pain, with consequent improvement in the movement of involved joints.

b. Homograft

(1) When applied on freshly excised wounds, a homograft may achieve temporary physiological wound closure (until rejection). It may provide time for a donor site to heal for reharvesting, while protecting the portion of the excised wound that might not have been covered with the autograft because of extensive full-thickness injury.

(2) May be used for testing of a granulating wound for readiness for autografting.

c. Synthetic dressings of several varieties have been produced in recent years, but their clinical usefulness remains to be established.

B. Nutritional support is a crucial factor in the care of a burn patient. The nutritional requirements for any given patient depend not only on the extent and condition of the burn but also on the patient's age, prior state of nutrition, and whether or not there are any metabolic or organic disorders. The patient who has sustained thermal injury is very different from other surgical patients in metabolic function and nutritional requirements.

1. Altered metabolism and nutritional needs of the burn patient. The metabolic rate can increase 100–120% above normal, depending on the extent of the burn injury. There is little opportunity to achieve adequate nutritional intake during the first week after injury, since fluid and electrolyte balance takes priority. In addition, gastrointestinal changes associated with the burn injury preclude normal oral alimentation during the first few days.

a. Fluid and oral electrolytes should be calculated by taking into account the patient's daily maintenance requirements, loss through the burn wound, loss due to elevated body temperature, and GI losses (nasogastric suction, vomiting, and diarrhea) (see Chap. 9).

b. **Calories.** The formula developed by Curreri can be used to estimate caloric requirements for burn patients:

Adult 25 kcal/kg body weight + 40 kcal/%burn
Child 35 kcal/kg body weight + 60 kcal/%burn

c. **Nitrogen.** Following major thermal injury, the loss of body protein, as evidenced by increased urine nitrogen, increases the daily protein needs by two to four times the amount required prior to injury (1.6–3.2 gm nitrogen/kg body weight). The calorie-nitrogen ratio is thought to be optimal at 130–150 kcal/gm nitrogen.

d. **Vitamins and trace elements.** Mere intake of food does not guarantee that the body will utilize the nutrients to the best advantage. A number of enzyme systems are deranged in the initial hypermetabolic state; these enzymes depend for their integrity on certain vitamins, particularly A, B complex, C, K, and folate. In addition, care must be taken to maintain normal levels of zinc, calcium, magnesium, and phosphorous.

2. **Methods of nutritional support**

   a. **Intravenous hyperalimentation**

      (1) **Peripheral vein.** 10% dextrose with 3.5% l-amino acids plus Intralipid, 10% (should be limited so that the fat source is only 25–30% of total calories).

      (2) **Central vein.** The details of catheter insertion and monitoring can be found elsewhere in this text (see Chaps. 10 and 25). Because of the exceedingly high frequency of catheter-related sepsis in burn patients, this type of alimentation should be reserved for those with severe burns whose caloric requirements cannot be met through the oral, enteral, or peripheral vein routes.

   b. **Enteral.** A number of enteral preparations are currently available. The calorie-nitrogen ratio and osmolarity should be noted prior to the selection of a particular diet. Continuous drip feeding given by nasogastric or nasojejunal tube is preferable to bolus feedings and will be better tolerated by the patient with fewer GI and biochemical complications. Situations in which enteral feeding is appropriate include the following:

      (1) A burn greater than 20%.

      (2) As a dietary supplement in patients with less than a 20% burn.

      (3) A patient unable or unwilling to take an adequate diet.

      (4) In endotracheal intubation or in unconscious patients (measure the gastric residue frequently).

   c. **Oral.** All patients who can consume and tolerate food orally should be started on an oral diet. Most patients with less than a 15% burn can be supported adequately on oral intake alone. Specifically, these patients should have a high-calorie, high-nitrogen diet. Oral supplements are given as needed to improve the calorie and nitrogen intake.

III. Complications of burns

A. Septic complications

1. **Invasive burn wound sepsis**

   a. **Definition.** Invasion of viable subeschar tissue by microorganisms.

   b. **Signs and symptoms.** Mental confusion, ileus, hypothermia, hemorrhagic spots within the burn wound, tachycardia, hypotension, and other signs of sepsis.

c. Diagnosis. Quantitative culture of biopsy specimen, including subjacent tissue (more than 100,000 bacteria/gm of tissue), and histological evidence of bacterial invasion.

d. Treatment. Excision of the involved wound. Ideally, the wound should have been excised before invasive burn wound sepsis developed. Therefore, frequent, careful inspection of the burn wound is critical in timing the excisional procedure.

e. The **prognosis** is extremely poor (mortality over 95% once invasive burn wound sepsis is established).

2. Suppurative thrombophlebitis

a. Occurs in 5% of burn patients (most often in the lower extremities).

b. The incidence is directly related to the duration of intravenous cannulation.

c. *Staphylococcus* is the most frequently recovered single organism.

d. The diagnosis is confirmed by the presence of intraluminal purulence.

e. Treatment is by excision of the entire length of involved vein.

B. Gastrointestinal complications

1. Ileus

a. Very common immediately following injury if the burn is over 25%. It usually resolves in 3–5 days.

b. Recurrence usually is a manifestation of sepsis. Ileus and gastric dilation may be the first clinical signs of sepsis.

c. When an ileus develops acutely, the patient may become hypovolemic because of a large volume of third-space fluid sequestration.

d. The gastric residue should be measured frequently, especially in patients receiving gastric tube feeding.

e. Check peritoneal signs and x-rays, to rule out an unrecognized acute abdominal disorder (e.g., perforated duodenal ulcer).

2. Gastroduodenal hemorrhage (Curling's ulcer)

a. Approximately 12% of burn patients develop upper GI tract hemorrhage from stress ulceration.

b. Mucosal erosions or sharply punched-out ulcerations without surrounding chronic inflammation predominate.

c. Endoscopic evaluation is the best means of diagnosis and localization.

d. Perforation can occur (in approximately 10% of patients) with Curling's ulcer, although it is more rare than the hemorrhagic complications.

e. The prophylactic use of cimetidine and antacids should be considered.

f. Initial nonoperative management and indications for surgical intervention are essentially the same as those for hemorrhage from peptic ulcer disease of the duodenum (see Chap. 6).

g. The operation of choice is vagotomy and resection.

C. Scarring and contracture of the burn wound

1. Pathophysiology

a. The process of burn wound healing, with a marked increase in vascularity, fibroblasts, myofibroblasts, collagen deposition, interstitial material, and edema, is conducive to the formation of hypertrophic scars and contractures.

   b. The burn wound will shorten because of the contractile force of the myofibroblasts.

   c. The position of comfort for the joint is the position of contracture, because the new collagen fibers will fuse together in that position.

2. Prevention

   a. Proper positioning of each joint.

   b. Splinting.

   c. Active and passive exercise to maintain full range of motion.

   d. Skeletal traction if necessary in the postgrafting period.

   e. Pressure dressing (more than 25 mm Hg) after completion of wound healing.

3. Late surgical correction

   a. Wait until after the scar has lost its activity and matured.

   b. Procedures (e.g., Z-plasty, rotational flap, excision and grafting) must be tailored to the individual and depend on the location and type of scar present.

   c. Late correction must be followed by an adequate combination of preventive measures, as described in **2**.

IV. Miscellaneous

A. Electrical injury

   1. The superficial appearance is deceptive; there is more extensive deep soft tissue damage.

   2. Check the electrocardiogram for cardiac irregularities.

   3. Initial fluid resuscitation may be begun by calculation according to the surface injury, but much more fluid is often required.

   4. Keep the urinary output at 1.0–1.5 ml/kg/hr to prevent renal tubular damage. Use mannitol if necessary. Sodium bicarbonate can be used to alkalinize the urine and may prevent the complications of hemoglobinuria and myoglobinuria.

   5. Monitor arterial blood gases, especially pH.

   6. Watch for edema. Escharotomy or fasciotomy may be needed.

   7. Watch for hemorrhage when necrotic tissue over blood vessels sloughs.

   8. Early debridement or excision, in multiple stages if necessary, helps control infection.

   9. Watch for such late complications as convulsions and cataracts.

B. Management of minor burns

   1. Small burns may be managed in an office or outpatient facility.

   2. The wound is cleaned with bland soap and water.

   3. Small blisters may be left intact.

   4. The wound may be left open if it is on an extremity, washing it twice a day. It may be covered with a nonadherent material (petrolatum gauze or Xeroform) and then further covered with dry gauze to provide protection and comfort.

   5. No prophylactic systemic or topical antimicrobial agents are necessary. If they are needed, the patient needs hospitalization.

Suggested Reading

Artz, C. P., Moncrief, J. A., and Pruitt, B. A. *Burns: A team approach*. Philadelphia: Saunders, 1979.

Pruitt, B. A. The burn patient: I. Initial care. *Curr. Probl. Surg.* 16:April 1979.

Pruitt, B. A. The burn patient: II. Later care and complications of thermal injury. *Curr. Probl. Surg.* 16:May 1979.

Shires, G. T., and Black, E. A. Consensus development conference: Supportive therapy in burn care. *J. Trauma* 19:855, 1979.

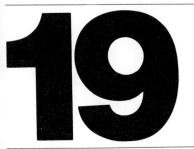 **Pediatric Surgery**

Recent advances in the management of the pediatric patient—especially the neonate—such as blood gas monitoring, respiratory support by mechanical ventilators, total parenteral nutrition, better heat control with Servo-Control beds and Isolettes, improved surgical techniques, and better understanding of neonatal pathophysiology have greatly increased the survival rate of neonates and children with major, potentially fatal congenital anomalies, malignant tumors, surgical infections, and traumas. Just as important are improved techniques in anesthesia and the increasing number of pediatric anesthesiologists.

I. General considerations. During the first 4–6 days of life, the full-term infant is particularly hardy and will withstand a major operation well, provided the unique physiology of the infant is taken into account.

A. Fluids and electrolytes

1. Because of high total body water content (700 ml/kg body weight; blood volume 88 ml/kg), the newborn infant needs minimal maintenance fluids during the first days of life.

2. Beyond the immediate postnatal period, infants normally exchange water and metabolites rapidly. Abnormal losses through the GI tract may result in dehydration and electrolyte depletion within a few hours. Replacement of these losses is calculated by reference to Table 19-1.

3. Fluid administration during an operation should be no more than 5 ml/kg/hr, up to a maximum of 15 ml/kg.

4. As a rule, the use of 10% dextrose in 0.2 normal saline, with adequate potassium, as shown in Table 19-2, is sufficient for maintenance fluid and electrolyte therapy.

5. IV fluid orders for children are written on an hourly basis and should be reviewed and changed if necessary q4h in a critically ill patient.

6. Fluid deficit is estimated by observation of (a) body weight, (b) tissue turgor, (c) sunken eyes, (d) mucous membrane moisture, (e) quality of pulse, and (f) urine output. An infant in shock from dehydration, blood loss, or sepsis will be pale, listless, and hypothermic.

7. Blood volume must be expanded rapidly in severely dehydrated infants, using plasma, electrolyte solution, or blood; 20 ml/kg can be safely "pushed" rapidly IV. Further therapy is calculated by estimation of the degree of dehydration and observation of improvement of the infant measured by pulse, respiration, skin color, urine output, electrolytes, and weight.

8. Losses from suction, fistulas, or diarrhea are measured q4h and replaced promptly.

9. Parenteral alimentation. An infant or child who needs IV fluids for more than 1 wk (e.g., chronic ileus, obstruction, sepsis), one in whom protein losses will continue for an indefinite period (e.g., fistulas, peritonitis, burns, ileitis), or an infant recently operated on in whom these conditions are apt to occur (e.g.,

Table 19-1. Composition of Abnormal External Fluid Losses in Infants

Fluid	Sodium (mEq/liter)	Potassium (mEq/liter)	Chloride (mEq/liter)	Protein (gm/100 ml)
Gastric	50	10	100–150	. . .
Pancreatic	130	10–15	90–120	. . .
Small intestinal	120	5–15	90–120	. . .
Bile	130	5–15	90–120	. . .
Ileostomy	100–300	5–15	50–100	. . .
Diarrhea	10–90	10–80	20–100	. . .
Sweat				
Normal	10–30	3–10	10–35	. . .
Cystic fibrosis	50–130	5–25	50–110	. . .
Burns	140	5	110	3–5

gastroschisis, massive intestinal resection) is started on parenteral hyperalimentation to reduce protein depletion and susceptibility to infection.

    a. A Silastic IV catheter is inserted into the superior vena cava via the jugular or subclavian vein. Enough protein, nonprotein calories, electrolytes, vitamins, and minerals are given to maintain positive nitrogen balance and to replace previous and continuing losses. Maintenance of asepsis in the infusion system is of critical importance.

    b. Total parenteral nutrition can now be achieved by administration of 10% dextrose, together with proteins, vitamins, electrolytes, and minerals, given by the peripheral route and supplemented with 10% Intralipid solution. This supplies adequate nutrition and obviates the chance of infection associated with central hyperalimentation.

10. Plasma or albumin is used more frequently in infants and small children than in adults for conditions such as shock, sepsis, and burns. Plasma loss is tolerated poorly by infants, owing to their rapid metabolic rate and relatively large body surface area. Albumin maintains colloidal osmotic pressure. There is suggestive evidence that plasma proteins are utilized for nutrition to a greater extent than in adults. Albumin usually is replaced in amounts of 10–20 mg/kg/day, but amounts of 50–75 mg/kg/day have been given in severe situations.

11. Blood replacement is necessary when there is acute or chronic blood loss.

    a. Normal blood volumes are: infant, 85 ml/kg; child, 75 ml/kg.

    b. Acute blood loss is replaced in appropriate amounts to maintain normal vital signs, good skin color, normal temperature, and alertness and to restore a normal blood count.

    c. Chronic blood loss in newborns is replaced when hemoglobin drops below 8 gm/100 ml. Replacing blood at higher levels suppresses the normal bone marrow response of newborns, who have physiological hemolysis in the first week of life.

    d. Chronic blood loss in older infants and children is replaced when the hemoglobin drops below 9 gm/100 ml. Anemic patients are susceptible to infection, their wounds heal poorly, they do not feel well, and they eat poorly. Packed red cells, 10–15 ml/kg, are given slowly, followed by a blood count. Since infants often are severely vasoconstricted, they may need more blood than originally estimated.

Table 19-2. Maintenance IV Fluid Therapy (Newborn and Older Children)

Condition and Weight	Water (ml/kg/24 hr)	Calories (Cal/kg/24 hr)	Sodium (mEq/kg/24 hr)	Potassium (mEq/kg/24 hr)	Chloride (mEq/kg/24 hr)	Expected Urine Output (ml/kg/24 hr)
Newborn						
<1000 gm Average	150	50	3	1	3	30 ml total in first 24 hr
1000–1500 gm Average	120	100	3.5	1	3.5	50–100
1500–2500 gm Average	100	100–110	3.5	1–1.5	3.5	50–100
Older infants						
1–10 kg	100	100	3.5	1–1.5	3.5	50–100
11–20 kg	1000 ml + 50 ml/kg for wt > 10 kg	1000 Cal + 50 Cal/kg for wt > 10 kg	…	…	…	…
21 kg and over	1500 ml + 20 ml/kg for wt > 20 kg	1500 Cal + 20 Cal/kg for wt > 20 kg	…	…	…	…

12. Hypoglycemia is a frequent problem in newborn infants following trauma, operation, or sepsis. Blood sugar is measured whenever irritability, twitching, or convulsions occur. Postoperatively, neonates are maintained on a 10% glucose solution for several days to prevent hypoglycemia.

13. Hypocalcemia: a serum calcium concentration below 7 mg/100 ml requires treatment with an IV drip of 200 mg calcium gluconate/kg/day, with one fourth the total given in the first 30–60 min.

B. Temperature control

1. Hypothermia may develop rapidly, particularly in premature infants. Infants respond to cooling with increased heat production, but their relatively large surface area and minimal subcutaneous fat permit excessive heat loss.

   a. Shock, sepsis, anesthesia, and application of surgical preparation solutions accentuate heat loss.

   b. Hypothermia produces increased oxygen need; if not corrected, it results in acidosis, hypoglycemia, and hyperkalemia.

   c. If severe hypothermia is present postoperatively, respiratory depression or arrest may occur.

   d. An incubator set at 32°C (90°F) is used during diagnostic and therapeutic procedures in premature infants.

   e. During operation, warming pad is used, and the temperature is monitored; skin preparation is limited and is followed by prompt draping.

2. Sudden hyperthermia under anesthesia, leading to convulsions, is potentially fatal. All-out efforts (e.g., iced alcohol bath) to reduce the temperature are indicated. Most commonly, hyperthermia occurs in a febrile infant whose dehydration was inadequately corrected preoperatively; in rare instances, hyperthermia occurs without clues to its cause. Adequate attention to preoperative rehydration and to reduction of fever and tachycardia decreases the incidence and severity of this problem.

C. Respiratory problems

1. The airway of an infant is small, the tidal volume may be only 15 ml, and the upper airway dead space is proportionately large (2 ml/kg). Thus, the infant has a narrow margin of respiratory reserve.

2. Small amounts of laryngeal edema or mucus may cause serious obstruction. Attempts to compensate through tachypnea soon result in fatigue and combined respiratory and metabolic acidosis.

3. *Never restrain an infant flat on his or her back*; the hazard of aspirating saliva or vomitus is great.

4. Every half hour postoperatively, **change the infant's position**, and stimulate a cry and cough with pharyngeal suctioning. Direct tracheal suctioning with use of a laryngoscope sometimes may be necessary.

5. High humidity generated by an ultrasonic nebulizer is effective in thinning tracheobronchial secretions and reduces insensible water loss. Ultrasonic nebulization requires special monitoring in premature infants. Infants may "soak up" water in a humid atmosphere and develop water intoxication. **Weigh** the infant periodically and use **ultrasonic nebulization** intermittently.

6. Laryngeal edema following prolonged endotracheal intubation may result in hoarseness or stridor. This is treated with humidification and parenteral corticosteroid therapy. Skillful use of a **Silastic endotracheal tube** may obviate the need for tracheostomy.

7. Tracheostomy is performed for retraction, restlessness, or air hunger that cannot be managed by intubation.

Table 19-3. Endotracheal Tube Sizes for Infants, According to Age

Age	Internal Diameter (mm)
Small newborn	3.0
Large newborn	3.5
6–24 months	4.0
24–36 months	4.5
4 years	5.0
5 years	5.5
6 and 7 years	6.0
8 and 9 years	6.5
10 and 11 years	7.0
12 and 13 years	7.5
14 and 15 years	8.0
16 and beyond	8.5

  a. Tracheostomy in a small infant is a difficult procedure and must be done with adequate exposure, assistance, and equipment in the operating room. Passage of an endotracheal tube allows control of the airway and facilitates location of the small, soft trachea.

  b. Ordinary silver tracheostomy tubes are not suitable for small infants because they often are too long, occlude the carina, and have a high-resistance narrow bore. (Table 19-3 shows endotracheal tube sizes.) Plastic or Silastic tubes can be cut to the appropriate length and are well tolerated.

  c. If respiratory distress occurs after a tracheostomy, immediately take a chest x-ray to rule out pneumothorax or pneumomediastinum.

D. Gastrointestinal tract

  1. A newborn infant normally passes a large meconium stool within the first few hours of life. Swallowed air reaches the rectum within 12–18 hr; a prolongation of this time is expected in premature infants and in any infant who has an anoxic episode during delivery. Plain x-rays of the abdomen normally demonstrate the presence of gas throughout the gastrointestinal (GI) tract. Paucity of gas shadows and dilated loops of bowel with evidence of air or fluid should alert the examiner to possible mechanical bowel obstruction or abdominal masses.

  2. Infants under 1 yr of age swallow a considerable amount of air during feedings and sucking; it is normal to see air in the small intestine on abdominal x-rays.

  3. Hypoglycemia resulting from a prolonged period during which the patient takes nothing PO may result in irritability, twitching, or convulsions. IV fluids should be started in any infant in whom absence of oral intake is required for more than 3 hr.

E. Indications for antibiotics. See Table 19-4.

  1. Sepsis, suspected sepsis, peritonitis, pneumonitis, meningitis, and wound infections.

  2. Thoracic and cardiac operations, intestinal resection or anastomosis, gastroschisis and ruptured omphalocele, and genitourinary procedures when infection is present.

  3. Patient on a respirator.

  4. Prophylaxis preoperatively in rheumatic heart disease, cystic fibrosis, and immunological disorders (e.g., Wiskott-Aldrich syndrome, agammaglobulinemia).

  5. Antibiotics are not used routinely in full-term healthy infants undergoing clean upper abdominal operations (e.g., duodenal obstruction), repair of unruptured omphalocele with primary closure, gastrostomy, nephrectomy, or resection of intra-abdominal cysts and tumors.

Table 19-4. Antimicrobial Drugs Frequently Used in Pediatric Surgery

Drug	Dosage	Comments
Aqueous penicillin	Newborn: 60,000 units/kg/ day IV q12h Older infant: 25,000–50,000 units/kg/day IV or IM q4–6 h	Single most useful agent for gram-positive cocci and enterococci.
Ampicillin	50–200 mg/kg/day IV or IM q4–6h (oral use causes diarrhea in very young)	Gram-positive cocci, **Hemophilus influenzae**, some strains of **Escherichia coli**, salmonella, shigella; use with kanamycin or gentamicin in sepsis and peritonitis.
Cephalothin	50–100 mg/kg/day IV or IM (painful) q4–6h	Gram-positive cocci, including coagulase-positive staphylococci, **E. coli, Klebsiella, Proteus mirabilis**; use with kanamycin or gentamicin in sepsis and peritonitis.
Methicillin	100–200 mg/kg/day IV or IM q4–6h	Coagulase-positive staphylococci.
Oxacillin	50–100 mg/kg/day PO q6h	Coagulase-positive staphylococci.
Kanamycin	15 mg/kg/day IM q12h	Many gram-negative organisms except **Pseudomonas**; use with penicillin or ampicillin.
Gentamicin	Premature and first 5 days of life: 3–5 mg/kg/day IV or IM q12h After 5 days of life: 3–7.5 mg/ kg/day IV or IM q8h	**Pseudomonas**, gram-negative rods, gram-positive cocci; use with penicillin or ampicillin in sepsis and peritonitis.
Erythromycin	25–40 mg/kg/day PO	Use in patients allergic to penicillin.
Clindamycin	10–40 mg/kg/day IV or IM q6h	Primary drug for **Bacteroides** infections.
Chloramphenicol	50–100 mg/kg/day IV q6h	Use in life-threatening infections when another effective drug not available.
Ticarcillin disodium	Neonates, first week: 75 mg/kg IM or IV q6h; after 1 week, 600 mg/kg/day q4h. Infants: 200–300 mg/kg/day IV or IM q4–6h	**Pseudomonas** infections.
Neomycin	50–100 mg/kg/day PO in 6 divided doses	Bowel preparation; necrotizing enterocolitis in newborn.
Sulfisoxazole	150–180 mg/kg/day PO q4–6h; 100 mg/kg/day IV or IM q8–12h	Do not use in patients under 2 mo of age; urinary tract infections.
Nitrofurantoin	6 mg/kg/day PO q6h	Urinary tract infections.
Nystatin	2 ml (200,000 units) PO qid	Oral **Candida** infections (thrush).

II. Surgical conditions in the newborn

A. Airway or pulmonary emergencies. See Tables 19-5 and 19-6.

1. Cyanosis with tachypnea, dyspnea, stridor, intercostal retraction, or nasal flaring is cause for alarm and indicates a need for prompt diagnosis and treatment.

2. **Diagnosis of an airway problem** involves the following routine:

   a. Place the infant in an Isolette with oxygen and high humidity. Start 10% glucose in water IV. Oral and tracheal suctioning is used as necessary. With respiratory arrest or pending arrest, the infant requires assisted ventilation.

   b. Observe the infant's breathing pattern. Measure vital signs. Auscultate the chest. Examine the head, neck, abdomen, and neurological system.

   c. Pass a catheter into each nostril and down the esophagus into the stomach.

   d. Take a portable upright chest x-ray including the abdomen.

   e. Measure blood gases and do a complete blood count. Correct severe acidosis with sodium bicarbonate.

   f. Electrolyte, blood urea nitrogen, blood sugar, calcium, and bilirubin determinations are obtained, and an electrocardiogram is done if indicated.

   g. Blood, cord, and tracheal cultures are obtained.

   h. A careful review of the family history and the course of the mother's pregnancy, labor, and delivery is obtained.

   i. The diagnosis is usually obvious by this time unless an unusual cardiac or vascular lesion is present. Cardiac catheterization and urgent surgical therapy may be necessary.

3. **Esophageal atresia** with or without a tracheoesophageal fistula is suspected when excessive salivation is present at birth and persists. Feedings produce coughing, choking, or cyanosis. A catheter passed into the nares meets an obstruction 8–10 cm from the lips and will not pass into the stomach. A chest x-ray demonstrates the catheter in the neck and upper chest. Air injected through the catheter in most instances outlines the proximal atretic pouch. The catheter should be irrigated every hour with normal saline and placed on constant suction to aspirate saliva. Air in the GI tract confirms the presence of an associated tracheoesophageal fistula. The absence of air suggests atresia without a fistula.

   The infant should be placed in a semisitting position. A small constant suction catheter is placed in the proximal esophageal pouch to remove saliva. Humidity, oxygen, and antibiotics are used to treat pulmonary infection. An operation is performed as soon as pulmonary sepsis has cleared.

4. **Diaphragmatic hernia** is particularly serious in an infant because the mediastinum is mobile and readily displaced, causing severe respiratory and circulatory embarrassment.

   a. Suspect a diaphragmatic hernia in a newborn with respiratory distress, a scaphoid abdomen, and a shifted apical cardiac impulse. A chest x-ray will demonstrate air-filled loops of intestine in the pleural cavity, with mediastinal displacement. Rarely, this lesion may be confused with a congenital lung cyst.

   b. If the patient is cyanotic and dyspneic, an endotracheal tube is inserted and respiration assisted with gentle positive pressure, no greater than 10–15 cm H_2O. The patient usually has both metabolic and respiratory acidosis. An attempt at resuscitation should be made, and immediate surgical repair

Table 19-5. Respiratory Distress in the Newborn

Condition	Symptoms	Physical Findings	X-ray Findings	Comments
Airway obstruction				
Choanal atresia	Apnea and cyanosis at rest, relieved with crying	Catheter will not pass nose.		Early operative correction.
Pierre-Robin syndrome	Retraction, choking with feedings	Small jaw, midline cleft palate, retrodisplaced tongue.		Prone position, tube feeding.
Lingual thyroid or cyst	Tachypnea, retraction	Palpable mass at base of tongue, head retracted.		May need temporary tracheostomy; excise mass.
Macroglossia	Noisy obstructive breathing	Large tongue (actual) or small mouth.		Suspect Down's syndrome, cretinism, Beckwith's syndrome. Treat primary condition; partial glossectomy occasionally required.
Vocal cord paralysis	Tachypnea, retraction, stridor, poor cry	Laryngoscopy is diagnostic.		Tracheostomy if bilateral.
Subglottic stenosis	Wheeze, poor cry, retraction	May be visible on laryngoscopy.	Stenosis seen on xeroradiograms of neck	Tracheostomy, dilation, endoscopic cautery or laser resection.
Vascular ring	Wheezing, choking on feeding	Head may be retracted.	Indented esophagus on barium swallow, aortography	Divide anomalous artery.
Neck mass (cystic hygroma, hemangioma)	Tachypnea, retraction, stridor, poor cry	Laryngoscopy is diagnostic.		Excision.
Esophageal atresia, with or without tracheoesophageal fistula	Choking on feeding, excessive salivation	Unable to pass nasogastric tube into stomach.	Blind pouch (contrast medium); gas in stomach with fistula	Repair.

Tension lesions (pulmonary displacement)

Pneumothorax	Progressively severe tachypnea, cyanosis, tachycardia, retraction	Absent breath sounds, mediastinal shift.	No lung markings on affected side	Needle aspiration; may need chest tube if condition persists after aspiration.
Pneumomediastinum	Complication of ventilator therapy, cyanosis	May have subcutaneous emphysema.	Air in mediastinum, pericardium	May need pericardiocentesis.
Pneumopericardium	Same as above	Muffled heart sounds.	Same as above.	Same as above.
Pneumoperitoneum	Increasing abdominal distention; complication of ventilator therapy	Abdomen distended, but not tense.	Free air in peritoneum	Needle aspiration. *Must be distinguished from necrotizing enterocolitis* (see Table 19-10) or *perforation of GI tract*.
Diaphragmatic hernia	Severe dyspnea, tachypnea, cyanosis, tachycardia, retraction	Scaphoid abdomen; no breath sounds on side of hernia.	Intestine in chest on affected side	Nasogastric tube; endotracheal tube with positive pressure; O_2, IV $NaHCO_3$; immediate operation.
Congenital lung cyst; lobar emphysema	Same as above	Mediastinal shift.	Radiolucency, possibly with air-fluid level on affected side	Thoracotomy and excision (lobectomy)
Empyema or pyopneumothorax	Same as above	Fever, absent breath sounds, dullness.	Opacity or air-fluid level	Diagnostic thoracocentesis, then chest tube; specific antibiotics (organism usually *Staphylococcus*)
Eventration of diaphragm	Same as above	Dullness, absent breath sounds on affected side.	Elevated diaphragm	Thoracotomy and repair if condition is severe.

Table 19-5 (Continued)

Condition	Symptoms	Physical Findings	X-ray Findings	Comments
Pulmonary insufficiency				
Atelectasis or pneumonia	Progressively severe tachypnea, cyanosis, tachycardia, retraction	Dullness, absent breath sounds on affected side.	Opacification of involved lung	Tracheal suction, antibiotics, humidity.
Hyaline membrane disease	Same as above	Rales, rhonchi, diminished breath sounds.	Ground-glass appearance, air bronchograms	Same as above; may need assisted ventilation; measure blood gases as needed.
Wilson-Mikity syndrome	Same as above	Same as above.	Same as above	Same as above; appears after prolonged course of respiratory distress and oxygen therapy.
Cardiac failure	Same as above	Same as above.	Rales, enlarging liver, diminished urinary output, edema	Digitalis, diuretics; cardiac surgery may be necessary.
Abdominal distention (e.g., intestinal obstruction, peritonitis, sepsis, paralytic ileus)	Respiratory distress with grunting respirations; vomiting bile	Abdominal distention; scanty diarrheal stools or obstipation.	Elevated diaphragm; dilated loops of intestine with air-fluid levels	Antibiotics, nasogastric tube; fluid replacement; operation, if indicated.

Table 19-6. Drugs Frequently Utilized in Cardiopulmonary Resuscitation in Children

1. Sodium bicarbonate: several vials, 1 mEq/ml (usual initial dose 2–4 mEq/kg repeated q10 min until arterial pH is measured)
2. Epinephrine: several vials, 1:10,000 concentration, 0.1 mg/ml (usual dose 0.1 ml/kg by IV push)
3. Isoproterenol: 0.2–0.4 mg/100 ml (usual initial dose 1–2 ml, then continuous slow infusion)
4. Calcium chloride: 10% concentration, 100 mg/ml (usual dose 0.2 ml/kg)
5. Solutions: 5% serum albumin, 6% dextran (70,000 daltons), 10% dextran (40,000 molecular weight), Ringer's lactate, normal saline, dextrose, and water

Source: R. L. Replogle and H. M. Reyes. Management of Trauma and Shock in the Pediatric Patient. In C. A. Smith (ed.), *The Critically Ill Child: Diagnosis and Management* (2nd ed.). Philadelphia: Saunders, 1977.

is required. An abdominal approach is preferred. The viscera are reduced into the abdomen, the diaphragm is repaired, and any rotational anomaly of the intestine is corrected.

B. Intestinal obstruction in the newborn

1. Any infant who **vomits bile-stained material** in the first days of life has intestinal obstruction unless it can be absolutely ruled out.

2. Failure to pass normal meconium stool, passage of bloody stool, and abdominal distention are other features strongly suggestive of intestinal obstruction in a newborn.

3. If intestinal obstruction is suspected, a systematic plan of diagnosis should be followed.

   a. Pass a **nasogastric tube**, and note the amount and character of the aspirate.

   b. Do a complete **physical examination**, including a rectal examination. The history and physical findings may suggest a cause other than obstruction (e.g., sepsis, birth anoxia, hypothyroidism, or intracranial hemorrhage) for which an appropriate workup is done.

   c. Begin **IV fluids** calculated to include fluid sequestered in the intestine. Determination of electrolyte and acid-base balance is made.

   d. Obtain a **flat plate of the abdomen** and **upright x-rays of the abdomen and chest**. If air is seen only in the stomach or duodenum but not more distally, duodenal atresia, tight duodenal stenosis, or a rotational abnormality with midgut volvulus is present. Prompt operation is indicated without further studies.

   e. If distention is present and x-rays show multiple intestinal loops with air-fluid levels, a gentle **barium study of the colon** is indicated.

      (1) A tiny unused colon seen on contrast enema indicates small-bowel obstruction due to atresia, stenosis, meconium ileus, or, rarely, an internal hernia. Urgent exploration is indicated except in meconium ileus, which may be treated by Gastrografin enemas.

      (2) A normal or slightly distended colon may indicate congenital aganglionosis, meconium plug syndrome or, rarely, a rectal or low colonic stenosis, or a condition not requiring operation. The surgical conditions in which a normal or dilated colon is present do not require urgent operative correction. Meconium plugs commonly pass when the barium is expelled. Hirschprung's disease and its accompanying obstructive

symptoms can be controlled by saline irrigation of the colon; a colostomy and biopsy confirmation of the diagnosis is performed electively. Low colonic or rectal stenosis may be amenable to dilation; if not, an operation can be done electively.

C. Anorectal malformation

1. Careful **inspection** of the perineum and genitalia provides correct diagnosis of most anomalies.

2. The critical decision in the newborn is to determine if the anomaly is a "low" or a "high" lesion.

3. **Low lesions in boys** invariably have a fistula opening in the midline of the perineum, either at the usual site of the anus or anterior to it. A limited anoplasty in the newborn period, followed by persistent dilations for a month or more, provides good results.

4. **Low lesions in girls** usually present with a fistula to the perineum or to the vaginal fourchette. Dilation usually is adequate initial treatment, although a limited "cutback" procedure may be necessary to give a functionally adequate although ectopic opening. The decision about a later procedure to place the anus in a normal position need not be made until the child is 4–6 yr of age.

5. When no perineal fistula is present in boys, the likelihood is great that the lesion is a high one. With high lesions, a fistula into the urethra or, rarely, into the bladder, is always present.

6. After 24 hr of age—longer if required for the abdomen to begin to show mild distention—**inverted lateral x-rays** help to define the level of the anomaly. High lesions are indicated by gas only above a line drawn from the pubis to the sacrococcygeal junction.

7. In high lesions a **colostomy** is indicated. Definitive reconstruction is technically difficult and is best done when the child is between the ages of 18 and 24 mo.

D. Abdominal wall defects

1. **Omphalocele** is the result of embryonic arrest during the period when the GI tract is herniated into the umbilical cord. The clinical presentation is a mass of viscera herniated through the umbilical ring and covered by a membranous sac.

2. Small omphaloceles will close spontaneously if kept protected and painted several times with 0.5% silver nitrate solution. Early operation is also satisfactory if no concurrent problems exist, e.g., prematurity, severe congenital anomaly (especially cardiac), pulmonary problems, or sepsis.

3. Large omphaloceles are more difficult problems. The abdominal cavity is underdeveloped; forceful return of the viscera and complete closure of the abdomen may elevate abdominal pressure, resulting in respiratory insufficiency, impaired venous return, and even compromised circulation to the intestine. **Immediate primary closure** by full-thickness, uniform manual stretching of the abdominal wall has been used successfully by the authors for the last few years, even with large omphaloceles. An alternative is to cover the viscera with a Silon sheet sutured to the full thickness of the abdominal wall. The sac is reduced in size every day and after 7–10 days is completely removed and the abdominal wall closed.

4. Omphalocele may rupture prior to or during delivery. In this event, immediate closure must be carried out. Primary closure is done only if possible without tension; a staged closure using a Silon sheet is very satisfactory.

5. **Gastroschisis** differs etiologically from a ruptured omphalocele but presents much the same problem. In most instances, primary closure by full-thickness

gentle, manual circumferential stretching of the abdominal wall closes the defect and permits reduction of the viscera into the peritoneal cavity. This affords shorter duration of respiratory embarrassment and ileus and less infection. In some instances, staged closure with a Silo-Sac is used.

E. Abdominal masses in infants and children. See Tables 19-7 and 19-8.

    1. Abdominal masses in the newborn or very young infant are often asymptomatic and usually benign, but all masses must be considered to be malignant until proved otherwise. Early diagnosis and treatment are essential.

    2. The leading cause of death in infants and children is trauma; malignancy is second in frequency. The most common malignancies are Wilms' tumor and neuroblastoma.

    3. Transillumination of a flank mass by a powerful light may indicate hydronephrosis.

    4. Diagnosis is facilitated by a complete blood count, urinalysis, chest x-ray, and plain x-rays of the abdomen.

        a. An **intravenous pyelogram (IVP)** is the most important diagnostic study in evaluating abdominal masses. Nonvisualization of the kidneys will require a voiding cystourethrogram and renal scan.

        b. A **liver scan** may localize an abdominal mass and will identify it as either cystic or solid. Rarely, aortography, inferior venacavogram, cystoscopy, retrograde pyelography, and barium studies are necessary.

        c. A **gallium-67 scan** is an essential study in lymphoma as well as in intraabdominal abscesses.

        d. A **bone scan** identifies metastatic bone lesions.

        e. A **24-hr urinary catecholamine** determination is essential in the diagnosis of neuroblastoma and is of prognostic significance in the follow-up of patients with this malignancy.

        f. A **bone marrow** study is mandatory in all patients with suspected malignant tumors.

    5. If the infant is healthy and full-term, prompt laparotomy can be undertaken.

        a. If urinary or intestinal obstruction is present, rapid intervention is required.

        b. If the infant is very premature or ill from another cause, operation should be delayed until improvement has been obtained.

        c. In **stage IV tumors**, initial management consists of chemotherapy and radiotherapy. At some time during the course of therapy, persistence of the primary lesion will require surgical excision. Solitary metastatic lesions to the lung should be approached aggressively by surgical excision.

F. Masses in the neck. See Table 19-9.

    1. Neck masses present at delivery only rarely require emergency treatment.

        a. Cystic hygroma (lymphangioma) is a soft mass in the anterior cervical triangle that may involve any portion of the neck, parotid region, and cheek and extend under the tongue and around the pharynx and larynx. Despite their alarming appearance, these masses usually do not cause respiratory or feeding problems. A period of observation, allowing the baby to grow, is worthwhile, since surgical excision is tedious and accompanied by many complications when done in a newborn.

        b. Masses in the **thyroid** are rare. Congenital goiter is the most frequent mass and usually is due to maternal medications during gestation; these goiters

Table 19-7. Abdominal Masses in Infancy

Organ or Area	Lesion	Diagnostic Studies	Treatment
Kidney	Unilateral multicystic kidney	IVP; renal scan (nonfunctioning kidney or obstruction with some function)	Resection
	Hydronephrosis (unilateral or bilateral)	IVP; renal scan; voiding cystourethrogram	Resection or pyeloplasty
	Polycystic kidney (bilateral)	IVP; renal function tests (large cysts)	Supportive
	Tumors (fibromas, mesoblastic nephromas, Wilms' tumor)	IVP; distortion and displacement of calices and pelvis	Resection
	Renal vein thrombosis	History of diabetic or toxemic mother and large baby; flank mass on examination; IVP: no visualization; hematuria, thrombocytopenia, anemia	IV therapy; no immediate operation; 5–10% may require later nephrectomy for renal hypertension
Extrarenal (retroperitoneal)	Neuroblastoma	IVP: displaced kidney	Resection; good prognosis if < 1 yr
	Teratoma (rare location)	IVP: displaced kidney	Resection
	Sarcoma	IVP; upper GI series: displaced kidney, stomach, duodenum	Resection; poor prognosis

Liver	Cysts	Hepatomegaly; liver scan for space-occupying lesions	Resection
	Hemangioma	Liver scan; arteriogram	Biopsy; may develop high output heart failure and thrombocytopenia
	Hamartoma	Liver scan	Resection
	Hepatoma	Liver scan	Hepatic lobectomy if localized
	Glycogen storage disease	Hepatomegaly; abnormal glucose tolerance test	Biopsy
	Hepatitis (neonatal)	Hepatomegaly; liver chemistries	Operative cholangiography and liver biopsy
	Choledochal cyst	Cholangiogram; upper GI series	
Intestinal and mesenteric	Duplication (large and small intestine)	Barium enema: obstruction or displacement; GI bleeding	Resection and anastomosis
	Mesenteric cyst	Examination (very mobile); barium studies (displacement)	Resection of cyst; may need bowel resection as well
Ovary	Cyst	IVP; barium enema (displacement); mass in lower abdomen	Resection
	Teratoma and other solid tumors	IVP; barium enema (displacement); mass in lower abdomen	Resection
Bladder	Bladder neck obstruction	Pass catheter; voiding cystogram; IVP	Vesicostomy; later definitive operation
	Neurogenic bladder	Infant with meningomyelocele	Usually does not require operation
Vagina and uterus	Hydrometrocolpos	Abdominal midline mass with bladder displacement on cystogram	Primary reconstruction

Table 19-8. Malignant Tumors in Infancy

Tumor	Age	Symptoms	Diagnostic Studies	Metastases	Catecholamine	Treatment	Prognosis of Cure
Wilms' tumor	1–4 yr	Abdominal mass, often found by mother; microscopic hematuria in 40%	IVP: calices distorted	Lung	Normal	Excision Irradiation (begin on day of operation) if lesion beyond capsule Actinomycin D and vincristine	70% 2-year survival if metastases present; 90% if no metastases present
Neuroblastoma	Less than 1 yr (may appear up to teens)	Abdominal mass; bone pain or proptosis secondary to metastases may be first symptom. Usually crosses midline of abdomen. Also occurs in posterior mediastinum	IVP: kidney or ureter displaced by tumor; bone and chest x-rays show metastases	Bones, liver, skin, bone marrow and lymph nodes.	Elevated (diagnostic after operation)	Excision when possible; biopsy when nonresectable	75% cure under 1 yr; overall survival over 1 yr less than 20%

Teratoma	Newborn to 5 yr	Sacrococcygeal, ovarian, or mediastinal mass	Chest x-ray	Generalized	...	Total excision	Good if excised in newborn period; prognosis poor in older child
Hepatoma	Newborn to teens (usually before 2 yr of age)	Upper abdominal mass	Liver scan: space-occupying lesion	Generalized	...	Hepatic lobectomy if localized to one lobe	Less than 10%
Genitourinary rhabdomyosarcoma (prostate, bladder, vagina, uterus)	Newborn to teens (usually early infancy)	Abdominal mass or external lesions	IVP and cystogram (obstruction may be present)	Generalized	...	Pelvic exenteration if localized; chemotherapy and irradiation pre- and post-operatively	20–50%, if localized (depends on site)

Table 19-9. Neck Masses in Children

Type	Location	Character	Workup	Treatment
Lymphadenitis	Primarily upper lateral neck	Firm, movable, and tender	ENT examination, PPD, chest film, throat culture	Treat primary lesion if present; 7–10 days of antistaphylococcal drugs; incision and drainage if fluctuance develops; biopsy if no response to antibiotics.
Lymphoma	Lateral neck, supraclavicular region	Multiple rubbery, nontender nodes	Hematological investigation, chest film	Biopsy and staging laparotomy followed by chemotherapy or irradiation, depending on staging.
Carcinoma of thyroid	In thyroid or lateral cervical nodes	Hard nodule	History of head or neck irradiation in infancy, chest film, thyroid scan	Total thyroidectomy; node dissection if indicated; thyroxine or ^{131}I.
Thyroglossal duct cyst	Midline	Moves with swallowing; "tug" when tongue is protruded	None	If cystic, exercise with midportion of hyoid bone; if solid, biopsy to identify midline ectopic thyroid.
Branchial cleft cyst	Lateral along anterior border of sternomastoid muscle	Cystic; sinus tract may be palpable	None	Excise with sinus tract.

usually subside spontaneously. Occasionally, congenital goiters cause severe respiratory obstruction; subtotal excision is required. Virtually all tumors in the neonatal thyroid are teratomas; they are very rare and require early excision.

2. Neck masses in older children are more common. Their diagnostic features are summarized in Table 19-9.

G. Hypertrophic pyloric stenosis

1. Pyloric stenosis usually manifests itself in infants 2–6 wk of age. The diagnosis should be considered in any infant who vomits, although faulty feeding practices account for most instances of vomiting.

2. An infant with pyloric stenosis is hungry and will take a feeding immediately after vomiting. Vomiting ranges from mild to forceful and rarely is bile-stained.

3. Give the infant a bottle and observe the abdomen. Peristaltic waves across the upper abdomen from left to right are frequently seen. This sign is highly suggestive but not pathognomonic of hypertrophic pyloric stenosis.

4. The sine qua non of diagnosis is **palpation of the enlarged pylorus**. It is most commonly felt just to the right of the midline, halfway between the xiphoid and umbilicus. Palpation is best done from the baby's left side using the left hand. If the mass is not palpated on the initial examination, the examination should be repeated after an interval. If the mass is not palpated after several attempts by experienced examiners, an upper GI series is obtained. If several examiners have failed to find the pyloric mass, the radiologist usually finds a hiatus hernia, chalasia of the esophagus, or pylorospasm rather than pyloric stenosis. Operation ordinarily should not be done unless a mass is palpated.

5. If vomiting has been prolonged, hypochloremic, hypokalemic alkalosis is common. A solution of 0.45% saline with 5% glucose is begun IV. After the baby voids, potassium chloride is added at a concentration of 40 mEq/liter. Hydration should be restored and acid-base balance brought within normal limits prior to operation.

H. GI bleeding in infants and children

1. Although GI bleeding is frightening in any age group, in children it rarely is life-threatening. The child's cardiovascular system will tolerate acute bleeding better than an adult's. Fifty percent of cases of GI bleeding in childhood will not be diagnosed and will not recur.

2. A child with acute GI bleeding should have blood drawn for a complete blood count, typing and cross matching, coagulation profile, and liver function studies. An IV infusion is started with Ringer's lactate or normal saline solution. A nasogastric tube is inserted into the stomach to see if blood is present in the upper GI tract. A bone marrow biopsy is performed if leukemia is suspected. Vitamin K, 1 mg, is given to newborns who have not already received it.

3. Barium studies in the acute phase rarely are helpful and will only jeopardize a patient who may become hypovolemic if prolonged studies are carried out.

4. Blood should be started if there is evidence of shock and a falling hematocrit.

5. A rule of thumb in acute GI bleeding in children is that surgical intervention is carried out when the patient has had one complete exchange of blood volume without cessation of bleeding and there is no evidence of blood dyscrasia or coagulopathy.

6. Acute GI bleeding in children is divided into three groups (Table 19-10):

Table 19-10. Gastrointestinal Bleeding in Infants and Children

Age	Peak Age	More Frequent and Common Causes	Other Causes	Clinical Manifestation and Character of Bleeding	Workup	Treatment
Newborn	1–2 days	Swallowed maternal blood		Vomiting bright red blood	Apt test positive	None.
		Hemorrhagic disease of newborn		Patient may be pale, listless	Apt test negative	Vitamin K.
		Gastroduodenal ulcer		Patient may be pale, listless	Apt test negative	Blood transfusion; nasogastric irrigation.
			Midgut volvulus	Vomiting bile; bloody stool; scaphoid abdomen	X-ray (intestinal obstruction)	Immediate operation.
			Duplication	Vomiting bile if obstructed, bloody stool	Barium studies	Operation.
			Reflux esophagitis	Vomiting blood	Barium studies	Keep child upright in infant seat; thicken feedings.
			Necrotizing enterocolitis	Vomiting bile, bloody stool, abdominal distention. Premature with anoxia or infant on respiratory assistance	Air in wall of intestine, ileus; air in portal vein and biliary tree	Conservative treatment requires IV fluids, antibiotics, both systemic and per Levin tube to GI tract; albumin; nasogastric suction; and operative intervention for evidence of peritonitis, perforation, gangrene, failure of medical management in 24 hr, unrelenting metabolic acidosis, or increasing thrombocytopenia.

Age	Lesion	Symptoms and Signs	Diagnostic Studies	Treatment
1 mo—2 yr	Anal fissure	Bright bleeding with hard stool	None	Stool softener.
1–6 mo	Intussusception	Colic; blood in stool (currant jelly); abdominal mass	Barium enema	Hydrostatic pressure with barium enema; operation if barium unable to reduce completely or symptoms longer than 12 hr.
6–12 mo	Meckel's diverticulum	Hematochezia; anemia	Barium studies normal; sodium pertechnetate scan may be helpful	Operate with second recurrence of massive bleeding and hemoglobin less than 8 gm/100 ml.
Over 4 mo	Peptic esophagitis	Poor feeder; vomiting; recurrent pneumonia	Upper GI series; esophagoscopy; manometry and pH studies	Antispasmodics; keep child in infant seat, especially after feeding. Anti-reflux operation may be necessary.
Over 2 yr	Polyp	Bright to dark rectal bleeding	Barium enema; proctoscopy	Remove via proctoscope; if massive bleeding, operate
2–4 yr	Polyp, Meckel's diverticulum, T&A, epistaxis			
Over 3 yr	Esophageal varices	Vomiting blood (usually with aspirin ingestion or viral infection)		Supportive therapy; occasionally, Sengstaken-Blakemore tube; shunt after 8 yr of age; generally improve with age (good liver function).
Over 5 yr	Peptic ulceration	Vomiting blood (usually with aspirin ingestion or viral infection)		Supportive therapy; usually operate if blood loss exceeds one blood volume.

a. Newborn (95% of causes are nonsurgical).

b. Age 1 mo–2 yr (33% are surgical or serious medical cases).

c. Age over 2 yr (high percentage of surgical or serious medical diseases).

7. When the patient's condition is stable, **definitive barium studies** (upper and lower GI series with small-bowel follow-through) are performed, along with proctoscopy. **Obtain stools** for specific pathogen culture and examination for parasites. Angiography is just beginning to be used commonly in pediatrics. **Technetium scan** after cleaning the colon may be helpful in the diagnosis of Meckel's diverticulum.

8. Gastroenteritis should not be considered a cause for GI bleeding until all other causes have been ruled out. Bleeding due to gastroenteritis is rare.

I. Umbilical hernia

1. The great majority close spontaneously. Incarceration and strangulation are rare complications.

2. Operation is not advised until age 3 if the defect is greater than 2 cm. If the defect is less than 2 cm, observation is continued until age 5. All defects in females should be repaired at age 5, since pregnancy may precipitate incarceration. In males, any defect less than 2 cm need not be repaired, since it will close further as abdominal muscles develop in adolescence.

J. Appendicitis. Children react with abdominal pain to a large variety of nonsurgical illnesses. However, the symptom complex of abdominal pain, vomiting, and fever requires that the diagnosis of appendicitis be a prominent consideration.

1. Remember that appendicitis progresses more rapidly in children than in adults.

2. If abdominal pain persists and there is localized lower abdominal tenderness with rebound, predominantly right-sided but occasionally midline or slightly to the left, that cannot be explained on the basis of another condition, **operation** for appendicitis must be undertaken.

K. Constipation in childhood, although usually not a serious organic problem, can become a serious social and psychological problem for both child and parents.

1. The common type of constipation is functional, without any known causes; motor dysfunction of the colon is suspected but not proved.

2. Onset of constipation occurs with toilet training at age 2–3 yr. The child has one to two massive stools a week and constant soiling due to fecal impaction and overdistention of the colon. Growth and development are normal. The rectal examination demonstrates stool impacted in the rectum.

3. Hirschsprung's disease, in contradistinction, begins in the newborn period, the rectum usually is empty of stool, and there is a failure of normal growth and development.

4. The **diagnosis** of functional constipation is made by history, physical examination, and a barium enema that demonstrates a uniformly distended colon without areas of narrowing.

5. **Treatment** consists of reassurance, keeping the colon relatively empty through daily bowel movements encouraged by stool softeners and suppositories (no laxatives), and prevention of fecal impaction. Suppositories are inserted when the child awakens in the morning in order that he or she can defecate before leaving for school. With constant treatment, most children develop proper bowel control in 6–18 mo.

Suggested Reading

Aperia, A., Broberger, O., Thodenius, K., and Zetterström, R. Renal control of sodium and fluid balance in newborn infants during intravenous maintenance therapy. *Acta Paediatr. Scand.* 64:725, 1975.

Firor, H. V. Omphalocele—An appraisal of therapeutic approaches. *Surgery* 69:208, 1971.

Gans, S. L. *Surgical Pediatrics.* New York: Grune & Stratton, 1973.

Kirtley, J. A., and Holcomb, G. W. Surgical management of diseases of the gallbladder and common duct in children and adolescents. *Am. J. Surg.* 111:39, 1966.

Krauss, A. N., and Auld, P. A. M. Metabolic requirements of low-birth-weight infants. *J. Pediatr.* 75:952, 1969.

Potts, W. J. *The Surgeon and the Child.* Philadelphia: Saunders, 1959.

Rowe, M. I., and Marchildon, M. B. Physiologic considerations in the newborn surgical patient. *Surg. Clin. North Am.* 56:245, 1976.

Roy, R. N., and Sinclair, J. C. Hydration of the low birth-weight infant. *Clin. Perinatol.* 2:393, 1975.

Stephens, F. D., and Smith, E. D. *Ano-Rectal Malformations in Children.* Chicago: Year Book, 1971.

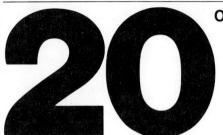

Organ Transplantation

I. **Kidney transplantation** is a well-established treatment for patients with end-stage kidney disease. It is the treatment of choice unless serious contraindications are present, such as severe chronic obstructive pulmonary disease, malignancy, active infections, or advanced age. Diabetes mellitus is not considered a contraindication. The greatest likelihood of success is with living-related donors, but cadaver kidney transplantation is desirable in many instances, necessitating the development of active regional programs for procurement and distribution of cadaver organs.

A. **Identification and evaluation of potential cadaver organ donors:**

1. **Identification of a potential donor**

   a. Arrives at hospital alive.

   b. Under age 65 yr, over 8 mo.

   c. Kidneys are functioning.

   d. Is unconscious and requires mechanical ventilation.

2. **Absolute contraindications to organ donation** are

   a. Malignancy (except for CNS tumors or basal cell carcinoma of the skin).

   b. Sepsis.

   c. Preexisting renal disease or known potential etiological factors of long standing (e.g., hypertension, diabetes mellitus).

3. In the **management of a potential donor,** vigorous measures are taken to resuscitate and maintain an optimal hemodynamic status and renal function. Colloids, crystalloids, and furosemide (40–200 mg by IV push) are used to expand plasma volume and induce brisk diuresis. The serum creatinine level should be 3.0 mg/100 ml or below, or if over 3.0 mg/100 ml, should decrease with the diuresis.

4. **Brain death** is customarily determined by a neurologist or neurosurgeon, as follows:

   a. Absence of spontaneous respiration.

   b. Absence of spontaneous movement; unresponsive to painful stimuli.

   c. Absence of pupillary and eye-globe (cephalo-ocular) responses.

   d. Confirmation of brain death by absence of brain blood flow (scintiscan or angiogram), or, if these tests are not available, a silent electroencephalogram.

5. **Permission** to remove kidneys (and possibly other organs) must be obtained from the next of kin. Legally, under the Uniform Anatomical Gift Act, permission is not required if the person carries a donor card, indicating his or her desire to donate organs at the time of death.

B. Procurement and maintenance of cadaver kidneys

1. The donor is taken to the operating room after brain death has been declared. Circulation and respiratory support must be maintained until organ procurement is under way.

2. Pretreatment of the donor with methylprednisolone (30 mg/kg IV) at 1 hr and with phenoxybenzamine (100 mg IV) a half hour before removal of the kidneys is helpful in averting agonal renal vasospasm and protecting functional integrity.

3. Heparin, 2 mg/kg IV, is administered to the donor prior to removal of the kidneys.

4. The kidneys are removed with care to ensure that arteries, veins, and ureters are of adequate length. Excessive manipulation must be avoided, and the en bloc technique (removal with a segment of aorta and inferior vena cava) is recommended for this reason. Lymph nodes and spleen are removed for tissue typing.

5. The kidneys are cooled immediately by submersion in iced saline solution and by intra-arterial flush with an iced crystalloid solution. An electrolyte solution for kidney preservation (Travenol, 930 ml) is the base solution used by the authors. Immediately before use, add heparin, 5000 units; 50% glucose, 50 ml; 50% magnesium sulphate, 24 mEq; and 25% mannitol, 25 ml.

6. Subsequent preservation of the kidneys may be carried out in 0–4°C cold storage if reimplantation is anticipated within 12–24 hr, or by continuous hypothermic perfusion with plasma-derived colloid perfusates for longer periods (up to 48–72 hr).

C. Evaluation of living donors

1. The donor must be a blood relative of the recipient, with an ABO blood group compatible with that of the recipient.

2. The donor must be healthy, as determined by the history and physical examination.

3. The **workup protocol** includes the following (all of which should be within normal range):

   a. Chest x-ray, electrocardiogram.

   b. Complete blood count, fasting blood sugar, serum electrolytes, blood urea nitrogen, creatinine, creatinine clearance, uric acid, calcium, phosphorus, liver function tests, prothrombin time, and partial thromboplastin time. A postprandial blood sugar or glucose tolerance test may be indicated in the related donor of a diabetic recipient.

   c. Urinalysis; three urine cultures.

   d. Intravenous pyelogram.

   e. Abdominal angiography (to determine the anatomy of the renal arteries). Kidneys with solitary renal arteries are preferred, although multiple (two or three) arteries can be successfully anastomosed.

D. Evaluation of recipient. The uremic patient is evaluated for dialysis or transplantation as follows:

1. **Renal function** is determined by clearance studies. Irreversible renal impairment must be confirmed. Renal biopsy often is desirable for this purpose and for diagnosis of the disease process.

2. **Lower urinary tract abnormalities** (e.g., obstruction, reflux, bladder residual) must be detected by history, voiding cystourethrogram, residual urine determination, cystoscopy, and retrograde pyelography, as indicated. If ab-

normalities are present, and appropriate surgical correction (e.g., bladder neck revision, construction of an intestinal conduit) may be indicated prior to transplantation.

3. The **chest x-ray** must be negative for active parenchymal disease.

4. Severe, uncontrolled **hypertension** with elevated plasma renin activity, or **urosepsis,** are the only strict indications for **pretransplantation nephrectomy.**

5. **Liver function tests** must reveal no evidence of active parenchymal disease. HB_s antigenemia requires appropriate precautions on the part of all dialysis and transplantation personnel but does not preclude transplantation.

6. Evaluation of **autoimmune disease** is made by determination of C3, C4, antinuclear antibody, LE cell preparations, and anti–glomerular basement membrane (anti-GBM) antibody. Active, progressive autoimmune disease usually delays transplantation. Anti-GBM antibody has been associated with recurrent disease.

7. **Symptomatic secondary hyperparathyroidism** is evaluated by a serum calcium determination, bone x-rays, and parathyroid hormone assays. Subtotal parathyroidectomy or total parathyroidectomy with autotransplantation may be indicated prior to transplantation.

8. **Social and pertinent psychological profiles** must be obtained to evaluate the ability of the patient to cooperate in the complex treatment regimen.

9. **Histocompatibility.** ABO compatibility between donor and recipient is requisite. Further typing for the HLA antigens is performed on all recipients and all donors (living-related and cadavers). Within families, it is done to guide in the choice of the most compatible donor.

   a. Two haplotype-matched (HLA-identical) siblings offer the best chance for a successful transplant. A mixed lymphocyte culture test is performed between all ABO compatible family members. The best donor is the least reactive with the recipient by mixed lymphocyte culture. HLA matching with cadaver kidneys is performed to select the best-matched recipient for a given donor. Matching donor and recipient for the DR antigens is currently advocated by some centers.

   b. A preoperative cross match (using recent sera as well as previous sera known to contain anti-HLA antibodies) must be performed routinely. The presence of circulating antidonor HLA antibodies (presensitization) will cause hyperacute kidney rejection.

E. **Preparation of a living donor.** In addition to the usual measures of preoperative preparation, the following must be accomplished:

1. Special **operative permits** must be signed, indicating the donor's knowledge of the possible consequences of his or her donation.

2. One unit of **autologous blood** is taken from the donor several days preoperatively for use during the nephrectomy procedure in lieu of banked blood.

3. The prospective donor is brought to the operating room 1 hr before induction of anesthesia, and **IV hydration** with 15 ml/kg of Ringer's lactate is begun.

4. An **indwelling catheter** is placed during the operation to permit free urine flow and to record urine output rate.

5. During anesthesia, strict attention is paid to maintenance of normal blood pressure and continuous good hydration.

6. Vasopressors cannot be used.

7. IV furosemide may be given to induce diuresis in the donor kidney prior to clamping of the renal artery.

8. Immediately prior to removal of the kidney, the donor is given an anticoagulant (2 mg/kg heparin). The left kidney is taken preferentially, all other factors being equal.

9. Following removal, the kidney is flushed by gravity flow (100 cm) with a crystalloid solution at 4.0°C (39.2°F) containing heparin (until the renal venous effluent is clear and the kidney is cooled) and transplanted immediately. The intracellular-type solution described in **B.5** is satisfactory.

F. Preoperative and operative management of the recipient

1. After an appropriate workup, the uremic patient is usually started on **hemodialysis** in anticipation of a renal transplant. Access to the arterial circulation for hemodialysis is achieved with external Silastic arteriovenous shunts or internal arteriovenous fistula formation by direct arteriovenous anastomosis or by interposition of an autologous vein, bovine heterograft, or prosthetic graft.

2. Baseline **hematological data** are obtained. If persistent leukopenia is detected, a bone marrow aspirate and a spleen scan are obtained. If significant splenomegaly and hypersplenism are detected, it is advisable to perform a splenectomy prior to transplantation to facilitate subsequent immunosuppression. Routine pretransplantation splenectomy is performed in many centers.

3. A **chest x-ray** and **bacterial and viral culture** of skin lesions and of the nose, throat, sputum, and urine are obtained.

4. Recipients of elective (living-related donor) transplants are given **daily baths** with germicidal soap for 1–2 wk preoperatively.

5. **Blood transfusions** are given preoperatively and intraoperatively as indicated. Routine pretransplantation transfusion is now recommended for all potential recipients, since it seems to confer an immunological advantage.

6. The **operative permit** signed by the recipient must include a special indication that he or she has been made aware of the possible consequences of transplantation.

7. **Immunosuppressive agents,** consisting of azathioprine (Imuran), 5 mg/kg PO, and prednisone, 5 mg/kg PO (or IV equivalent), is given immediately before transplantation. Methylprednisolone, 20 mg/kg IV, may be given during operation.

8. **Prophylactic antibiotic** treatment (a cephalosporin) is recommended in cadaver donor transplantation.

9. A catheter is placed for measurement of **central venous pressure,** and correct positioning of the catheter is verified by x-ray before induction of anesthesia. During operation, the central venous pressure is maintained at 8–10 cm saline by appropriate infusion of crystalloid or blood.

10. At operation, the kidney is placed in the iliac fossa of the recipient with the renal artery anastomosed to the internal or external iliac artery, and with the renal vein anastomosed to the common iliac vein. Customarily, the donor ureter is implanted into the bladder.

11. Postoperative immunosuppression

a. **Azathioprine,** 5 mg/kg, is given for 3 days, and then maintained at 1.0–2.5 mg/kg/day indefinitely. If, following transplantation, renal function is poor (serum creatinine > 3 mg/100 ml), the dose of azathioprine is reduced by 50%. If the patient develops leukopenia (white cell count < 6000/mm^3), the azathioprine dose is reduced or eliminated. If liver dysfunction occurs, cyclophosphamide is substituted for azathioprine.

b. **Prednisone.** The starting dose is 1–2 mg/kg/day. The dose is decreased in stepwise fashion to 20 mg/day at 6 mo. While on corticosteroids, the patient takes oral antacids.

c. **Methylprednisolone IV,** 20 mg/kg/day, may be given for the first 3 postoperative days.

d. **Antilymphocyte globulin** is not routinely used in all transplantation centers. It is administered IV or IM in doses ranging from 15 to 30 mg/kg on variable schedules.

e. **Other agents.** The following may be used:

(1) Local radiation to the graft (150 R, every other day × 4).

(2) Anticoagulants and antiplatelet drugs.

12. **Postoperative laboratory studies**

a. **Daily.** Serum electrolytes, fasting blood sugar, blood urea nitrogen, creatinine, complete blood count, urinalysis, urine culture.

b. **Weekly.** Calcium, phosphorus, serum proteins, uric acid, liver function tests.

c. **Renal scans.** On postoperative days 1, 3, and 7 and as needed.

d. **Ultrasound examination** is useful in determination of the presence of perirenal fluid collections and swelling of the kidney.

e. **Renal biopsy** is helpful in the diagnosis of rejection.

f. Intravenous pyelography and renal arteriography are rarely indicated; the contrast medium may cause renal dysfunction.

13. **Rejection episodes** are characterized by a decrease in renal function, proteinuria, swelling and tenderness of the kidney, fever, tachycardia, and hypertension. The diagnosis is confirmed by renal scan and closed renal biopsy. Treatment consists of reversion to the immediate posttransplantation schedule of prednisone; other adjuncts may include IV methylprednisolone, irradiation to the kidney, anticoagulation in the event of blood vessel involvement in the graft, and antilymphocyte globulin. Success in reversal of a rejection reaction will become apparent within 3–4 days.

II. Transplantation of other organs

A. Transplantation of **corneas** in selected patients with blindness due to certain varieties of corneal opacities is a well-established procedure. Corneal transplants have a high success rate, in part due to the restricted access of antigen from and antibody into the anterior ocular chamber.

B. Good clinical results are now being achieved with **allografts of the heart, liver, and bone marrow** performed at a few specialized centers where the effort is presently concentrated. **Lung** and **pancreas** transplants have had limited success.

C. **Skin allografts** and **heterografts** are being used with considerable success in several burn units, allowing good wound coverage for prolonged periods until autografts are available.

Suggested Reading

Jamieson, S. W., Stinson, E. B., and Shumway, N. E. Cardiac transplantation in 150 patients at Stanford University. *Brt. Med. J.* 1:93, 1979.

Jonasson, O., and Hoversten G. Replacement of pancreatic beta cells as treatment for diabetes mellitus. *Surg. Annu.* 1978:1, 1978.

Najarian, J. S., and Simmons, R. L. *Transplantation*. Philadelphia: Lea & Febiger, 1972.

Najarian, J. S., Sutherland, D. E. R., Simmons, R. L., Howard, R. J., Kjellstrand, C. M., Mauer, S. M., Kennedy, W., Ramsay, R., Barbosa, J., and Goetz, F. C. Kidney transplantation for the uremic diabetic patient. *Surg. Gynecol. Obstet.* 144:682, 1977.

Salvatierra, O., Potter, D., Cochrum, K. C., Amend, W. J. C., Duca, R., Sachs, B. L., Johnson, R. W. J., and Belzer, F. O. Improved patient survival in renal transplantation. *Surgery* 79:166, 1976.

Starzl, T. E., Porter, K. A., Putnam, C. W., Schroter, G. P. J., Halgrimson, C. G., Weil, R. III, Hoelscher, M., and Reid, H. A. S.. Orthotopic liver transplantation in 93 patients. *Surg. Gynecol. Obstet.* 142:487, 1976.

21

I. **General comments**. The development of new and more effective antineoplastic agents, as well as an increased understanding of older agents, has expanded the list of neoplastic diseases that respond to chemotherapy. In patients with certain tumors, treatment with chemotherapy can produce cure; in other patients, therapy may be palliative or ineffectual. It is now apparent that chemotherapy used in combinination with other therapeutic modalities (e.g., radiation and surgery) may effect further cures or significant prolongation of survival compared with single-modality therapy.

Along with new drugs and new treatment programs have come new and increased toxicities. Injudicious use of chemotherapeutic agents can lead to significant morbidity and mortality. Therefore, evaluation of the patient's condition becomes just as important as the selection of therapy. When there is a potential for cure, increased toxicity and risk are acceptable. When the aim is only palliation, drug toxicity becomes acceptable when some benefit accrues from therapy, e.g., prolongation of survival or relief of symptoms. Frequently, the final decision must be made between the patient and his or her physician.

Chemotherapy should be administered, or treatment supervised, by a specialist in cancer treatment.

A. **Principles of chemotherapy.** A large body of data on growth rate and drug responsiveness of normal hematopoietic tissue and of neoplastic growths has contributed to the development of certain simple concepts.

1. **Concept of "total cell kill"**

   a. A single viable clonogenic malignant cell can produce a lethal tumor.

   b. Immune mechanisms play a small role unless a small number of cancer cells is present.

   c. Cell kill by antineoplastic agents follows first-order kinetics; i.e., a constant fraction rather than a constant number of cells is killed by a given drug.

2. **The rate of tumor cell proliferation is a major determinant of therapeutic responsiveness.** Tumor growth rate is dependent on the average mitotic cell cycle time, the degree of cell loss, and the fraction of proliferating cells. In a tumor mass, only a fraction of the cells are rapidly proliferating; the remainder of the cells are out of cycle. As a tumor increases in mass, its growth rate decreases (Gompertizian function) mostly because of a decrease in proliferating cells. Most drugs have greater toxicity for cycling cells, with some variation in toxicity at different phases of the cell cycle. Nonproliferating cells can be recruited into the proliferating fraction after treatment with anticancer agents, or by reduction of the tumor mass surgically, or with radiotherapy. Thus, individual tumor sizes (metastatic tumor) and the total body burden of tumor cells influence responsiveness to chemotherapy.

3. **Combination chemotherapy** has been utilized in an effort to increase the magnitude of the cell kill. Successful combinations have been based on several general principles:

a. Use drugs that are active against the specific tumor when used alone.

b. Use drugs with different mechanisms of action.

c. Use drugs that produce toxicity in different organ systems or at different times following drug administration.

d. Use drugs in repeated, brief courses to minimize adverse host effects, e.g., immunosuppression.

4. Adjuvant chemotherapy is the term employed when chemotherapy is used as part of a multimodality treatment program after primary local therapy with radiation or surgery, or both. Local therapy is curative in less than half of all patients with cancer; the remainder have unrecognized metastases. The aim of adjuvant chemotherapy is destruction of micrometastases, prevention of clinical metastases, and achievement of cure. The basic principles of adjuvant chemotherapy are:

a. Surgery and radiation are limited by the extent of the tumor; chemotherapy is limited by the total cancer mass.

b. Chemotherapy is most effective at maximum tolerated doses and is ineffective at lower doses.

c. Adjuvant therapy should be given as soon as possible after surgery.

Since the use of chemotherapy in this setting does not guarantee cure, or even benefit, one must consider that adjuvant chemotherapy causes toxicity in asymptomatic patients who may already have been cured by prior therapy. Thus, this type of therapy should be supervised by a specialist familiar with the drugs, as well as with the disease being treated.

B. Classification of antineoplastic agents can be made according to their mechanism of action in the cell cycle and at the molecular or biochemical level.

1. There are **three classes** of agents based on cellular kinetic effects. They are cell cycle nonspecific (CCNS), cell cycle specific (CCS), and cell cycle stage specific (CCSS) agents. Most agents in the CCNS group are more active against proliferating cells than nonproliferating cells.

2. On a molecular basis, agents can be divided into those that bind to macromolecules other than enzymes (covalently or noncovalently), agents that are incorporated into a macromolecule, and agents that inhibit vital enzymatic reactions. This classification is based on the specific action of an agent that is thought to cause cell death. Some agents are still classified as "other" because the specific subcellular mechanism of action is not known.

II. Use of chemotherapeutic agents

A. Assessment of response. A data base evaluating all likely metastatic sites should be obtained prior to initiation of therapy. In addition to a physical examination, x-rays, and scans, tumor markers also may be required. In the case of gestational choriocarcinoma and testicular carcinoma, tumor marker alone is indicative of active disease.

1. A **complete response** requires complete resolution of all measurable disease.

2. A **partial response** is defined as a greater than 50% reduction in the sum of the products of the perpendicular diameters of marker lesions without progression of any other lesion or appearance of new lesions.

3. Stable disease refers to patients not demonstrating regression of disease but without a change in their performance status or progression.

4. Progression of disease is defined as an increase greater than 25% in the product of the perpendicular diameters of measurable lesions, the appearance of any new lesion, or a significant decline in performance status.

B. **Toxicity: principles of management and prevention.** While each drug has its own spectrum of toxicity, general knowledge of the nature and management of drug toxicity is essential to the proper administration of cancer chemotherapy.

1. **Bone marrow toxicity** is seen with almost all antineoplastic agents and often necessitates dose adjustment, or lengthening the interval between drug administration, or both.

   a. **Anemia** is usually mild but may become severe and symptomatic with prolonged therapy. This can be handled by red cell transfusions. Anemia is not a contraindication to further chemotherapy.

   b. **Leukopenia** is a frequent and serious problem. The timing (nadir) and duration of neutropenia induced by chemotherapeutic agents depends on the agent, dose, and schedule of administration. Leukopenia of between 2000 and 3000 white blood cells rarely causes significant difficulty. However, when the number of neutrophils drops below 500 cells/mm^3, serious infections can occur. A leukopenic patient with the most trivial symptoms suggesting infection may already have an overwhelming sepsis. Consequently, **fever in a leukopenic patient is an emergency**. Blood cultures and cultures of all possible sites of infection must be obtained promptly and broad-spectrum antibiotics administered. Adequate therapy would include an aminoglycoside and carbenicillin, or equivalent. Neutropenic patients with sepsis whose neutrophil count does not increase within 7–10 days generally die of overwhelming sepsis despite antibiotic therapy.

   c. **Thrombocytopenia** is also a serious but infrequent side effect of cancer chemotherapy and may be associated with life-threatening hemorrhage. Platelet counts are a necessity prior to administration of chemotherapy.

2. **Gastrointestinal toxicity** is frequently observed. Nausea and vomiting often occur within 2–8 hr after drug administration and may continue for 12–72 hr. These effects vary with the drug used, the dose administered, and the individual patient. Phenothiazenes, although of doubtful efficacy, may ameliorate these symptoms. Several cannabinoids, including delta-9-tetrahydrocannabinol, are undergoing clinical trial as antiemetics in patients receiving chemotherapy; the results to data are promising. Diarrhea or constipation may result from treatment.

3. **Mucocutaneous toxicity** is less common than the preceding effects but occurs frequently and may occur in the absence of other toxic reactions. Stomatitis is the most frequent side effect. **Alopecia** is common with some agents but may occur with almost any agent. Dry skin, eruptions, pigmentation and nail changes are included in the many possible side effects.

4. **Cardiac toxicity** was not a problem until the introduction of doxorubicin (Adriamycin) and other anthracycline analogues into clinical use. The use of prolonged Adriamycin therapy may be limited by the development of irreversible cardiomyopathy. Myocyte degeneration occurs with anthracycline therapy; it is a progressive subclinical injury to the heart eventually manifested by left ventricular dysfunction that may lead to clinically significant heart failure. Quantitative radionuclide angiocardiography should be used to estimate the left ventricular ejection fraction prior to and during anthracycline therapy. A decline in ejection fraction of 15% may be an indication to stop therapy and prevent congestive heart failure. Contributing factors to cardiomyopathy are the total dose of Adriamycin (limit to 550 mg/m^2) and radiotherapy to the mediastinum.

   Another cardiotoxic reaction can occur early during anthracycline therapy. This is a pericarditis-myocarditis that tends to affect patients with no previous history of cardiac disease and may lead to death. Arrhythmias may occur early during therapy. The most common is sinus tachycardia, but symptomatic supraventricular tachycardia, heart block, and ventricular arrhythmia can occur.

There is some evidence that administration of alpha-tocopherol may prevent cardiotoxicity without altering the antineoplastic effects of Adriamycin.

5. Drug-induced **pulmonary disease** is an infrequent, but clinically significant, manifestation of antineoplastic therapy. Although primarily associated with bleomycin therapy, pulmonary toxicity has been described with busulfan, cyclophosphamide, methotrexate, melphalan, chlorambucil, procarbazine, BCNU, methyl CCNU, and mitomycin C. The common pathological process is a fibrosing alveolitis. The onset may be insidious and nonspecific. Close clinical monitoring with early withdrawal of the drug is necessary to halt or reverse potentially lethal pulmonary disease. Aggressive, early evaluation is mandatory. A lung biopsy is almost always indicated.

6. **Nephrotoxicity** was found to be a complication of cancer chemotherapy infrequently until the advent of high-dose methotrexate therapy and the introduction of cisplatin as an antineoplastic agent. When using these agents, vigorous hydration should be assured. Caution should be exercised in the use of other nephrotoxic drugs, such as aminoglycoside antibiotics, concomitantly with these agents.

C. **Response to therapy**. Clinical studies of antineoplastic agents have identified specific drugs that are active in the treatment of various disseminated malignancies. The **individual agents and usual doses** are listed in Table 21-1. However, since it has been demonstrated that combination chemotherapy is superior to single-agent chemotherapy in many malignancies, both in response rate and duration of response, combination therapy should be used. The usual dose is frequently different from that used in combination chemotherapy.

A general **guide to the therapy of neoplastic diseases** is presented in Table 21-2. It is important to understand the disease being treated, the stage of the disease, and its therapy. Specific curative treatment programs must be closely adhered to in order to obtain curative results.

Response to any therapy will vary among patients. Careful pretreatment evaluation of a patient is needed to aid in administration of optimum therapy or, in some instances, withholding of therapy. Important factors to note are the patient's performance status, nutritional state, age, and history of prior therapy with alkylating agents or radiation to the pelvis.

D. **Means of administration**

1. **Systemic therapy** has proved to be the most useful and reproducible, whether administered IV or PO.

2. **Regional perfusion or infusion** techniques have not been proved superior to systemic therapy. Although studies have suggested that these techniques offer some benefit over systemic chemotherapy, prospective randomized studies have not been done.

3. **Intracavitary therapy** has proved to be of palliative benefit in the control of malignant pleural effusions. **Intrathecal** administration of antineoplastic agents may be the appropriate route in certain conditions.

E. **Perspectives on immunotherapy**. It has been well demonstrated that tumors elicit an immune response from the tumor-bearing host. In spite of this tumor-specific response, the host immune system fails to elicit tumor rejection, and progressive tumor growth continues in the face of demonstrable immunity.

Immunotherapy of cancer is being evaluated in the treatment of human tumors. The presence of tumor-specific antigens suggests that somehow this specificity can be utilized as a therapeutic advantage to the host. Since an adequate detailed understanding of the immunobiology of the tumor-bearing host is lacking, most clinical trials have adopted empirical approaches utilizing various adjuvants, e.g., BCG, levamisole, or **C. parvum** in order to stimulate specific or nonspecific immune responses to the tumor. No definite therapeutic recommendations can be

Table 21-1. Specific Agents Used in Cancer Chemotherapy

AGENTS THAT BIND TO MACROMOLECULES OTHER THAN ENZYMES

Drug	Route	Usual Dose	Toxicity		Comments
			Acute	Delayed	
Alkylating agents (CCNS)					
Mechlorethamine	IV	0.4 mg/kg or 10–15 mg/m² in single or divided dose	Nausea and vomiting	Leukopenia, thrombocytopenia	With prolonged administration, bone marrow toxicity is cumulative and irreversible except with cyclophosphamide. Gonadal dysfunction is common. All alkylating agents are mutagenic and carcinogenic. Cyclophosphamide is immunosuppressive.
Chlorambucil	PO	0.1–0.2 mg/kg/day 6–12 mg/day		Leukopenia, thrombocytopenia	
Melphalan	PO	0.1 mg/kg/day × 7 2–4 mg/day maintenance or 6 mg/m²/day × 5 days q6wk	Occasional nausea	Leukopenia, thrombocytopenia	
Cyclophosphamide	IV PO	1200 mg/m² q3wk 100–150 mg/day to keep WBC 2000–3000	Nausea and vomiting	Leukopenia, hemorrhagic cystitis, alopecia common; pulmonary toxicity possible; stomatitis	
Triethylenethiophosphoramide (Thiotepa)	IV IM	0.2 mg/kg/day × 5 days, or 0.6–0.8 mg/kg	Nausea and vomiting	Leukopenia, thrombocytopenia	

Table 21-1 (Continued)

Drug	Route	Usual Dose	Toxicity		Comments
			Acute	Delayed	
AGENTS THAT BIND TO MACROMOLECULES OTHER THAN ENZYMES					
Busulfan	PO	2–6 mg/day		Neutropenia, thrombocytopenia, pulmonary fibrosis, skin hyperpigmentation	
BCNU (carmustine)	IV	200 mg/m² × 1 q6wk; subsequent doses adjusted depending on blood count	Nausea and vomiting	Leukopenia and thrombocytopenia (prolonged); hepatotoxicity possible	
CCNU (lomustine)	PO	200–225 mg/m² q6–8 wk	Nausea and vomiting	Leukopenia and thrombocytopenia (prolonged); hepatotoxicity possible; stomatitis	
Dibromodulcitol	PO	2.5–3.5 mg/kg/day for 5–7 wk, or 4–5 mg/kg/day for 10–20 days every month	Nausea and vomiting, anorexia, diarrhea	Leukopenia, thrombocytopenia, alopecia, cutaneous lesions	Presently not available for general use.
Antibiotics (CCNS)					
Mitomycin C	IV	20 mg/m² IV q4–6 wk, or 0.06 mg/kg twice weekly	Nausea and vomiting	Leukopenia, thrombocytopenia, nephrotoxicity, pulmonary toxicity	
Actinomycin D	IV	0.01 mg/kg/day × 5, or 0.04 mg/kg/wk, or 1.2–1.8 mg/m² q3wk	Nausea and vomiting	Leukopenia, thrombocytopenia, stomatitis, diarrhea, alopecia, cutaneous lesions	Cumulative marrow toxicity with prolonged administration.

Drug	Route	Dose	Acute toxicity	Major toxicity	Comments
Doxorubicin (Adriamycin)	IV	60–75 mg/m² q3wk	Nausea and vomiting	Leukopenia, thrombocytopenia, GI disturbances, stomatitis, alopecia for all, cardiotoxicity	Limit total dose to 550 mg/m²; reduce usual dose by 25% for bilirubin over 1.2 mg/100 ml; by 50% if over 3.0 mg/100 ml.
Mithramycin	IV	0.025 mg/kg/day × 6–8 days, or 0.05 mg/kg every 2 days for 3–4 doses	Nausea and vomiting	Leukopenia, thrombocytopenia	Bleeding diathesis may occur and be lethal; may use drug in single dose for hypercalcemia.
Bleomycin (CCS agent)	IV	10–15 mg/m²/wk	Nausea and vomiting, chills, fever	Mucocutaneous ulcerations, alopecia, pulmonary fibrosis	IV infusion over 24 hr/dose may be less toxic.
	SC	10–15 mg/m², twice/wk or daily			
	IM	10–15 mg/m² q5–6 days			
Other agents					
Cisplatin (*cis*-diamine-dichloroplatinum)	IV	50–75 mg/m² q3wk, or 15–20 mg/m²/day × 5 q3–4 wk	Nausea and vomiting	Renal, auditory; leukopenia and thrombocytopenia not marked	Higher doses (80–100 mg/m²) may be given with IV hydration before and after dosing if urine output is 150 ml/hr.
Dacarbazine (DTIC)	IV	4.5 mg/kg/day q 28 days × 10, or 250 mg/m²/day q 21 days × 5	Nausea and vomiting; marked "flulike" syndrome	Leukopenia, thrombocytopenia	
Plant alkaloids (CCSS)					
Vinblastine	IV	0.1–0.2 mg/kg/wk, or 0.2–0.4 mg/kg/d q3wk	Nausea and vomiting, anorexia	Leukopenia, alopecia, neurological symptoms, stomatitis	

Table 21-1 (Continued)

Drug	Route	Usual Dose	Toxicity		Comments
			Acute	Delayed	
AGENTS THAT BIND TO MACROMOLECULES OTHER THAN ENZYMES					
Vincristine	IV	0.01–0.03 mg/kg/wk, or 1.0–1.4 mg/m²/wk until neurotoxicity develops		Peripheral neuropathy, paralytic ileus	
AGENTS INCORPORATED INTO MACROMOLECULES (CCS)					
6-Thioguanine	PO	2.0 mg/kg/day		Mild marrow depression	
6-Mercaptopurine	PO	2.5 mg/kg/day		Mild marrow depression; hepatotoxicity possible	
AGENTS THAT INHIBIT VITAL ENZYMATIC REACTIONS (CCS)					
Cytarabine	IV	2–3 mg/kg/day × 10–20 days, or 1–3 mg/kg/day over 24 hr for up to 10 days		Leukopenia, diarrhea, stomatitis	
5-Fluorouracil	IV	12.5 mg/kg/day × 4–5 days (limit 800 mg/dose), then ½ dose every other day until toxicity appears	Nausea		The "loading" course is repeated after 4 wk, or 15 mg/kg/wk is given.
Methotrexate (amethopterin)	PO IV	2.5–5.0 mg/day, or 40–60 mg/m²/wk		Anemia, leukopenia, thrombocytopenia, stomatitis, hepatotoxicity	Toxicity is enhanced by poor renal function.

OTHER AGENTS

	Route	Dose			
Procarbazine	PO	100 mg/m²/day	Nausea and vomiting	Leukopenia, thrombocytopenia, cutaneous lesions	Neurotoxicity may manifest itself by disorders of consciousness, peripheral neuropathy, or complications of enzyme inhibition and ataxia. **Note:** alcohol intolerance.
Hexamethylmelamine	PO	300 mg/m²/day	Nausea and vomiting, occasional cramps and diarrhea	Leukopenia, mild thrombocytopenia; neurological disturbances sometimes severe	Pyridoxine, 100 mg tid, may alleviate neurotoxicity and allow treatment to continue. Not available for general use.
Tamoxifen	PO	10 mg bid	Nausea and vomiting	Thrombocytopenia (transient), hot flashes, rash	Patients with estrogen receptor–negative tumor are unlikely to respond.

HORMONAL AGENTS

	Route	Dose			
Diethylstilbesterol	PO	15 mg/day (1 mg in prostate cancer)		Fluid retention, feminization, uterine bleeding	Hypercalcemia possible.
Fluoxymesterone	PO	10 mg bid		Fluid retention, masculinization	
Megestrol acetate	PO	40 mg qid			
Medroxyprogesterone	IM	400 mg twice/wk			
Prednisone	PO	10–100 mg/day		Fluid retention, hypertension, diabetes	

Table 21-2. Treatment of Neoplastic Diseases and Responses to Chemotherapy

Type of Cancer	Treatment of Primary (Local and Regional)	Active Agents	Treatment of Micrometastases (Adjuvant Therapy)	Treatment of Metastatic Disease
Cancers in which chemotherapy can be curative				
Gestational trophoblastic disease	Hysterectomy.	Methotrexate Actinomycin D	Chemotherapy given until HCG titer is normal for 6 mo.	Single agent curative unless liver or brain involved or large tumor burden—then triple agent therapy.
Testicular	Radical orchiectomy alone or with retroperitoneal node dissection.	Cisplatin Vinblastine Bleomycin Vincristine Cyclophosphamide Actinomycin D Adriamycin Methotrexate	Positive HCG or alpha fetoprotein indicates active disease. Treat with combination therapy: cisplatin, vinblastine, and bleomycin. Adjuvant therapy not recommended.	Combination chemotherapy; selective surgical "debulking" may be needed to obtain a cure.
Hodgkin's disease	Radiotherapy, staging laparotomy indicated only when findings will change treatment selection.	Mechlorethamine Vincristine Procarbazine Prednisone Adriamycin (doxorubicin) Bleomycin Vinblastine Dacarbazine (DTIC) Cyclophosphamide	Adjuvant to radiation therapy presently not indicated.	Stage IIIB and IV with MOPP or C-MOPP or ABVD for MOPP failure.
Diffuse histiocytic lymphoma	Radiotherapy if local disease only.	Cyclophosphamide Adriamycin Vincristine Prednisone Bleomycin High-dose Methotrexate Procarbazine		CHOP therapy.

Cancers in which response to chemotherapy improves survival				
Breast carcinoma	Mastectomy or radiotherapy with axillary node dissection.	Adriamycin Cyclophosphamide Methotrexate 5-Fluorouracil Dibromodulcitol Vincristine Prednisone Tamoxifen Megestrol Diethylstibesterol Fluoxymesterone	Treatment indicated for node-positive patients. Premenopausal patients benefit most from CMF. Postmenopausal patients may benefit from CMFVP.	Hormonal therapy for estrogen receptor–positive tumors. CAF, CMF combinations useful with and without hormones or vincristine.
Ovarian carcinoma	Bilateral oophorectomy with total hysterectomy and omentectomy and thorough exploration to stage and debulk all gross disease. Decreasing size of residual disease may allow cure.	Adriamycin Cisplatin Cyclophosphamide Hexamethylmelamine 5-Fluorouracil Methotrexate Melphalan Chlorambucil	Stage II disease; unknown whether radiotherapy to abdomen and pelvis is superior to chemotherapy with Hexa-CAF or CAP	Stage IIIB and IV treated with Hexa-CAF or CAP. Second-look operation indicated after six cycles. Stage IIIA radiotherapy versus chemotherapy?
Soft tissue sarcomas	Wide en bloc excision. Chemotherapy and radiotherapy before operation for advanced stages.	Adriamycin Actinomycin D DTIC Cyclophosphamide Methotrexate	Continued therapy with high-dose methotrexate, vincristine, and adriamycin may improve cure rate.	Combination therapy with Adriamycin-DTIC or Cy-VADIC
Osteogenic sarcoma	Radical surgery, or limb salvage and preoperative chemotherapy with vincristine, high-dose methotrexate, and Adriamycin.	Adriamycin High-dose methotrexate Actinomycin D Cyclophosphamide Bleomycin	Continued chemotherapy postoperatively may increase survival. No controls in reported studies.	Adriamycin, Cy-VADIC, or CAB

Cancers in which response to chemotherapy improves survival

Type of Cancer	Treatment of Primary (Local and Regional)	Active Agents	Treatment of Micrometastases (Adjuvant Therapy)	Treatment of Metastatic Disease
Adenocarcinoma of stomach	Cardia-esophagogastrectomy Palliative-total radical gastrectomy Distal-subtotal radical gastrectomy Palliative resection also indicated.	5-Fluorouracil BCNU Adriamycin Mitomycin C	Benefits from postoperative radiotherapy or chemotherapy unproved.	Radiation and 5-FU or BCNU for unresectable or local residual disease. 5-FU + BCNU, 5-FU + BCNU + Adriamycin, 5-FU + mitomycin C + Adriamycin, 5-FU + Adriamycin have had some success.
Small cell carcinoma of lung	Radiotherapy to primary.	Adriamycin Cyclophosphamide CCNU DTIC Hexamethylmelamine Methotrexate Procarbazine Vincristine	Chemotherapy with radiation to gross disease confined to thorax increases survival. Prophylactic radiation to brain of unknown benefit to overall survival.	VAC, COP, MACC, etc. Many polychemotherapy regimens reported.
Endometrial carcinoma	Surgery and radiotherapy, alone or together.	Progestins Adriamycin Cyclophosphamide 5-Fluorouracil		Progestins; other drugs may not prolong survival.
Prostatic carcinoma	Surgery and radiotherapy, alone or together.	Diethylstilbesterol Cyclophosphamide 5-Fluorouracil Adriamycin DTIC		Diethylstilbesterol; after failure, cyclophosphamide. Combination therapy not proved better than single agent.
Bladder cancer	Surgery and radiotherapy, preoperative or post-	Adriamycin Cyclophosphamide Cisplatin		Cisplatin is drug of choice. Adriamycin + 5-FU is an alternative

Cancer	Treatment	Drugs	Combinations / comments
Melanoma	Wide local excision and regional lymph node dissection for levels III, IV, and V.	DTIC BCNU CCNU Actinomycin D Vincristine Dibromodulcitol	DTIC. No combinations proved better. Completed trials show no benefit.
Malignant gliomas	Surgery and radiation.	BCNU CCNU 5-Fluorouracil Procarbazine	BCNU.
Cancers in which minimal or no palliation can be achieved with chemotherapy			
Squamous cell carcinoma of head and neck	Surgery and radiotherapy, alone or together.	Adriamycin Bleomycin Cisplatin Cyclophosphamide Dibromodulcitol Hexamethylmelamine Methotrexate Vinblastine Vincristine	Cisplatin and bleomycin; methotrexate; high response rates of short duration. Poor responses in local recurrence in site previously irradiated.
Carcinoma of lung (other than small cell)	Surgery for resectable disease; radiation for node-positive resections, nonsurgical candidates, and unresectable disease.	Adriamycin CCNU Cisplatin Cyclophosphamide Dibromodulcitol DTIC Hexamethylmelamine Methotrexate Procarbazine Vinblastine Vincristine	CAP, CAMP.
Carcinoma of esophagus	Surgery and radiotherapy, alone or together.	Bleomycin Cisplatin CCNU Cyclophosphamide	Cisplatin and bleomycin.

Table 21-2 (Continued)

Cancers in which response to chemotherapy improves survival

Type of Cancer	Treatment of Primary (Local and Regional)	Active Agents	Treatment of Micrometastases (Adjuvant Therapy)	Treatment of Metastatic Disease
Carcinoma of pancreas	Total pancreatectomy versus Whipple procedure.	Adriamycin BCNU 5-Fluorouracil Mitomycin C Streptozotocin	5-FU and radiation may improve results of Whipple procedure; chemotherapy and radiation improve survival of locally advanced unresectable disease over radiation alone.	5-FU; 5-FU and BCNU; FAM.
Carcinoma of colon and rectum	Wide resection to include all lymph nodes draining the primary tumor.	5-Fluorouracil? Methyl-CCNU?	Proof of benefit from adjuvant therapy lacking.	No increase in survival with chemotherapy.
Renal cell carcinoma	Radical nephrectomy.			

MOPP = mechlorethamine, vincristine, prednisone, procarbazine
C-MOPP = cyclophosphamide, vincristine, prednisone, procarbazine
ABVD = Adriamycin, bleomycin, vinblastine, dacarbazine
CHOP = cyclophosphamide, Adriamycin, vincristine, prednisone
CMF = cyclophosphamide, methotrexate, 5-fluorouracil
CMFVP = CMF, vincristine, prednisone
CAF = cyclophosphamide, Adriamycin, 5-fluorouracil
Hexa-CAF = hexamethylmelamine, cyclophosphamide, amethopterin, 5-fluorouracil
CAP = cyclophosphamide, Adriamycin, cisplatin
Cy-VADIC = cyclophosphamide, vincristine, Adriamycin, DTIC
CAB = cyclophosphamide, actinomycin D, bleomycin
VAC = vincristine, Adriamycin, cyclophosphamide
COP = cyclophosphamide, vincristine, procarbazine
MACC = methotrexate, Adriamycin, cyclophosphamide, CCNU
CAMP = cyclophosphamide, Adriamycin, methotrexate, procarbazine
FAM = 5-fluorouracil, Adriamycin, mitomycin C

made at this time despite promising, positive data using BCG as an adjuvant to surgery of stage I lung cancer, and of melanoma with positive regional lymph nodes.

Future clinical trials will involve more specific therapies. Antineoplastic agents can be specifically directed to a tumor by linking the drug with antibodies to tumor-specific antigens. Other efforts are directed at enhancement of tumor cell antigenicity through alteration of cell surface antigens by enzymes. Response to any new immunotherapies will ultimately depend on the immune status of the host. The general immunocompetence of the host is effected by multiple factors, which include tumor burden, age, nutritional state, and prior or concomitant therapy with immunosuppressive or antineoplastic agents and with radiation.

Suggested Reading

Brodsky, I., Kahn, S. B., and Conroy, J. F. (eds.). *Cancer Chemotherapy III*. New York: Grune & Stratton, 1978.

Chabner, B. A., Myers, C. E., Coleman, C. N., and Johns, D. G. Clinical pharmacology of antineoplastic agents. *N. Engl. J. Med.* 292: 1107, 1159, 1975.

Jelsema, C. L., Killion, J. J., and Winkelhake, J. L. Enzymatic Alteration of Cell surface Antigenicity. In J. Holcenberg and P. Robbins (eds.), *Enzymes as Drugs*. New York: Academic, 1980. Chap. 7.

Legha, S. S., Slavik, M., and Carter, S. K. Hexamethylmelamine. An evaluation of its role in the therapy of cancer. *Cancer* 38: 27, 1976.

Levine, N., and Greenwald, E. S. Mucocutaneous side effects of cancer chemotherapy. *Cancer Treat. Rev.* 5:67, 1978.

Mischler, N. E., Earhart, R. H., Carr, B., and Tormey, D. C. Dibromodulcitol. *Cancer Treat. Rev.* 6:191, 1979.

Mouridsen, H., Palshof, T., Patterson, J., and Battersby, L. Tamoxifen in advanced breast cancer. *Cancer Treat. Rev.* 5:131, 1978.

Rozencweig, M., VonHoff, D. D., Slavik, M., and Muggia, F. M. Cis-diamminedichloroplatinum (II). A new anticancer drug. *Ann. Intern. Med.* 86:803, 812, 1977.

Silver, R. T., Young, R. C., and Holland, J. F. Some aspects of modern cancer chemotherapy. *Am. J. Med.* 63:772, 1977.

Weiss, H. D., Walker, M. D., and Wiernik, P. H. Neurotoxicity of commonly used antineoplastic agents. *N. Engl. J. Med.* 291:75, 127, 1974.

Weiss, R. B., and Muggia, F. M. Cytotoxic drug-induced pulmonary disease: Update 1980. *Am. J. Med.* 68:259, 1980.

Willson, J. K. V. Pulmonary toxicity of antineoplastic drugs. *Cancer Treat. Rep.* 62:2003, 1978.

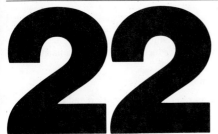

Venous Disorders of the Lower Extremities

I. Facts and definitions

A. Anatomy. The venous drainage from the lower extremity is by three systems: superficial, perforator, and deep.

1. The **superficial** system includes all the subcutaneous venous vessels. The major superficial channels are the greater and lesser saphenous veins. The greater (long) saphenous system drains the superficial tissues of the medial and posterior aspects of the lower leg and thigh and empties into the common femoral vein at the groin. The short saphenous system drains the superficial lateral aspect of the leg and empties into the popliteal vein.

2. The **deep** venous system is composed of thin-walled channels that follow the arteries and their branches. In the calf, these veins are paired. In addition to the paired veins, there are venous sinuses within the soleus muscle. Above the knee, the deep veins usually are not paired.

3. Connecting the superficial and deep systems are the communicating **perforator** veins. The majority of these channels join the greater saphenous system and are found in a regular series on the medial aspect of the lower extremity. There are usually one or two perforators above the knee, three or four between the knee and the ankle, and one perforator (the arch vein) just below the medial malleolus. In a functional sense, the greater and lesser saphenous veins are perforators.

B. Physiology. All three parts of the venous system contain one-way valves favoring blood return to the heart. Perforator valves favor flow from superficial to deep veins. In the upright position, hydrostatic venous pressure is limited by competent venous valves. Venous flow is maintained through the presence of these valves, cardiac perfusion, and lower extremity muscle contraction. Of these, the **muscle pump** is the greatest contributor.

C. Pathology

1. **Primary varicose veins** are manifested by dilation and elongation of the superficial system. The deep and perforator venous systems are normal; i.e., their valves are competent and functioning.

2. **Secondary varicose veins** also involve dilation and elongation of the superficial venous system. The perforator and deep venous systems are incompetent.

3. **Venous thrombosis**

   a. **Elements promoting venous thrombosis (Virchow's triad)**

      (1) **Hypercoagulability** is associated with malignant disease, blood dyscrasias, or trauma or may be present for undetermined reasons.

      (2) **Venous stasis** can occur in the intraoperative and postoperative period. It occurs in pregnancy, in the postpartum period, in heart disease, dehydration, immobilization from chronic disease or acute injury, and in patients with an incompetent venous system.

    (3) Endothelial injury results from trauma, venipuncture, IV infusion, or infection. Intimal injury causes a reduction in fibrinolytic activator activity within the vessel wall and reduces the intrinsic capacity of the vessel to inhibit thrombus formation.

b. Classification of venous thrombosis

    (1) Superficial thrombophlebitis refers to inflammation and thrombosis of subcutaneous veins. The perforator and deep venous systems are not involved.

    (2) Deep thrombophlebitis refers to inflammation and thrombosis of the deep venous system. The perforator veins sometimes are also involved. The superficial system usually is not involved.

    (3) Phlebothrombosis refers to thrombosis of the deep venous system not accompanied by immediate signs or symptoms of inflammation. The superficial veins are usually not involved.

    (4) To produce classic milk leg, or **phlegmasia alba dolens**, the common femoral vein above the deep femoral vein must be thrombosed. The external iliac vein up to and including the junction of the internal iliac vein is sometimes involved. The leg is swollen, pale or mottled, and cool. Although the main deep venous channels are occluded, small veins in the lower extremity remain patent, so that some routes of venous drainage from the limb via collateral channels are available. Phlegmasia alba dolens usually does not carry a risk of gangrene.

    (5) In **phlegmasia cerulea dolens,** nearly the entire venous collateral bed of the leg is thrombosed in addition to thrombosis of the iliofemoral system. Drainage of blood from the leg is seriously impeded. The leg is massively swollen, exquisitely tender, cold, and deeply cyanotic. Gangrene is an imminent threat.

    (6) Suppurative thrombophlebitis, or infection with suppuration of a previously cannulated vein, requires surgical excision of the involved vein.

II. Primary varicose veins

A. Incidence and etiology

    1. Primary varicose veins constitute the most common venous disorder of the lower extremity, affecting 10% of the population, three fourths of the patients being young women.

    2. Varicosities result from incompetence of proximal valves in the affected veins. Dilation of the vein prevents the valve cusps from meeting, allowing increased hydrostatic pressure to be transmitted to the next lower segment of vein. Progressive distal dilation and valve incompetence result in the varicosity.

3. Factors predisposing to varicose veins are:

    a. Hereditary defects in the venous structure.

    b. Occupations requiring standing in place for long periods.

    c. Pregnancy and other conditions causing increased intra-abdominal pressure.

    d. Old age, resulting in loss of tissue elasticity.

    e. Obesity.

B. Clinical features

    1. Symptoms usually are minimal. Cosmetic appearance is the most common reason for consultation. Symptoms, when present, usually include aching, tiredness, a sense of fullness in the leg when the person is upright for long periods, and nocturnal muscle cramps.

    2. The major sign of primary varicose veins is the presence of tortuous, dilated venous channels. These most commonly involve the posterior communicating arch joining the greater and lesser saphenous systems.

    3. Complications of long-standing varicosities are:

        a. Venous thrombosis.

        b. Edema.

        c. Stasis dermatitis (brawny induration and pigmentation).

        d. Ulceration, usually in the area of the medial malleolus (rare).

        e. Hemorrhage.

C. Diagnosis

    1. Evaluation begins with a thorough history and physical examination. Special attention should be given to the peripheral arterial system in complicated cases.

    2. Trendelenburg's test is useful in distinguishing primary from secondary varicose veins (Fig. 22-1).

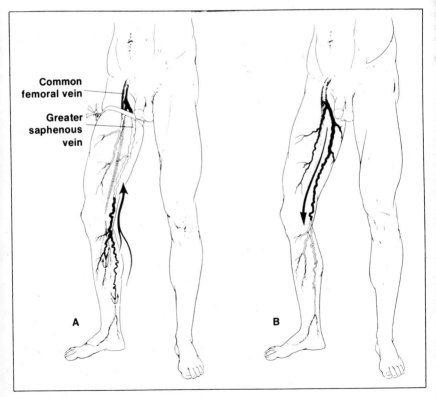

Figure 22-1. Trendelenberg test. Rapid filling of varicose veins from the calf when the superficial venous system is occluded at the groin indicates incompetent perforator veins (A). Rapid filling of the superficial venous system from above when the tourniquet is removed indicates saphenous venous valve incompetence (B). Both abnormalities may be present in the same extremity.

   a. With the patient supine, elevate the limb to 65 degrees, and allow the veins to empty by gravity aided by gentle manual milking. Apply a rubber tourniquet high on the thigh to occlude superficial vein flow.

   b. Have the patient stand; record the time and direction in which the veins fill.

   c. If the varices remain empty for more than 20 sec, valves in the communicating veins are competent. If the veins fill rapidly with the tourniquet in place, there is incompetence of valves in the communicating veins. If, when the patient is standing, the tourniquet is removed and rapid filling of veins from above is noted, incompetence of valves of the greater saphenous vein is confirmed.

   d. The same test may be applied to the lesser saphenous system using a tourniquet or manual compression just below the popliteal fossa.

  3. Patency of the deep venous system may be clinically evaluated by placing a tourniquet at the groin level and elevating the limb. Patency is assured by rapid emptying of the superficial system.

  4. The location of **perforating veins** can best be determined by palpation of the leg in the elevated position, looking for fascial defects that normally are present but are enlarged where dilated imcompetent veins penetrate the fascia.

  5. Noninvasive vascular laboratory testing usually is not necessary in the evaluation of uncomplicated cases of varicose veins; however, the tests are accurate and are useful when physical examination is inconclusive. **Doppler ultrasound** and **photoplethysmography** are used in perforator localization and the differentiation of primary from secondary varicose veins. **Phleborheography, impedance plethysmography,** and **Doppler ultrasound** are also accurate in the confirmation of deep system patency.

  6. Venography. Contrast venography generally is not required in patients with uncomplicated varicose veins, since it is not usually more accurate than a thorough physical examination or noninvasive testing. Venography, however, should be performed prior to removal of congenital varicose veins to document the presence of a deep venous system; such patients also should be evaluated for the presence of congenital arteriovenous fistulas.

D. Nonoperative treatment. Conservative treatment for varicose veins should be employed first, unless the chief complaint is cosmesis.

  1. The principles of nonoperative treatment are:

   a. Have the patient wear firm elastic support when in an upright position. Elastic stockings should be put on before getting out of bed in the morning.

   b. Instruct the patient to avoid prolonged periods of standing or sitting.

   c. Have the patient avoid circular constricting garments, such as tight girdles and circular garters.

   d. Instruct the patient to elevate the legs above the level of the heart for 20 min tid.

  2. Sclerotherapy of varicose veins is performed by the injection of a sclerosing agent (e.g., sodium tetradecyl sulfate or sodium morrhuate) into the appropriate veins, followed by compression using elastic wraps. Although this method has been used successfully for sclerosing of the entire superficial system, in the hands of the inexperienced sclerotherapist it is probably best limited to the treatment of minimal varicosities or varicosities remaining after superficial venous stripping.

E. Operative treatment

  1. Indications

   a. Cosmesis.

   b. Symptomatic varicosities.

    c. Anatomical or symptomatic progression of varices while the patient is receiving nonoperative therapy.

    d. Stasis ulceration if due solely to superficial venous insufficiency; i.e., the deep venous system is competent (stasis ulceration is seldom seen with only superficial venous incompetence).

    e. Recurrent varicosities not responsive to sclerotherapy.

2. Varicosities and perforator sites should be marked the evening before operation. A **marking solution** that will not come off during skin preparation can be made by the pharmacist: pyrogallol (500 mg), 40% ferric chloride solution (4 ml), acetone (5 ml), and alcohol, qs up to 10 ml. The solution is applied with an applicator stick and darkens as it dries.

3. **Standard operative treatment** of varicose veins is high ligation at the saphenofemoral junction and stripping of the greater saphenous system from the saphenofemoral junction to the ankle. If the short saphenous system is involved, it is ligated at the saphenopopliteal junction and stripped from the external malleolus to the point of ligation. All perforating veins also should be ligated at the fascial level. Dilated tributaries of the long or short saphenous trunks also should be stripped, or, alternatively, may be sclerosed postoperatively.

4. **Postoperatively,** pressure bandages are applied from the toes to the groin and are maintained for 7–10 days. An elastic stocking should be worn until 3–4 weeks after the operation.

5. **Ambulation** with assistance is begun the day of operation. While the patient is walking, leg movement is to be constant. Sitting or standing promotes venous stasis and should be discouraged.

6. **Discharge** from the hospital is usually on the third postoperative day.

7. **Complications** of stripping and ligation

    a. Hematoma can be prevented by placing the patient in the Trendelenburg position, by expressing blood from the wound before closure, and by using an elastic bandage. Drainage usually is not needed. Postoperatively, the foot of the bed should be elevated to reduce venous pressure when the patient is in bed.

    b. Infection, skin necrosis, and wound breakdown. Careful operative technique is imperative. Avoidance of thin skin flaps is important to avoid skin necrosis.

    c. Patchy numbness. Superficial nerves are sometimes interrupted during stripping. If the saphenous and sural nerves are spared, minimal numbness will result. Restoration of sensation usually occurs in 6–12 mo.

    d. Early recurrence may be caused by:

        (1) Failure to recognize and strip an accessory saphenous vein joining the common femoral vein.

        (2) Failure to recognize and strip an incompetent small saphenous vein.

        (3) Failure to deal adequately with incompetent perforator veins.

    e. Ligation of the femoral artery occurs in inexperienced hands but can be obviated by adequate knowledge of groin anatomy.

    f. Deep venous thrombosis and pulmonary embolism occur rarely.

III. Secondary varicose veins

    A. Secondary varicosities are caused by **high venous pressure** applied to the superficial venous system as a result of:

1. **Deep venous insufficiency with incompetence of the perforator veins** (see Fig. 22-1).

2. **Congenital or acquired arteriovenous fistula.**

B. There is often a **history of thrombophlebitis or trauma.** Usually, there will be clinical signs of deep venous insufficiency (edema, dermatitis, stasis ulcer), as well as the presence of superficial varicosities.

C. **Nonoperative therapy** is instituted (see **II. D.1**) with the use of elastic support. Since the patient requires elastic stocking support because of deep venous insufficiency, stripping of superficial varicosities is not necessary in most cases. In patients who are not responsive to conservative treatment or who do not comply with conservative measures, operative therapy may be required (see **VI. B. 2**).

D. **Post-traumatic arteriovenous fistulas** are treated by resection of the fistulous communication. Congenital fistulas usually are multiple and respond poorly to operative intervention; varicosities should be treated nonoperatively in most cases.

IV. Superficial venous thrombosis

A. **Phlebitis migrans** is a disorder characterized by recurrent attacks of thrombophlebitis involving segments of previously normal superficial veins. The cause is unknown. The typical patient is a man under 45 yr of age who complains of pain, redness, tenderness, and swelling of a segment of superficial vein, usually in the leg but sometimes on the trunk or arm. After an acute episode, remission may last several years. Many cases of Buerger's disease (thromboangiitis obliterans) begin with this disorder. This condition also may be associated with collagen vascular diseases (particularly systemic lupus erythematosus) and gastrointestinal malignancy. **Treatment** is symptomatic; elastic support of inflamed leg veins is helpful. Smoking should be discouraged. In persistently active cases, long-term anticoagulant therapy may be required.

B. **Thrombophlebitis in varicose veins** usually presents as firm, tender, reddened cords or as red streaks overlying varicosities that were previously soft and painless. Treatment consists of the following:

1. Medication for pain and active use of the leg as soon as pain permits. Bed rest is not advised in this situation, since it only promotes venous stasis. Antibiotics and anticoagulants are not needed. Some physicians recommend anti-inflammatory agents, such as aspirin or phenylbutazone.

2. When there is involvement of the greater saphenous system at the saphenofemoral junction, **anticoagulation** or **division of the saphenous vein** is indicated to prevent extension as a femoral thrombophlebitis.

V. Deep vein thrombosis. Deep vein thrombosis may occur with (thrombophlebitis) and without (phlebothrombosis) an associated inflammatory reaction.

A. **Incidence.** The incidence of deep venous thrombosis in the general population has not been accurately determined. The incidence in postoperative patients has been shown, using ^{125}I-fibrinogen uptake, to be 30% in patients over 40 yr of age.

B. The **etiology** of deep venous thrombosis in a given patient is not always evident. Certain **risk factors** have been identified; these include congestive heart failure, advanced age, malignancy, trauma, obesity, the postoperative state, immobility, and pregnancy. In most of these conditions one can identify at least one element of Virchow's triad. Venous stasis and intimal injury are fairly easily identified. Hypercoagulability has an elusive definition; no specific coagulation factor abnormalities have been identified to correlate with a hypercoagulable state with the possible exception of antithrombin III deficiency and such factors as elevated plasma procoagulants in postoperative patients and alternative fibrin polymerization reactions in animal neoplasms. Certain serum and blood element abnormalities that may predispose to hypercoagulability include thrombocytosis, polycythemia, and hyperproteinemias.

C. **Pathophysiology.** When intimal injury is the cause, thrombosis probably begins at the site of injury. When stasis or hypercoagulability is at fault, thrombus is thought to form in the venous valve sulci and then to propagate. Although thrombosis frequently starts in the calf veins it does not always do so; isolated iliac or femoral thrombosis is not uncommon. Thrombus behavior is variable. Spontaneous lysis is seen in 80% of calf vein thromboses; complete superficial and deep venous occlusion occurs in phlegmasia cerulea dolens.

D. **Clinical findings.** Deep venous thrombosis is both overdiagnosed and underdiagnosed on the basis of clinical findings. The classic **signs and symptoms** of deep venous thrombosis include edema, diffuse pain and tenderness, cyanosis, increased warmth, and superficial venous distention. Tenderness on compression of the posterior calf muscles (Pratt's sign) or forceful dorsiflexion of the foot (Homans' sign) may be seen. Unfortunately, these signs and symptoms may be entirely absent in many patients with deep venous thrombosis, and only half of patients with these signs and symptoms can be found to have deep venous thrombosis when tested objectively.

E. **Differential diagnosis. Edema** may be secondary to lymphedema, congestive heart failure, or hypoalbuminemia. **Pain** may be associated with lymphangitis, ruptured muscles or tendons, peripheral neuritis, sciatica, arthritis, bursitis, soft tissue injuries, infection, and neoplasia.

F. **Diagnosis.** The most important aspect of diagnosis is a high index of suspicion. Although not conclusive, the presence of classic signs and symptoms should lead to further attempts at objective diagnosis. A high index of suspicion of deep venous thrombosis also should follow certain operative procedures that are associated with a high risk of deep venous thrombosis, e.g., abdominoperineal resection, open prostatectomy, open reduction and internal fixation of the hip. Screening of these high-risk patients for deep venous thrombosis may be indicated, especially if there is a prior history of venous disease.

1. **Noninvasive techniques.** Several noninvasive techniques (**Doppler ultrasound, impedance plethysmography, phleborheography**) that are nearly as accurate as contrast venography are now available for the diagnosis of deep venous thrombosis. These techniques are not only accurate but also are without risk, enabling them to be repeated many times. For this reason, they are excellent screening studies. Radioactive ^{125}I-fibrinogen uptake studies are best applied to epidemiological studies, since they are not accurate for deep venous thrombosis proximal to the mid-thigh. In many institutions, initiation or withholding of therapy is now based on the results of noninvasive techniques alone.

2. **Contrast venography.** In certain situations, noninvasive testing may not be applicable or available, and contrast venography is required. This test is especially useful in patients with a history of previous deep vein thrombosis, since noninvasive testing will not differentiate between old and new thrombi. Sometimes venography cannot make this distinction either, and ^{125}I-fibrinogen, if applicable, may be employed to detect ongoing thrombosis.

G. **Treatment**

1. **Prophylaxis** is employed primarily in hospitalized patients and constitutes such general measures as early postoperative ambulation, elevation of the legs, and adequate hydration. Specific measures such as compression stockings also may be used; their efficacy is controversial. The most frequently employed prophylaxis is minidose heparin (5000 units SC q8–12h). This regimen has been shown by many, although not all, investigators to decrease the incidence of deep venous thrombosis in postoperative patients. To be effective, heparin is best started 2 hr prior to operation.

2. **Anticoagulation** to prevent thrombus extension is the preferred method of therapy for deep venous thrombosis. Continuous IV heparin infusion is begun following an initial loading dose of 5000 units. The infusion is regulated to keep the partial thromboplastin time at 1½–2 times control. Heparin should be

continued for a minimum of 7 days. Warfarin should be started orally during heparin therapy and regulated to maintain the prothrombin time at 1½–2 times control. In addition to anticoagulation, the patient should be put on complete bed rest with the lower extremity elevated to avoid embolic complications and to treat edema. Oral anticoagulation should be continued for 4 mo following the first episode of deep venous thrombosis; recurrent episodes require a longer course of therapy. Recurrent thrombosis (particularly migratory) should alert the physician to the possibility of an ongoing general stimulus to thrombosis (e.g., vasculitis, gastrointestinal neoplasm.)

3. **Thrombolytic therapy** consists of using plasminogen-activating substances such as streptokinase or urokinase. Delayed approval of these substances by the FDA has prevented a large experience in this country with these agents. European data suggest that the incidence of venous valvular damage may be less with this form of therapy, although this is controversial.

4. **Venous thrombectomy** usually is not performed because of the high operative blood loss and high rethrombosis rates. It may be indicated, however, in cases of plegmasia cerulea dolens unresponsive to anticoagulation.

H. Complications of deep venous thrombosis

1. Pulmonary embolus with acute respiratory failure.

2. Venous valvular damage resulting in the postphlebitic state.

3. Chronic pulmonary hypertension secondary to repeated small pulmonary emboli.

4. Gangrene secondary to massive deep venous thrombosis (phlegmasia cerulea dolens).

5. Increased incidence of future deep venous thrombosis.

VI. Postphlebitic syndrome.
The postphlebitic syndrome is caused by sustained venous hypertension in the distal lower extremity. The hypertension may be secondary to continued thrombotic occlusion, or to recannulization following clot lysis through damaged venous valves, resulting in increased hydrostatic venous pressure. The increased pressure may be transmitted to the superficial system through incompetent perforator veins. The onset may occur a few weeks to many years following deep venous thrombosis.

A. Components of the postphlebitic syndrome

1. **Edema** is secondary to fluid transudation secondary to increased venous pressure.

2. **Pigmentation** is secondary to hemosiderin deposition from broken-down, extravasated red blood cells.

3. **Stasis dermatitis** is an exczematous condition with cutaneous weeping of serum.

4. **Panniculitis,** as evidenced by woody induration about the ankles following fat necrosis secondary to local adipose tissue ischemia, is due to sustained venous hypertension and poor cellular perfusion.

5. **Ulceration** is ischemic in nature, as evidenced by a buildup of anaerobic metabolic end products secondary to decreased cellular perfusion resulting from venous hypertension. These ulcers most commonly are present about the medial malleolus, corresponding to the normal location of perforating veins.

B. Treatment

1. **Nonoperative treatment** with good patient compliance is adequate for most cases of postphlebitic syndrome. These measures consist of elevation of the legs higher than the heart whenever possible and elastic graded pressure stockings.

Antibiotics occasionally may be needed to combat secondary infection. Corticosteroid creams are sometimes of benefit in treating stasis dermatitis. Weight loss is helpful in obese patients.

Ulceration may be treated on an ambulatory basis in many cases. Leg elevation coupled with zinc oxide–impregnated gauze wraps may be used on an outpatient basis to heal ulcers. When this is not successful, hospitalization, with constant leg elevation will heal any simple stasis ulcer. Split-thickness skin grafting may be added to hasten wound closure, but recurrence will be the rule if measures are not subsequently taken to combat venous hypertension. Compression stockings can be used for this purpose if they have not been employed previously. Ulcers that appear during adequate compression therapy usually will require operative management.

2. **Operative therapy** is primarily aimed at preventing transmission of the deep venous hypertension to superficial levels. This may be done in a limited fashion by perforator ligation limited to the area of the ulcer, or by more extensive approach of subfascial ligation of all perforators below the knee. Removal of the incompetent saphenous systems, if present, usually should accompany perforator ligation unless there is extensive occlusion of the deep venous system, in which case any operative approach probably is contraindicated.

Newer surgical techniques have been described that address the primary problem of valvular incompetence. These procedures include venous valve repair and valve transfers; their place in the surgical treatment of postphlebitic syndrome has yet to be determined. When sustained venous hypertension unresponsive to nonoperative measures is due primarily to venous occlusion from nonrecannulized thrombi, venous bypass techniques may be employed in certain situations.

Suggested Reading

Bergan, J. J., and Yao, J. S. T. *Venous Problems.* Chicago, Year Book, 1978.

Cranley, J. J. *Vascular Surgery: Peripheral Venous Disease.* Hagerstown, Harper & Row, 1975. Vol. 2.

Flanigan, D. P., Goodreau, J. J., Burnham, S. J., Bergan, J. J., and Yao, J. S. T. Vascular laboratory diagnosis of clinically suspected acute deep vein thrombosis. A diagnostic and therapeutic schema. *Lancet* 2:331, 1978.

Hobbs, S. T. *The Treatment of Venous Disorders.* Philadelphia: Lippincott, 1977.

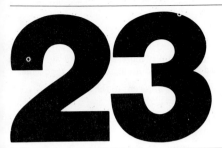

Common Anorectal Disorders

I. Clinical examination

A. The history

1. The patient comes in fear or pain, or both. Be reassuring and gentle.

2. Pay particular attention to the following:

   a. **Pain.** Type? During, before, or after bowel movement? Itching?

   b. **Change in bowel habits.** Diarrhea? Constipation? Combination of both?

   c. **Protrusion.** When? Is underclothing soiled? Is protrusion constant? After staining or defecation? Does prolapsed tissue reduce spontaneously? With manipulation? Not at all?

   d. **Bleeding.** Bright? Dark? Pink on the paper? Mixed with stool? Dripping after defecation?

B. Preparation

1. The outpatient should be prepared for examination with a Fleet enema administered in the knee-chest position the night before; another enema should be given 1–2 hr prior to examination.

2. Preparation for immediate examination requires two Fleet enemas administered with the patient in the knee-chest position. This enema may cause increased secretion of mucus. If the patient is apprehensive or in extreme pain, diazepam (Valium), 5–10 mg, or meperidine (Demerol), 50 mg, or both, can be given parenterally 1 hr prior to examination.

3. **Position** of patient

   a. **Knee-chest position.** The patient's left arm is folded across the chest; the left shoulder is touching the table; the head is turned to the right; and the knees are slightly apart, allowing the sigmoid colon to hang free. Tilt the proctoscopic table into a head-down position.

   b. **Sims' position.** The patient lies on the left side, with buttocks over the edge of the bed or table and the right leg drawn up.

C. Examination of the patient involves the following steps:

1. **External examination.** Try to localize any point of tenderness that might indicate a deep-seated infection; look for fissures, fistula tracts, excoriations, skin tags, hemorrhoids, or other abnormalities.

2. Digital examination

a. Using a lubricated finger cot, note the size of the prostate or position of the cervix; the amount of redundant internal hemorrhoidal tissue, as well as the presence of polypoid or hard masses; and areas of pain or tenderness.

b. The posterior quadrant of the rectum just internal to the anal canal is often overlooked; be sure to examine this area.

c. *Never use an instrument before performing a digital examination of the anal canal and rectum.*

3. Anoscopic examination. Insert the instrument and check all four quadrants of the anal canal, particularly posteriorly and anteriorly.

4. Proctoscopic examination

a. Insert the sigmoidoscope to 24 cm, watching carefully for abnormalities. *Never force the scope,* particularly in patients with previous pelvic operations.

b. During withdrawal, rotate the eyepiece end of the scope in a wide circle to visualize all the bowel mucosa. Be prepared to do a biopsy of mucosa or excise a polyp and to fulgurate with cautery. *Never take a biopsy specimen of a "polyp" without first applying pressure to its base;* it might be an inverted diverticulum.

II. Anorectal disorders

A. Anal fissure

1. **Acute severe pain begins during defecation,** usually with passage of a bulky or hard stool. The pain will last from a few minutes to several hours. The episode may be accompanied by slight bleeding, but the predominant symptom is pain.

2. An acute fissure will appear as a **narrow V-shaped raw split** in the mucosa of the anal canal. The apex of the mucosal split is in the rectum. Eighty percent of acute fissures are located posteriorly and can be seen readily on external examination if lateral traction is placed on the buttocks.

3. There is marked **spasm** of the anal canal and exquisite pain when a digital examination is performed.

4. The initial therapy consists of a trial of stool softeners, sitz baths, and Proctofoam-HC enemas. Patients with early acute symptoms respond well.

5. **Chronic and fissure** presents as a diagnostic triad of an enlarged anal papilla, generally a midline linear anal ulcer, and a sentinel pile. Surgical correction consists of a superficial transection of the external sphincter and excision of the hypertrophied papilla and skin tag.

6. **Pruritus ani** is a very common anal problem frequently associated with poor hygiene, excessive alkalinity of the stool, fistulas, fissures, anal warts, and hemorrhoids. Other etiological factors may be parasites, fungal infections, allergies to nylon and Dacron, and metabolic disorders such as diabetes. **Treatment** consists of elimination of the etiological factor and the use of topical hydrocortisone (Cort-Dome ½%).

B. Hemorrhoids

1. Acute thrombotic hemorrhoids

a. There is an acute onset of pain, unrelated to the patient's activity. A mass outside the anus can be felt by the patient.

b. A small vessel at the mucocutaneous junction has ruptured, causing hemorrhage into the subcutaneous tissues of the anal canal.

c. Inspection shows an extremely tender, dark, purplish nodule at some point on the anal verge. If present for more than a few hours, the overlying skin may be necrotic.

d. Treatment. The mass should have an ellipse of skin excised to evacuate the clot. Local anesthesia may be used, but in many cases pain is so intense that incision without an anesthetic causes no increase in pain. Relief of most of the pain occurs rapidly following evacuation of the clot. Hemostasis is achieved by pressure. If necessary, cautery or catgut sutures may be used. Apply ice bags for 24 hr; then begin sitz baths, compresses, and stool softeners.

2. Acute prolapsing edematous hemorrhoids

a. There usually is a history of symptomatic hemorrhoids in the past. Following defecation or straining, a prolapsed mass of hemorrhoids can be felt outside the anus. Digital reduction of the hemorrhoids, if attempted, is unsuccessful.

b. The prolapsed hemorrhoids become progressively more engorged, edematous, and extremely painful.

c. Inspection shows an edematous purplish mass surrounding the anus.

d. Treament consists of rest in bed in the prone position. If possible, the bed should be tilted 15 degrees head down, so that the buttocks and legs are elevated. Compresses are applied to the prolapsed hemorrhoids and adequate doses of analgesic drugs administered. When the acute episode has subsided, hemorrhoidectomy usually is indicated.

3. Internal hemorrhoids are the common chronic variety of hemorrhoids. They are varicose veins of the submucosal internal hemorrhoidal plexus. As the varices enlarge, the overlying mucosa becomes redundant. Enlargement may progress to involve the submucosal venous channels of the anal canal and perianal skin (external hemorrhoids).

a. The cause of hemorrhoids is unknown but may be related to chronic constipation, pregnancy, the human bipedal upright position, or the great American habit of reading in the bathroom.

b. Complaints are of protrusion during defecation producing discomfort; of protrusion with straining, coughing, lifting, or other daily activity, producing soiling of undergarments and pruritus ani; or of bleeding during defecation. Symptoms in a given patient are not constant but tend to come and go intermittently. The protruding hemorrhoids cause irritation and discomfort but usually not pain.

c. Frequently, the patient will describe manually reducing the hemorrhoidal tissue following defecation, coughing, or lifting heavy objects. Examination will reveal markedly redundant external hemorrhoidal tissue, and the examining finger will feel redundant internal tissue. Anoscopic examination reveals marked dilation of the internal hemorrhoidal vessels.

d. Hemorrhoids are common. **Therapy** is directed at regulation of bowel habits and perianal hygiene; operation is reserved for persistently and chronically symptomatic patients. Constipation is to be avoided. The patient should drink plenty of fluids. Prescribe a stool softener, such as dioctyl sodium sulfosuccinate (Colace) or dioctyl calcium sulfosuccinate (Surfak), and, if necessary, a bulk laxative. A sitz bath or use of Tucks pads for thorough cleaning of the perianal skin should follow every defecation.

e. Outpatient or office treatment by the application of elastic bands (Barron ligator) and the use of cryosurgery are useful methods in skilled surgical hands.

    f. Hemorrhoidectomy is reserved for those patients who have constant rather than episodic complaints, whose symptoms cannot be managed on the nonoperative regimen outlined in **d,** and who demonstrate a nearly complete rosette of hemorrhoidal prolapse on straining.

C. Prolapse

1. **Mucosal prolapse** is often an extension of hemorrhoidal disease. It also occurs, without large hemorrhoids, in debilitated elderly patients. Only the mucosa prolapses, so that the walls of the prolapsed mass are thin. The prolapse is circumferential, the anal opening is located centrally, and the prolapse is rarely larger than 10 cm even with straining. Excision of the redundant mass with end-to-end approximation of the mucosa is indicated.

2. **Intussusceptive rectal prolapse.** This type of prolapse involves all layers of the rectal wall, not just the mucosa. It starts as an intussusception of rectum into itself; on straining, the mass protrudes out of the anal canal. This type of prolapse is also circumferential, but there is a palpable groove between the prolapsed mass and the wall of the anal canal. The rectal opening is located centrally. The walls of the prolapsed mass are thicker than in simple mucosal prolapse.

   a. In patients who are acceptable operative risks, exicision of the prolapsed tissue and end-to-end approximation of each layer of the rectum should be done.

   b. In older and debilitated patients, use of a Thiersch wire is advised. A #20 silver wire is placed subcutaneously, approximately 3 cm around the rectum, the prolapse is reduced, and the wire is tightened sufficiently to prevent recurrence of the prolapse but not the passage of stool. The wire seldom becomes infected, but if it does, it can be removed in the surgeon's office without any great difficulty.

3. **Sliding rectal prolapse (complete rectal procidentia)** is really a sliding hernia of the pouch of Douglas into the rectum and then out of the anal canal. As the hernia protrudes, it turns the anterior wall of the rectum and canal inside out. The anterior wall of the prolapse is much thicker than the posterior wall since it contains the sliding peritoneal sac. Because of its asymmetrical development, the rectal opening points posteriorly.

   Operative repair of this type of rectal prolapse is a major undertaking whether done through the abdomen, through the perineum, or by a combined approach. The underlying cause is a defect in the pelvic diaphragm (levator ani) that must be repaired. The redundant bowel sometimes needs to be excised; if not, it should be anchored intra-abdominally.

D. Cryptitis

1. The patient complains of discomfort in the anal area following defecation.

2. Digital examination usually yields negative results. Anoscopic examination shows a markedly dilated V-shaped anal crypt without ulceration. Eliminate constipation, and use Proctofoam-HC. This condition does not need operative treatment, but if symptoms persist, biopsy of the crypt should be done to rule out a malignancy.

E. Perirectal abscesses

originate as infections in anal glands or crypts. A break in the mucosa, caused by necrosis resulting from the infection or trauma, permits the infection to extend into the perirectal tissues.

1. The abscess may be situated in one of the following areas:

   a. Beneath the anorectal mucosa or the perianal skin but superficial to the anal sphincter muscles: submucosal, subcutaneous, and mucocutaneous abscesses.

b. Betwen the internal and external sphincters: intermuscular abscess.

c. Lateral to both sphincters and below the levator ani muscle (pelvic diaphragm): ischiorectal abscess.

d. Above the levator ani muscle: pelvirectal abscess.

2. The main symptom is pain. Examination reveals a tender mass, usually fluctuant, with edema and inflammation of the overlying tissues.

3. Treatment involves incision and drainage. If the patient has signs of systemic toxicity (chills, fever, leukocytosis), administer a broad-spectrum antibiotic. Except for small submucosal and subcutaneous abscesses, incision and drainage should be performed in the operating room under general or regional anesthesia. Local anesthesia is never sufficient to permit adequate exploration of a significant perirectal abscess. A linear or cruciate incision is made over the area of maximum tenderness and fluctuance. A sample of the pus should be obtained for culture and antibiotic sensitivity tests. An instrument or a finger is inserted into the abscess cavity; all internal loculations are broken up, and the inital incision is extended so that the cavity is wide open. The cavity is then lightly packed with gauze. The patient is placed on ice packs and pain-relieving drugs for 24 hr and then given routine sitz baths. In the great majority of cases (95%) the abscess resolves, leaving an anal fistula.

F. Anal fistula. Fistula means "pipe" or "reed"; in this case, it refers to the narrow sinus tract left behind by a resolving perirectal abscess.

1. There is an internal opening in the base of an anal crypt. The external opening is in the perianal skin.

2. Fistulas with posterior external openings have their internal orifice in the posterior midline; fistulas with anterior external openings have radially located internal openings or may run as a horseshoe fistula to open internally in the posterior midline.

3. Anal fistulas must be either unroofed or excised in toto. Otherwise, the perirectal abscess will recur.

G. Condylomata acuminata (venereal warts) are moist, warty, whitish lesions situated at the anal verge. Additional lesions may be located within the anal canal or rectum. They grow very rapidly and cause a great deal of local irritation.

1. These lesions occasionally are mistaken for carcinoma; a specimen taken for biopsy will settle this issue.

2. Small lesions may be treated with podophyllum resin. Cover the surrounding normal skin with petroleum jelly, then paint the condyloma with 20% podophyllum resin in tincture of benzoin. Repeat this treatment weekly until the lesion is obliterated.

3. Skillfully performed cryosurgery has shown promising results.

4. Larger lesions should be excised. There will be a surprisingly large artery supplying the condyloma. Be prepared. Following excision, the base of the lesion should be fulgurated or ligated.

H. Hidradenitis suppurativa

1. Perianal glands become chronically infected with staphylococci, leading to persistent drainage, maceration, and scarring. The process is similar to that seen in the axillae.

2. Wide excision of the involved skin and subcutaneous tissues is required.

I. Pilonidal cyst and sinus is an **acquired, not an embryological, condition** in nearly every case. The process is a foreign body reaction to an ingrown hair in the intergluteal cleft complicated by secondary infection.

1. The patient complains of pain and drainage. Affected patients are usually men who are hairy, overweight, and have a job that necessitates sitting.

2. This lesion is commonly overtreated. Proper treatment can be carried out in the surgeon's office or outpatient clinic. A generous area around the sinus should be shaved. Local anesthesia is used, with 1% or 2% lidocaine (Xylocaine) with epinephrine infiltrated over the sinus tract. The tract is probed and incised to unroof the entire sinus. There invariably is a collection of hair and debris that should be removed. The wound is packed open and kept packed until healed.

3. In recurrent cases, excision of the sinus tract is required. Following excision, the wound is packed open and allowed to granulate and close secondarily. Only in an exceptional case, with multiple burrowing sinus tracts, will radical excision of all the tissues of the intergluteal cleft be required. Such operations are associated with considerable morbidity and are not needed for most cases of pilonidal sinus.

J. Carcinoma of the anus

1. **Squamous carcinoma** usually presents as an ulcer. The patient notices a little blood on the paper or feels a lump. There is little pain. Tuberculous and syphilitic ulcers should be differentiated by biopsy.

2. The skin surrounding the ulcer usually is indurated because of intracutaneous lymphatic spread of the cancer or because of inflammation from infection.

3. Metastases occur via the lymphatics both laterally to the iliofemoral nodes and upward to the perirectal and mesocolic nodes with equal frequency.

4. **Basal cell carcinoma** and **melanoma** also may originate in the perianal epidermis or in the anal canal. Primary adenocarcinoma arising in rectal mucosa below the anorectal ring frequently spreads downward and may appear clinically as carcinoma of the anus.

K. Radiation proctitis

1. Bright red bleeding and tenesmus may occur early following radiation treatment involving the pelvis. Low colonic obstruction caused by fibrous rectal stricture appears later.

2. Proctoscopic examination in the early stages will show irritable, friable mucosa at 6–18 cm from the anal verge. In later stages there may be marked stenosis, usually about 12–14 cm from the anus.

3. **Early treatment** consists of corticosteroid retention enemas at bedtime each evening for 1 wk; then the proctoscopic examination is repeated. In patients with late proctitis with stricture, colostomy may be necessary if the stricture cannot be resected.

L. Fecal impaction is the most common cause of obstructive bowel symptoms in elderly patients. Impaction also occurs in patients following rectal surgery, in orthopedic patients in traction or body casts, and in some neurotic children and adults.

1. Paradoxical diarrhea may occur around an obstructing impaction.

2. A digital examination quickly confirms the diagnosis.

3. **Treat** by manual digital breakdown of the bolus. Pass a rubber catheter beyond the mass and administer an oil-retention enema. Follow with Fleet enemas until the rectum is clear.

4. Acute impaction in elderly patients can be treated with caudal anesthesia—but stand clear!

M. Benign polyps

1. Any lesion that projects into the lumen of the bowel is a polyp. Polyps with a stalk are pedunculated; those without a stalk are sessile.

2. About 75% of all polypoid lesions of the entire large bowel can be seen through a 20-cm sigmoidoscope.

3. About 10% of patients over 45 yr of age harbor one or more polyps.

4. Less than 1% of adenomatous polyps contain a focus of true (i.e., invasive) carcinoma. Up to 40% of villous adenomas, on the other hand, will contain foci of invasive carcinoma.

5. Polyps seen through the sigmoidoscope should be biopsied.

    a. First, be sure the lesion is a polyp and not an inverted diverticulum. Push on the base; an inverted diverticulum can be returned to an everted position.

    b. Polyps that lie above the peritoneal reflection (12 cm from the anal verge) should be biopsied only by a skilled operator.

    c. Excise the polyp in toto, including all the stalk, together with a small rim of surrounding normal mucosa. Bleeding can usually be controlled by maintaining pressure on the biopsy site with a cotton pledget for 3 or 4 min. If bleeding continues, cauterize the bleeding point.

    d. A barium enema examination of the colon, using air contrast technique, should be carried out in every patient. Polyps will be found proximally in up to one of every four otherwise normal patients and in every patient with Gardner's syndrome and familial polyposis. The barium enema should be done either before or 10 days after excision biopsy of a polyp. Spasm, edema, or blood clots may confuse interpretation of any x-rays done in conjunction with the biopsy.

III. General principles of treatment

A. Always check the results of current therapy.

B. Sitz bath. Not more than 6 in. of comfortably warm water in a tub, three or four times a day for not more than 15 or 20 min.

C. Compresses. A wet cloth over the anal area with a hot water bottle or covered heating pad. If neither a bottle nor a pad is available, taping a piece of plastic across the buttocks will contain body heat.

D. If warm compresses do not produce improvement, use an **ice bag** or homemade ice pack (three cubes of ice wrapped in a wet facecloth).

E. For pain, use one of the compounds combining aspirin and codeine.

F. Suppositories are seldom of any value in rectal conditions, except psychologically. An anesthetic suppository with hydrocortisone will, in rare instances, be of benefit in a patient with extremely large, edematous internal hemorrhoids.

G. Diet is an important element of management. The foods listed in Table 23-1 should be avoided until the wound is healed and the patient is symptom-free.

IV. Preoperative and postoperative care

A. Preoperative orders are generally left by the anesthesiologist. If not, meperidine, 100 mg, and atropine, 0.4 mg, usually are given 1 hr prior to operation. The patient should fast from bedtime the evening before. A Fleet enema administered

Table 23-1. Foods to Avoid in Anorectal Disease

Nuts	Citrus fruits and juices
Fatty foods	Corn
Coffee	Any foods with seeds
Alcohol, including beer and wine	Popcorn
Spices	Excessive amounts of cheese and milk

with the patient in the knee-chest position is given at bedtime and repeated 2 hr before the operation.

B. Postoperative management

1. **Drains**. Occasionally, it may be necessary to place a small, lubricated rubber drain in the anal canal to give warning of hemorrhage.

2. **Diet**. Fluids are restricted until the patient voids. After voiding, the patient may progress to a liquid diet and usually to a general diet the following morning.

3. **For pain**. Dihydromorphinone (Dilaudid), 1–2 mg q3–4 hr for several days. Acetaminophen (Tylenol) with 30 mg of codeine q3–4 hr may be used for less severe pain.

4. **For sleep**. Secobarbital (Seconal), 100 mg.

5. A **tranquilizer**, such as chlordiazepoxide HCl (Librium), 10 mg qid, is started immediately.

6. **Metamucil**, 1 tablespoon with water bid, for 2 wk.

7. **Petrogalar**, 30 ml bid, until the first bowel movement, then once daily for 2 wk, unless the patient has diarrhea.

8. If **urinary retention** occurs, use a Foley catheter for a minimum of 48 hr. Cranberry juice, 240 ml bid, will help keep the urine pH acidic.

9. The day following the operation, the patient is given warm **wet compresses**. **Sitz baths** are given the next day.

10. **Avoid enemas and rectal examinations**; they produce pain.

11. Surfak, 1 or 2 capsules hs, is helpful in producing a soft, formed stool. If by the end of the fourth postoperative day a bowel movement has not occurred, insert a pediatric Fleet enema; repeat if necessary.

12. The patient should be seen weekly until the wound is healed. Keep the patient on sitz baths and Proctofoam-HC tid.

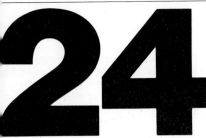

Cutaneous and Subcutaneous Tumors

I. General comments. Every physician should recognize most of the benign and malignant tumors of the skin. Obviously, all cutaneous tumors do not require excision. However, when it is decided to remove a lesion, a biopsy should be performed even if inspection alone by an experienced physician presumes a high degree of accuracy in diagnosis. Simple destruction of a small and innocuous-appearing lesion may be insufficient treatment.

II. Biopsy (meaning "vision of life") is the removal of tissue for examination under the microscope for the purpose of diagnosis. Various terms are used to describe biopsies, and they are helpful in detailing the techniques that are important in the diagnosis and management of cutaneous tumors.

   A. Excisional biopsy. When a cutaneous lesion is relatively small, it may be completely excised in a double convex design. Depending on requirements for the release of tension of the skin margins, these margins can be approximated by suture. The specimen is submitted to the pathologist for examination. A small tumor that has a sessile or pedunculated base can be sliced off with a scalpel or cut off with a small pair of scissors. This part of the tumor is the biopsy specimen, and the base of the lesion is cauterized prudently to destroy the "root" of the lesion. If the lesion should be malignant, and the pathologist finds that the tumor abuts on or extends into the margins, the surgeon can remove more tissue later.

   B. Biopsy for diagnosis to determine definitive surgical treatment and management is performed prior to definitive excision. An immediate examination (frozen section) may be prepared by the pathologist. If the pathologist finds it possible to make an accurate diagnosis after examination of the frozen section, the surgeon is then prepared to carry out the additional operative procedure that may be required for complete surgical removal of the cutaneous or subcutaneous tumor. Some wide excisions may require a skin graft or a local flap for closure.

   C. Elective biopsy is performed as a separate procedure specifically for establishing a diagnosis. A wedge of normal and abnormal tissue is removed. Later, after the pathology report is received, decisions are made about treatment of the tumor, e.g., operation, irradiation, cauterization, chemotherapy, cryotherapy, or appropriate combination therapy.

III. Anesthesia. Most cutaneous and subcutaneous tumors can be comfortably excised after administration of a local anesthetic. Lidocaine (Xylocaine) 0.5% with epinephrine 1:200,000, or 1% with epinephrine 1:100,000, or bupivacaine (Marcaine) 0.25% or 0.5% with or without epinephrine 1:200,000 are ideal local anesthetics. Local anesthetics without epinephrine are recommended in patients with severe cardiac disease or hypertension. The epinephrine additive is not always desirable in some metabolic diseases. It should be injected with caution into the hands and feet and used in the fingers and toes only by the very experienced clinician.

IV. Special considerations. Some tumors of the cutaneous or subcutaneous regions of the body may represent only a small part of what lies beneath or extends into other regions. It behooves the clinician to exercise sound judgment (common sense). For example, one should not attempt to remove a pulsating vascular lesion or a superficial-appearing cyst of the neck. These procedures should be performed by a qualified surgeon in an operating room.

A complete classification of cutaneous and subcutaneous tumors cannot be attempted here. Moreover, data are still being accumulated on many of these tumors, especially those of connective tissue origin, and there is not complete agreement on classification, therapy, and prognosis. Careful handling of the specimen, an adequate histological examination, and good communication with the pathologist should establish a reasonable diagnosis, adequacy of excision, and a plan for further therapy when indicated. Among the tumors that will not be considered individually because of their complexity or infrequency of occurrence are the histiocytoses, myomas, myxomatoses, leiomyomas, granular cell myoblastomas, desmoids, and certain fibromatoses.

V. Benign tumors. Benign tumors are removed because they interfere with function or with the patient's appearance. Also, although clinically they may appear benign, they may be premalignant or malignant lesions.

A. Tumors of the epidermis

1. **Verrucae (warts)** are caused by a virus and may occur on any skin surface, especially on the sole of the foot. Treatments that have been successful include excision, irradiation, electrocoagulation, and vaccinia virus injection beneath the lesion. Recurrence locally or at an adjacent site is common.

2. **Keratoses**

   a. **Senile keratoses.** See **VI**.

   b. **Seborrheic keratoses** are sharply marginated, brown, slightly raised, and usually only a few millimeters in diameter and have a "stuck-on" appearance. They are found on the trunk, face, and extremities (but not on the palms or soles) and usually do not occur before middle age. They are uniformly benign and should be treated by excision or electrodesiccation.

3. **Cysts**

   a. **Epidermal inclusion cysts** are elevated, firm, slow-growing, intradermal or subcutaneous tumors that develop into small, hard nodules. They are situated most frequently on the face, scalp, neck, and trunk and may be excised. If excised, the overlying skin pore and the entire cyst lining must be removed to avoid recurrence.

   b. **Sebaceous cysts** are retention cysts arising from plugged sebaceous glands about hair follicles. They commonly are found on the scalp and may become infected. They should be treated by excision of the entire lining of the sac and the skin pore. When the cyst is infected, preliminary incision and drainage is desirable, followed by excision a few weeks later. These cysts are less commonplace than epidermal inclusion cysts.

   c. Rarely, **dermoid cysts** occur in the skin or subcutaneous tissue. The most common site is the face, especially around the eyes, where they may be adherent to contiguous periosteum. These cysts are about 1–4 cm in diameter and usually are present at birth. Treatment is by excision.

4. **Keratoacanthomas.** These lesions may be solitary (the more common form) or multiple. They consist of a firm, dome-shaped nodule, 1–2 cm in diameter, with a central horn-filled crater. They are similar in appearance to squamous cell carcinoma both clinically and microscopically. The most common sites are exposed areas. The lesion usually grows for only a few weeks and involutes spontaneously within a few months. Sometimes, particularly if the lesion is located on the face, it increases in size for a longer period and may recur after treatment.

B. Tumors of vascular origin

1. **Hemangiomas.** Three types of congenital hemangiomas are generally recognized: nevus flammeus, capillary hemangioma, and cavernous hemangioma.

   a. **Nevus flammeus,** the so-called port-wine nevus, exhibits one or more dull red or bluish red patches, irregular in outline and flush with skin level. It usually is found on the side of the face or on the extremities and is frequently associated with vascular anomalies in other regions of the body. Cosmetic materials can sometimes be used to cover these unsightly spots.

   b. **Capillary hemangioma,** the so-called strawberry mark, is characterized by one or more bright red, soft, lobulated patches. The lesion first appears between the third and the fifth week of life. After growing in size for a period of months, it often begins to regress spontaneously and involutes, sometimes completely, within a few years. Surgical excision should be attempted in cases of ulceration but not for aesthetic reasons, since spontaneous regression frequently results in less deformity.

   c. **Cavernous hemangioma** is a large, purple to blue, subcutaneous mass, frequently underlying a capillary hemangioma. A large cavernous hemangioma sometimes is associated with thrombocytopenia and purpura as a form of consumption coagulopathy (Kasabach-Merritt syndrome) in infants and, rarely, in adults. Large hemangiomas are raised above skin level. Their removal, if they are extensive, may be difficult or impossible.

2. Lymphangiomas. There are three principal types of lymphangioma: simplex, circumscriptum, and cavernous.

   a. **Lymphangioma simplex** is a single, small, soft nodule, grayish pink in color and often less than 1 cm in diameter. It usually appears in adulthood.

   b. **Lymphangioma circumscriptum** consists of one or several patches, often extensive, opalescent, and verrucous in appearance. Diffuse swelling of the subcutaneous tissue may be present. These lesions appear at birth or in childhood.

   c. **Cavernous lymphangioma** causes diffuse and deformed enlargement of the region affected. It appears predominantly in the neck, mediastinum, and axilla. The vast majority of these tumors appear before the age of 2 and disappear during late childhood. If they become infected or interfere with breathing or swallowing, they may be excised. The difficulty of excision depends on the location.

3. Glomus tumors may be solitary (the more common type) or multiple. The solitary glomus tumor is characterized by a small, purple nodule that may be tender or extremely painful. The most common sites are the extremities, particularly a nail bed. Total excision is necessary. Multiple glomus tumors usually are small and asymptomatic, although occasionally they may reach a diameter of several centimeters.

C. Dermal tumors (tumors of subcutaneous or subepidermal origin). There are many dermal tumors that depend on microscopic examination for identification. Some respond to local excision, whereas others may require extensive surgical procedures and proper postoperative evaluation.

   1. Lipomas are single or multiple and are the most common subcutaneous tumors. They may be round, ovoid, or lobulated and are movable against the overlying skin. They occur most frequently on the upper back and shoulder. If they are superficial, they usually can be "shelled out" through a small incision.

   2. Fibromas may be pedunculated or have a sessile base. They are removed for diagnostic and aesthetic reasons.

   3. Keloids are fibrous tissue growths that are characterized by excessive scar tissue proliferation. They appear after injury (abrasions, lacerations, or incisions) and subsequent healing of the skin. Blacks are particularly susceptible. Corticosteroid injections and irradiation are sometimes helpful in conjunction with excision.

4. Palmar fibromatoses (Dupuytren's contracture) are most common on the palmar surfaces of the hands or plantar surfaces of the feet. These fibromatoses may be associated with Peyronie's disease. The complexities of the disease, especially in the hand, require treatment by a competent surgeon.

5. Ganglia are cyctic lesions thought to originate adjacent to or from synovial tissue of tendons or joints. They occur most commonly on the hand, wrist, fingers, palm, or dorsum of the foot, often as a result of trauma. They should be excised when they interfere with function or cause pain. An accomplished surgeon with special knowledge of the hand should perform the operation.

6. Xanthelasma is a slightly raised, yellow or tan skin lesion, often appearing on the eyelids. It is produced by cholesterol deposits in the tissues and may be associated with diabetes mellitus or atherosclerosis. Occasionally, the lesion may disappear in a person whose serum cholesterol levels have been lowered. Surgical treatment is indicated for aesthetic reasons.

7. Neurinoma (neurilemoma [schwannoma], neurofibroma). Neurilemoma and neurofibroma are both of nerve sheath origin and can occur in any nerve. The neurilemoma or schwannoma is usually solitary, benign, and encapsulated. Neurofibromas are nonencapsulated and occur as either solitary or multiple cutaneous lesions of varying sizes. When multiple, they may be accompanied by café au lait skin spots. The tumors are soft, globular, and easily deformed by pressure. They may be pedunculated. They are widely distributed throughout the body. Single neurofibromas usually arise in adult life, whereas multiple tumors appear in childhood or adolescence. The lesions are most characteristically seen in the Mendelian dominant syndrome of multiple neurofibromatosis (Recklinghausen's disease). Neurinomas that show signs of malignant degeneration or those that interfere with function should be excised.

D. Nevi exhibiting changes in pigmentation or increases in size should be excised with ample margins and to a reasonable depth.

1. Intradermal nevi are small skin tumors, usually benign, pigmented or nonpigmented, elevated or flat, with or without hair growth. They are usually excised for aesthetic reasons.

2. Junctional nevi are deeply pigmented and originate in the epidermal-dermal junction. They may develop into malignant melanoma and should be excised.

3. Compound nevi. Histologically, these nevi contain features of both junctional and intradermal nevi. They may or may not be pigmented.

VI. Premalignant tumors: senile keratoses. Senile keratoses, found in the aged, consist of patches of rough skin covered with crusts or scales or a thick keratin overgrowth (cutaneous horn). They occur on exposed sites, and there is an established relationship to solar exposure, especially in light-complexioned persons. There is familial susceptibility. These lesions have been called "farmer's skin," "sailor's skin," and "Texas skin." Senile keratoses are considered premalignant and occasionally degenerate into carcinoma. If malignancy is suspected, the lesions should be excised.

VII. Malignant tumors. Malignant tumors of the skin occur with greater frequency than any other malignant neoplasms. These tumors are removed because they are a threat to the life of the patient.

A. Tumors of the epidermis. Carcinoma of the epidermis occurs as basal cell carcinoma, squamous cell carcinoma, or as Bowen's disease. Basal cell carcinomas rarely metastasize. Squamous cell carcinomas metastasize infrequently, but when they do, it is usually to the regional lymph nodes. Bowen's disease may behave like squamous cell carcinoma. Predisposing factors are solar exposure, large doses of irradiation, burn, and other scars.

1. Basal cell carcinoma occurs particularly on skin exposed to sunlight. This carcinoma is usually a single, discrete lesion with raised, firm, gray margins.

Treatment consists of excision or x-ray therapy unless the skin has been previously irradiated. Five-year cure rates run as high as 95% when the condition is recognized early and treated adequately.

2. **Squamous cell carcinoma** may occur anywhere on the skin or mucous membranes. Most commonly, it is found on the head and neck, particularly in exposed areas. It may also arise in areas damaged by chemical irritants, scars, chronic ulcers, etc. Liberal excision is called for.

3. **Bowen's disease** (noninvasive squamous cell carcinoma of the skin) usually is a solitary lesion of sharp but irregular outline, with superficial, salmon-pink margins. It may be disseminated. It can occur on exposed skin (sun-damaged) or on nonexposed areas. The most common sites are the chest wall and face. (Noninvasive squamous cell carcinoma of mucosal surfaces occurs but is not classified as Bowen's disease.) Treatment is surgical excision or irradiation.

B. **Tumors of vascular origin: Kaposi's disease** (idiopathic hemorrhagic sarcoma) is most common in males and occurs most often on the legs and feet. It is characterized by one or more bluish to red nodules or macules. Small lesions may be excised and closed, but large, disseminated lesions will require skin grafting or skin or muscle flaps.

C. **Dermal malignancies**

1. **Fibrosarcoma** occurs most frequently on the extremities but may arise anywhere. Subcutaneous fibrosarcomas begin with one or more nodules on tendons or fasciae, eventually causing ulceration of overlying skin. Growth is slow and usually painless. Metastases occur late and may involve regional lymph nodes and visceral organs. Wide resection is indicated. Surgical excision gives slightly more than a 50% 5-yr cure rate.

2. **Liposarcoma** usually arises in an intermuscular fascial plane, particularly in the thighs, presenting as a diffuse, nodular infiltration of subcutaneous tissue. Liposarcomas metastasize late, especially to the visceral organs. Very wide and deep excision is necessary.

3. **Rhabdomyosarcoma** is of two varieties: one in children and one in adults. Most tumors in **children** are in the head, neck, or urogenital tract; in **adults,** they are most likely to develop in the extremities and torso. The tumor is usually deeply seated in the musculature and may involve skin and present as a soft mass. As it grows through the skin, it produces a red, fungating, lobulated mass. Both varieties have a high death rate.

D. **Malignant melanoma** is the most deadly of the skin tumors, with unpredictable growth patterns. The tumor is characterized by one or more flat or slightly raised lesions having a blue or brown to black color, by ulceration and bleeding, or by rapid increase in size of a pigmented nevus. Occasionally, faintly pigmented or nonpigmented melanomas may occur. The lesion may metastasize early through both the lymphatics and the bloodstream.

When a lesion is suspected of being a malignant melanoma, histological examination is mandatory. If the lesion **is** a malignant melanoma, its **depth of invasion** and its **thickness** should be determined. A definitive surgical operation should not be done in all cases prior to obtaining a reliable histological diagnosis. An excisional biopsy of a small lesion avoids an aimless extensive resection if the lesion is benign or even if it is the kind of malignancy that does not require wide resection. Furthermore, if the biopsy reveals malignant melanoma, another operation may or may not be desirable because of the location, depth of invasion, and thickness of the tumor. There is no unanimity of opinion now on the exact treatment for malignant melanoma. Consultations should be sought from an experienced surgeon, a chemotherapist, a radiotherapist, and an immunotherapist. Often, treatment is a team endeavor.

1. A **classification** of malignant melanoma has been established by Clark (see Suggested Reading) on the basis of **depth** of the tumor, divided into five levels.

   a. **Level 1**. In situ melanoma. All demonstrable tumor is above the basement membrane.

   b. **Level 2**. Melanoma has extended into the papillary dermis. At this level the tumor extends through the basement membrane and into the papillary dermis but does not fill the papillary dermis.

   c. **Level 3**. The tumor fills the papillary dermis and extends to the reticular dermis but not into it.

   d. **Level 4**. The tumor extends into the reticular dermis.

   e. **Level 5**. The tumor extends into the subcutaneous fat.

   Levels 1 and 2 have been termed **superficially invasive,** while levels 3, 4, and 5 have been termed **deeply invasive.** The superficially invasive tumors show about a 10% mortality at the end of 5 yr, while the deeply invasive tumors show more than a 50% mortality.

2. Studies by Breslow (see Suggested Reading) show that **tumor thickness** is important in predicting the outcome of the disease. Maximal tumor thickness is a reliable prognostic guide, with survival for 5 or more yr (free of tumor) for all patients whose tumors are less than 0.76 mm thick (measured by an ocular micrometer), regardless of level of invasion. Further, the incidence of metastatic disease is directly proportional to tumor thickness.

3. **Staging of malignant melanoma.** No tumor-node-metastases (TNM) classification is accepted at this time, although one has been proposed. As described, **depth of tumor** (Clark) and a measurement of the **tumor thickness** (Breslow) are important in determining definitive treatment for malignant melanoma. Another means is the **staging classification**, of which there are several. The New York University classification is recorded in Table 24-1.

E. **Lentigo maligna (Hutchinson's freckle)** is an irregularly pigmented, light brown to black macular lesion usually seen in the upper part of the face but may occur elsewhere, even on mucous membranes. The lesion may become a malignant melanoma and should be surgically excised.

Table 24-1. New York University Melanoma Cooperative Group Staging System

---

Stage I: Local disease

  IA Primary lesion alone
  IB Primary and satellites within 5 cm
  IC Local recurrence within 5 cm of primary site
  ID Spread more than 5 cm from primary site but within primary lymphatic drainage area

Stage II: Nodal disease (regional draining nodes)

  IIA Regional lymph nodes; clinically positive, histology not done
  IIB Regional lymph nodes; clinically negative, histology positive
  IIC Regional lymph nodes; clinically positive, histology positive

Stage III: Disseminated disease

  IIIA Remote cutaneous or subcutaneous melanoma
  IIIB Remote nodal involvement only
  IIIC Both of above
  IIID Visceral spread

Source: From A. W. Kopf, R. S. Bart, R. S. Rodríguez-Sains, and A. B. Ackerman. *Malignant Melanoma.* New York: Masson Publishing USA, 1979. Copyright © by Masson Publishing USA, Inc., New York.

F. Metastatic tumors. Various malignant neoplasms metastasize to the skin via the lymphatics or the bloodstream. When the primary tumor has been present for a long time, lymphatic dissemination is usually late. Dissemination through the bloodstream may occur early. Skin metastases most often contraindicate surgical excision. However, if a histological diagnosis is required, a biopsy may be performed. When a metastatic skin or subcutaneous tumor causes ulceration, excision with either primary closure or skin grafting will provide the patient more comfort and better hygiene.

Suggested Reading

Breslow, A. Thickness, cross-sectional areas and depth of invasion in the prognosis of cutaneous melanoma. *Ann. Surg.* 172:902, 1970.

Breslow, A. Tumor thickness, level of invasion and node dissection in stage 1 cutaneous melanoma. *Ann. Surg.* 182:572, 1975.

Breslow, A. Problems in the measurement of tumor thickness and level of invasion in cutaneous melanoma. *Hum. Pathol.* 8:1, 1977.

Clark, W. H., Jr. A Classification of Malignant Melanoma in Man Correlated with Histogenesis and Biologic Behavior. In W. Montagna and F. Hu (eds.), *Advances in Biology of the Skin*, Vol. 8, *The Pigmentary System*. Oxford: Pergamon, 1967.

Kopf, A. W., Bart, R. S., Rodríguez-Sains, R. S., and Ackerman, A. B. *Malignant Melanoma.* New York: Masson Publishing USA, 1979.

Stout, A. P., and Lattes, R. *Tumors of the Soft Tissues.* Washington, D.C.: Armed Forces Institute of Pathology, 1967.

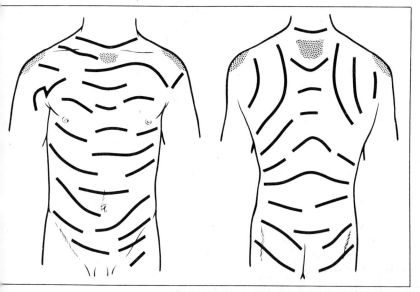

Figure 25-1. Placement of elective skin incisions. When making an elective incision for the removal of a skin or subcutaneous lesion, a better cosmetic result is obtained if the incision is placed in the lines of skin tension. The shoulder cape, just below the suprasternal notch, and the upper back just below the neck, as indicated by the areas of shading, are zones in which widening of the scar is likely to occur due to motion and tension in multiple directions.

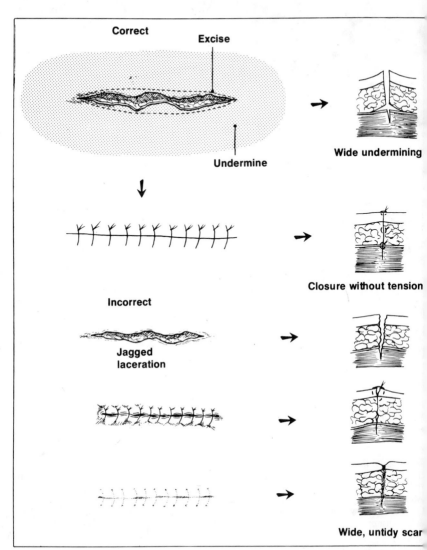

Figure 25-2. Suture of scalp and skin lacerations. *Never shave eyebrows or the scalp*; it is usually not necessary to shave around any laceration. Smear sterile lubricating jelly or the hair to hold it away from the wound. Wear cap, mask, and gloves. Gently wash the skin surrounding the laceration with chlorhexidine or iodophor solution. Use sterile towels to set up a sterile field. Establish anesthesia by infiltration of the wound margins, or use a field block. Clean the wound, remove foreign matter, excise irregular wound margins, and debride all nonviable tissue. Undermine all but superficial lacerations to reduce tension. Undermine on the trunk and extremities in the plane between subcutaneous fat and superficial fascia; in the scalp, undermine in the plane just external to the galea; in the face, undermine in the midst of subcutaneous fat. Suture each layer of the wound with fine sutures. Remove skin sutures as soon as possible.

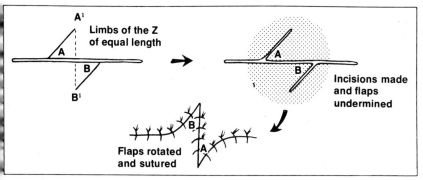

Figure 25-3. Technique of a Z-plasty. If there is tension along the length of a clean lacer-ation, or if the wound crosses a flexion crease, a Z-plasty may be a helpful maneuver to relieve tension.

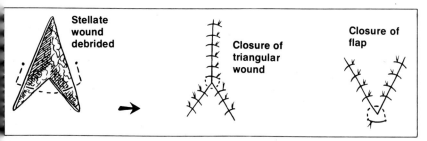

Figure 25-4. Suturing flaps and tips. Necrosis of the tip of a flap is avoided by use of the "tip stitch," a modified mattress suture that is brought subcutaneously away from the tip, so that pressure is not exerted on the tip when the suture is tied.

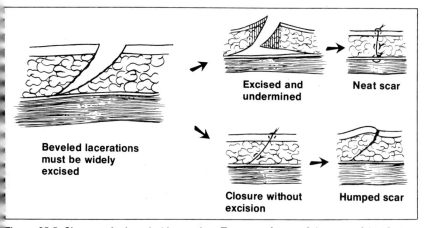

Figure 25-5. Closure of a beveled laceration. To avert a hump of tissue resulting from contraction of scar, excise a beveled wound to create vertical wound margins, and undermine it widely before closure. If the laceration is very deep, excise it in steps at each major layer of the wound.

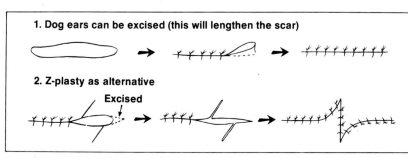

Figure 25-6. Closure of round and ovoid wounds. Direct suture closure of an ovoid wound sometimes results in a "dog ear." Excision of the dog ear will make the wound longer. Alternatively, a Z-plasty can be used to manage the dog ear; this makes the wound area wider.

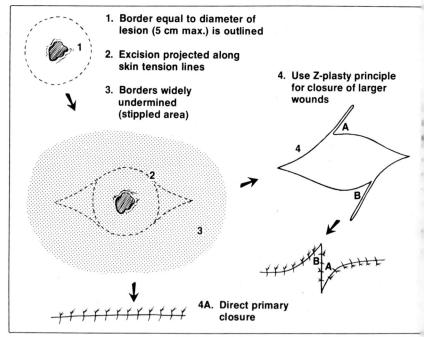

Figure 25-7. Excision of a suspected malignant skin tumor. Benign skin lesions can be excised with little or no margin. Lesions suspected of being malignant should be excised with a margin equal to the diameter of the tumor, up to a maximal margin of 5 cm. Prolongation of a circular wound by excision of small triangles at either end, together with wide undermining, often permits primary closure. Alternatively, use a Z-plasty.

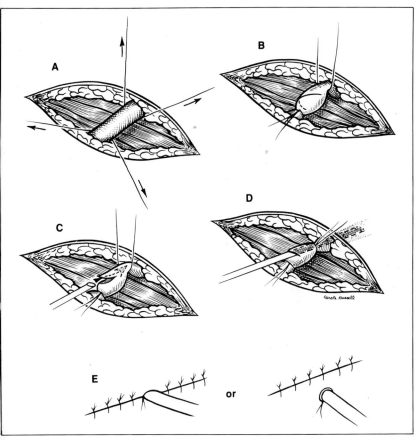

Figure 25-8. Venous cutdown. In infants, the great saphenous vein just anterior to the medial malleolus and the external jugular vein in the neck are the preferred sites for a cutdown. In adults, the antecubital vein at the elbow or the cephalic vein in the upper arm is preferred, although any accessible vein may be used. Apply a tourniquet proximal to the cutdown site. Prepare a sterile field; incise the skin transversely, dissect out the vein, and pass two ligatures around it (A). Tie the distal ligature (B), and place it on gentle traction. Make a beveled transverse incision halfway through the vein (C); release the tourniquet. Insert the venous catheter; tie the proximal ligature around the vein and catheter (D). Suture the wound, tying the catheter in place (E), and apply a dressing.

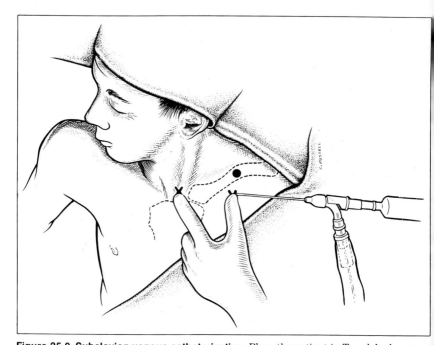

Figure 25-9. Subclavian venous catheterization. Place the patient in Trendelenburg position, prepare the skin, and set up a field using sterile towels. Observe strict aseptic techniques through the catheterization. Place a small button of local anesthetic at the skin puncture site; deeper tissues are not anesthetized. Insert the needle-catheter assembly through a point 3 cm below the middle of the clavicle, aiming at the center of the suprasternal notch. Keep the needle horizontal, and advance it while maintaining slight suction in the syringe. Entry into the subclavian vein is signaled by the abrupt appearance of blood in the syringe; advance the needle an additional 2–3 mm. Confirm the presence of the needle tip in the vein by ability to aspirate freely, then reinject blood. Hold the outer sheath in position, withdraw the needle, and advance the inner catheter into the superior vena cava. Spray the skin surrounding the puncture site with tincture of benzoin. Dress the catheter with antibacterial ointment and several layers of gauze covered completely with adhesive tape. Anchor the catheter to the external surface of the dressing with additional adhesive tape.

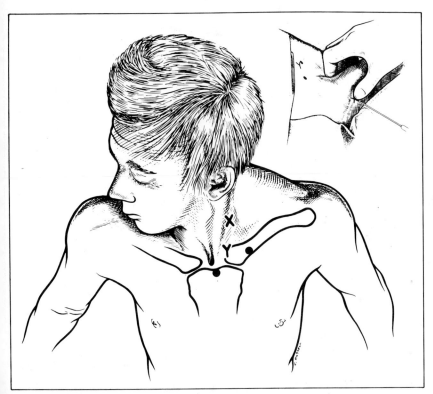

Figure 25-10. Internal jugular venous catheterization. The landmarks are indicated in the main drawing. The sternocleidomastoid muscle is grasped firmly, as indicated in the inset, and elevated slightly to fix the internal jugular vein. The needle is inserted at the posterior border of the sternocleidomastoid muscle, halfway between the mastoid process and the head of the clavicle (X) and is directed between the clavicular and sternal heads of the muscle (Y). The needle-catheter assembly is passed deep (posterior) to the sterno-cleidomastoid muscle to enter the vein. Other details of technique are identical with those for subclavian venous catheterization (see Fig. 25-9).

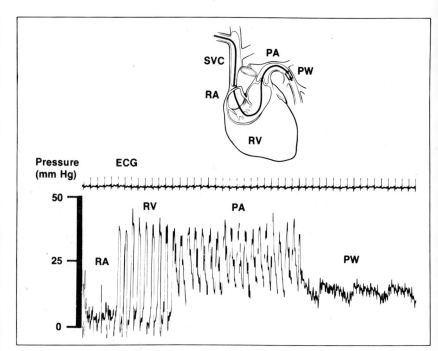

Figure 25-11. Insertion of Swan-Ganz catheter. Prime the catheter with heparinized saline (1 unit/ml), insert it via an antecubital vein cutdown (see Fig. 25-8), and pass the catheter via the brachial (medial) branch to the subclavian vein. Initial passage is facilitated by facing the curved tip of the catheter toward the humerus. Advance the catheter to the superior vena cava (SVC), rotate it 180 degrees so that the curved tip faces the midline, then half-inflate the balloon with air. Connect the primed catheter to a pressure transducer, and monitor pressure on an oscilloscope or recorder. Gently advance the catheter, observing the pressure tracing to identify the location of the catheter tip.

With the catheter tip in the superior vena cava (SVC), the pressure is low (usually less than 20 mm Hg); deflections are negative and coincide with respiration. When the right atrium (RA) is entered, pressure is unchanged, but deflections become positive and correspond with the heartbeat. Complete the inflation of the balloon, then continue advancing the catheter through the right ventricle (RV) and into the pulmonary artery (PA). Watch the ECG for premature ventricular contractions (PVCs) that result from impingement of the catheter tip in the myocardium; if PVCs occur, withdraw the catheter a little, then gently advance it again. After the catheter tip enters the pulmonary artery, advance it to a wedge position (PW), then deflate the balloon.

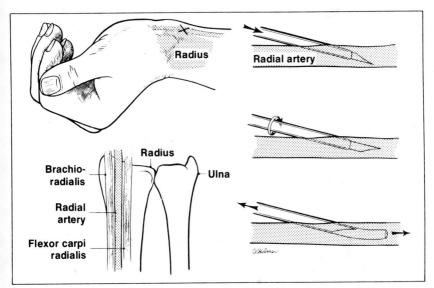

Figure 25-12. Insertion of radial artery catheter. The nondominant (usually left) upper extremity is preferred. The wrist is fully extended, supported on a towel roll and taped to a board. The radial artery is easily palpated between the tendons of the brachioradialis and flexor carpi radialis. The point of entry into the artery should be about 4 cm proximal to the main wrist flexion crease; the point of skin puncture is somewhat more distal. The skin is prepared with an antibacterial solution, the plastic-sheathed needle is inserted through the skin and into the artery with the needle bevel up. After entry into the artery, the needle is rotated 180° to turn the bevel down, the plastic catheter is advanced, the needle withdrawn and the arterial cannula connected to a transducer.

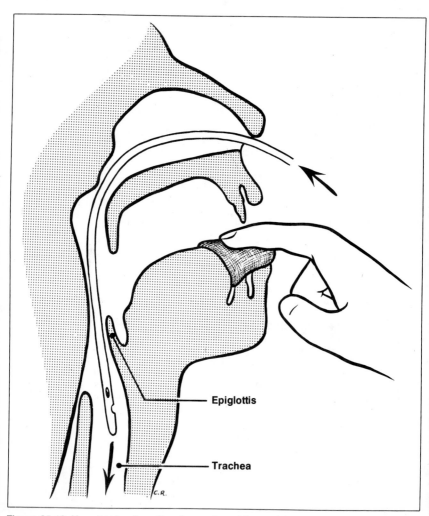

Figure 25-13. Nasotracheal suction. Insert the rubber catheter through the nose, extend the head, pull the tongue gently forward to open the epiglottis, and advance the catheter while the patient takes a deep breath. Sometimes a coudé tip catheter is needed.

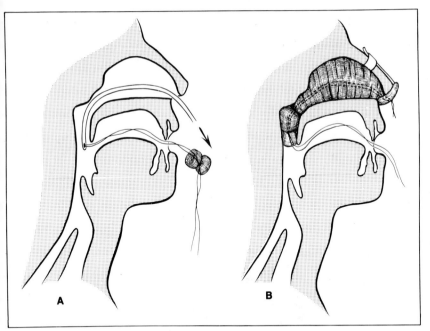

Figure 25-14. Nasal packing. A gauze roll is drawn into the nasopharynx as a posterior pack (A). Alternatively, a Foley catheter is used, the inflated balloon acting as the posterior pack. Then the anterior pack is placed, filling the nose (B).

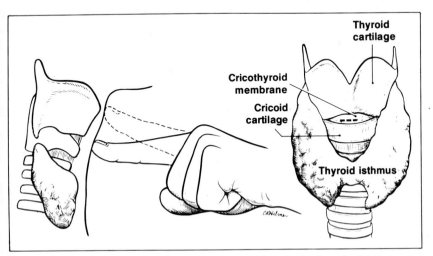

Figure 25-15. Cricothyrotomy. An airway can be established quickly and safely by puncture of the cricothyroid membrane (broken line). In an emergency, it is faster than a tracheostomy.

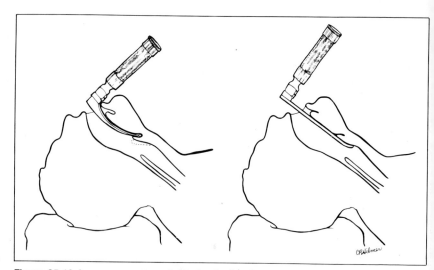

Figure 25-16. Laryngoscopy; endotracheal tube placement. Either a curved or a straight blade may be used. The tip of the curved laryngoscope blade is inserted **anterior** to the epiglottis, between the epiglottis and the base of the tongue. The straight blade is passed **posterior** to the epiglottis. In both cases, the entire laryngoscope is then **lifted straight anteriorly** to expose the larynx. An endotracheal tube can then be passed between the vocal cords through the posterior half of the larynx under direct vision.

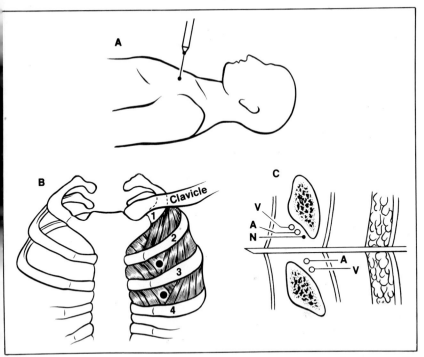

Figure 25-17. Needle thoracentesis (air). In suspected **tension pneumothorax,** a needle is inserted anteriorly (A) through the second or third interspace in the midclavicular line (B). The needle should pass through the middle of the interspace to avoid intercostal blood vessels (C).

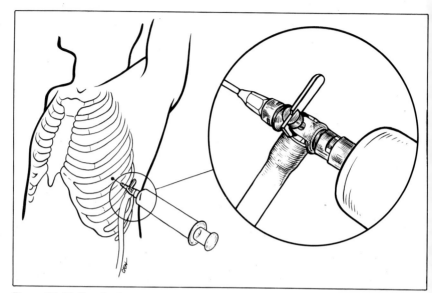

Figure 25-18. Needle thoracentesis (fluid). To remove an effusion, the patient sits upright; the needle is passed through the seventh or eighth interspace in the midposterior axillary line. Since the intercostal blood vessels in this part of the thorax all are in relation to the inferior border of the rib, the needle should pass immediately above the next lower rib.

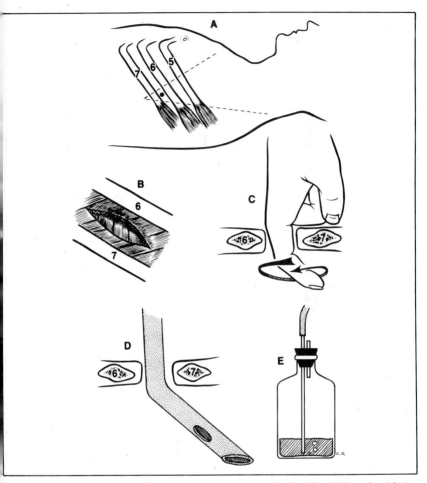

Figure 25-19. Insertion of a chest tube. A chest tube can be placed quickly and safely in an emergency through the sixth intercostal space in the midaxillary line (A). This location avoids major nerves and overlying muscles. A 2- to 3-cm incision is made in the mid-interspace and carried partially through the intercostal muscles (B). Entry into the pleural space is completed by blunt dissection with a clamp. A sterile gloved finger is inserted into the chest to clear adhesions, clots, etc. (C). The finger is withdrawn and a 32-35 Fr chest tube is inserted (D) and connected to water-seal drainage (E). The wound is sutured. The small induced pneumothorax clears immediately. The major advantage of this method is its safety in inexperienced hands.

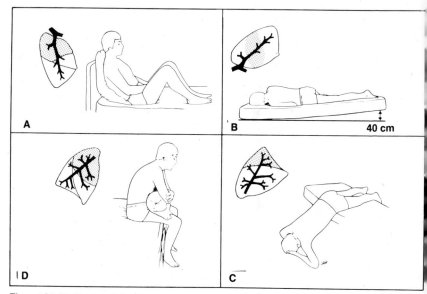

Figure 25-20. Postural drainage. Positioning of the patient to promote drainage from lung segments. A. Drainage of right upper apical segments. B. Drainage of right middle and lateral segments. C. Drainage of left apical segments. D. Drainage of basilar segments and trachea. The latter is most needed in postoperative patients and usually is difficult to arrange.

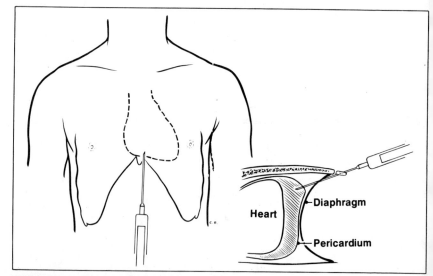

Figure 25-21. Needle pericardiocentesis. A 14- or 16-gauge Angiocath needle is inserted between the xiphoid and the left costal margin at an angle of about 30 degrees from the body wall and is advanced straight superiorly while suction is maintained on the syringe. ECG lead II can be connected to the steel needle and will accurately indicate when the epicardium is touched. If blood returns from the pericardial sac, leave the outer plastic cannula in place.

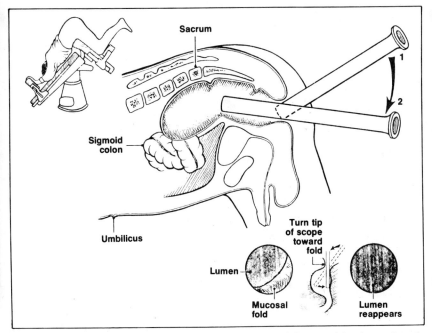

Figure 25-22. Sigmoidoscopy. Place the patient in the head-down position (*upper insert*). Digital rectal examination always is done as the first step.

Insert the sigmoidoscope through the anus, aiming at the patient's umbilicus (1). Advance only 3–4 cm, stop, rotate the scope (2), remove the obturator, and insert the eyepiece. Advance the scope under direct vision, turning the tip slightly toward each successive mucosal fold (*lower insert*). If the lumen is not apparent, withdraw the scope a little. Avoid insufflating air unless absolutely necessary. At about 15 cm the sigmoid colon curves to the left,; because of this angulation, or fixation of the bowel by disease, it is not possible to pass the scope beyond this point in about 30% of patients.

Attention during insertion is directed to safe, smooth passage of the sigmoidoscope. Attention during withdrawal is directed to careful scrutiny of the mucosa; use a rotary or spiral motion as the sigmoidoscope is slowly withdrawn.

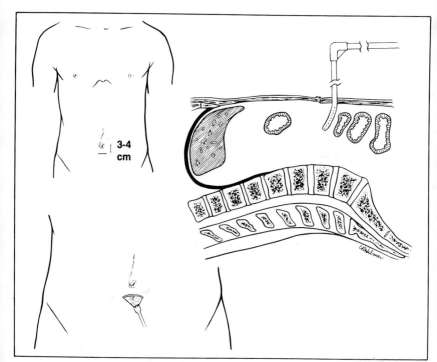

Figure 25-23. Abdominal diagnostic paracentesis. An 18-gauge IV catheter or a peritoneal dialysis unit is used. The peritoneum is exposed by dissection, under local anesthesia, in the midline, about 4–5 cm below the umbilicus. Alternatively, a blind percutaneous puncture can be made in the same location. The needle just enters the peritoneal cavity; the inner catheter then is advanced into the peritoneal cavity. If fluid does not return immediately, 100–200 ml of normal saline solution is run into the abdomen over 5 min using an IV drip set. The IV tubing and bottle are then lowered to the floor to siphon fluid from the abdomen.

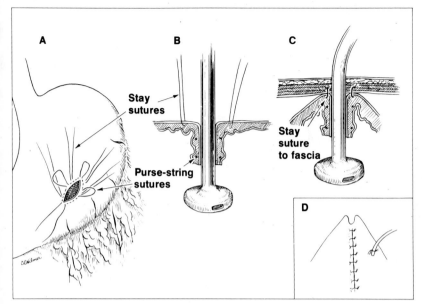

Figure 25-24. Stamm gastrostomy. The gastrostomy site is selected close to the greater curvature in the mid-body of the stomach. Stay sutures are placed as shown (A), with an absorbable purse-string suture within them. A small stab is made within the purse string suture and enlarged bluntly with a hemostat. The gastrostomy tube (usually a 24 Fr open-tip latex Pezzar catheter) is inserted into the stomach, and the purse-string suture is tied. A second purse-string suture is placed about the gastrostomy tube, about 1.5 cm from the first purse-string suture but still within the stay sutures, and tied, further inverting the gastric wall about the tube (B). The end of the gastrostomy tube is withdrawn through a stab wound (D), and the stay sutures are sutured to the posterior fascia (C).

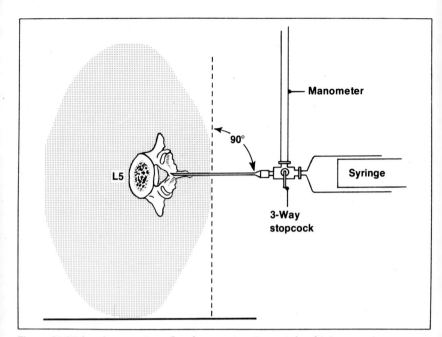

Figure 25-25. Lumbar puncture. Lumbar puncture in acute head injury requires precautions to prevent loss of fluid or a sudden drop in cerebrospinal fluid pressure. The needle is passed through the skin with the bevel facing the patient's side. When the needle engages the interspinal ligament, the obturator is withdrawn, and a saline-filled manometer and syringe are connected. When the subarachnoid space is entered, only a small volume of fluid will enter or leave the manometer; there is no change in the cerebrospinal fluid pressure.

Index

Because this book is a reference manual, the authors wished to provide complete and direct access to information. Therefore, the indexer has included alternate terms for main entries as separate entries in their own right; for example: Breathing/Respiration; Trauma/Wounds; Bicarbonate/Sodium bicarbonate. Standard abbreviations are indexed both under the abbreviation and the full term; for example, ECG (Electrocardiogram) and Electrocardiogram (ECG); CT scans (computed tomography) and Computed tomography (CT scans). Drug names are indexed by both the generic and proprietary names.

A Little, Brown

Spiral™ Manual

Manual of Surgical Therapeutics

Fifth Edition

**Departments of Surgery
The Medical College of Wisconsin
and University of Illinois**

**Edited by Robert E. Condon, M.D.
and Lloyd M. Nyhus, M.D.**

In each of its previous editions, **Manual of Surgical Therapeutics** was acclaimed as an "ideal pocket reference" and a "mass of information useful to surgeons of any age or degree of experience." A review in *New Physician* said, "This book should take its place alongside the tourniquet, bandage, scissors, and stethoscope as standard equipment in the pockets of the surgical house officer's white coat." *Gastroenterology* said it was characterized by "conciseness, completeness, and clinical pertinence." Now in a totally revised and updated edition, **Manual of Surgical Therapeutics,** Fifth Edition, maintains the high standards upon which its reputation is based.

Manual of Surgical Therapeutics, Fifth Edition, is the work of house officers and attending surgeons from the Departments of Surgery at The Medical College of Wisconsin and University of Illinois College of Medicine. Each contributor describes the management he finds most useful to bring together in a single volume straightforward clinical information about the successful nonoperative care of surgical patients.

Maintaining the popular outline format of previous editions, the fifth edition completely updates chapters and sections on general principles in the management of acute injury, together with specific features of the management of chest, vascular, extremity, and hand injuries, as well as infection. Sections relating to the evaluation of the body's "survival systems" — the renal, cardiac, and pulmonary systems — have been completely revised. Chapters on fluid and electrolyte therapy, coagulation disorders, and cancer

chemotherapy were rewritten to reflect current procedures. An entirely new section on stings and bites has been added to this edition. In fact, **Manual of Surgical Therapeutics,** Fifth Edition, has been revised, reviewed, updated, and rechecked in its entirety by contributors, old and new.

Spiralbound to lie flat, and organized in an accessible, outline format, **Manual of Surgical Therapeutics,** Fifth Edition, is still the perfect complement to its renowned partner in the **Little, Brown SPIRAL™ Manual Series,** the Washington University **Manual of Medical Therapeutics.** In the tradition of earlier editions, **Manual of Surgical Therapeutics,** Fifth Edition, will be used every day by clinicians who treat surgical patients.

Little, Brown and Company
Boston, Massachusetts 02106